Third Edition

Basic Clinical Pharmacokinetics

Michael E. Winter, Pharm.D.
Professor of Clinical Pharmacy
School of Pharmacy
University of California, San Francisco
and
Director
Clinical Pharmacokinetics Consultation Service
University of California Hospitals and Clinics
San Francisco, California

Edited by:
Mary Anne Koda-Kimble, Pharm.D.
Professor of Clinical Pharmacy
Chairwoman, Division of Clinical Pharmacy
School of Pharmacy
University of California
San Francisco, California

Applied Therapeutics, Inc.
Vancouver, WA

Applied Therapeutics, Inc.
Post Office Box 5077
Vancouver, Washington 98668-5077
(206) 253-7123

Library of Congress Catalog Card Number 94-70212
ISBN 0-915486-22-9

First Printing, July 1994
Second Printing, August 1994

For my family. For the Specialty Practice residents who have worked with me in the Clinical Pharmacokinetics Consultation Service at the University of California San Francisco: Theresa A. Salazer, Gene D. Mason, Elizabeth A. Stubits, Scott M. Fields, Dayna L. McCauley, Maureen S. Boro, Patrick R. Finley, Kevin Y. Ohara, Donna Jean Carroll, Paul M. Beringer, Melissa M.L. Choy, and Laura M. Morodomi.

Thank you to the Applied Therapeutics staff including: Nannette Naught, Lois Mullins, Billy Good, Rick Walsh, Heidi Whyms, Linda McCarley, and Pam Uthe for their hard work and support in making the third edition of this book a reality.

Notice to Reader

Drug therapy information is constantly evolving. Our ever-changing knowledge and experience with drugs and the continual development of new drugs necessitates changes in treatment and drug therapy. The editors, author, and the publisher of this work have made every effort to ensure the information provided herein was accurate at the time of publication. *It remains the responsibility of every practitioner to evaluate the appropriateness of a particular opinion or therapy in the context of the actual clinical situation and with due consideration of any new developments in the field.* Although the author has been careful to recommend dosages that are in agreement with current standards and responsible literature, the student or practitioner should consult with several appropriate information sources when dealing with new and unfamiliar drugs.

Contents

Introduction

Since the publication of the first edition of **Basic Clinical Pharmacokinetics**, the use of serum drug concentrations as a guide for monitoring drug therapy has continued to gain increased acceptance. The use of pharmacokinetic and biopharmaceutic principles in predicting plasma drug concentrations, as well as the changes in plasma drug concentrations which accrue over time, are now widely accepted as useful adjuncts in patient care. With the advancement of analytical technology every health care institution and practitioner has ready access to drug concentration assays and for some drugs (e.g., aminoglycosides, digoxin, phenytoin) monitoring serum drug concentrations has become the standard of practice. Appropriate use of serum drug concentrations, however, continues to be a major problem in the clinical setting. Basic pharmacokinetic principles must be applied rationally to specific patients. As a result, this book has been written to help the clinician apply pharmacokinetics and therapeutic drug monitoring to patient care.

The book is divided into two parts: the first reviews basic pharmacokinetic principles, and the second illustrates the clinical application of pharmacokinetics to specific drugs through the presentation and solution of common clinical problems. Part I is divided into sections which describe major pharmacokinetic parameters and their clinical applications. Equations which express the relationships between the various parameters and the resultant plasma concentrations are presented and discussed. A number of physiological and mathematical assumptions have been made. This is a common practice in the clinical setting and an attempt has been made to alert the reader to these assumptions. There are a large number of texts and articles that present a much more detailed and in-depth analysis and explanation of the pharmacokinetic principles being discussed. It is not the intent of this book to explore all of these issues. Rather it is the goal of this book to simplify pharmacokinetics so that it can be understood and visualized by practitioners so that the use of pharmacokinetic principles can become part of their professional practice. In the third edition a number of sections in Part I have been expanded. For example, the section on Selecting the Appropriate Equation now includes an algorithm to help guide the reader in a logical stepwise approach to choosing pharmacokinetic equations. The section on Interpretation of Plasma Drug Concentrations was expanded to help the reader understand more fully how and why to choose a pharmacokinetic revision model and how to evaluate the usefulness or validity of the pharmacokinetic predictions. A brief review of the principles associated with drug elimination in patients receiving peritoneal dialysis was added to the section on Dialysis of Drugs. The reader is strongly urged to read each section in the order that it appears in the text because many of the concepts discussed in the latter portions of the text are based on an understanding of those presented earlier.

Many individuals feel overwhelmed by the apparent complexity of some of the equations used to describe pharmacokinetic behavior of drugs. Therefore, extensive explanations which emphasize major concepts accompany the more complex equations. Figures are provided to help the reader visualize the concepts which are being reviewed. The principles discussed in Part I will give the clinician the basis for manipulating the dosing regimens and interpreting plasma drug concentrations for the drugs discussed in Part II of this text.

The drugs discussed in Part II were selected because their clinical assays are widely available and because an understanding of their pharmacokinetic and biopharmaceutic properties can substantially aid clinicians in dosing them more rationally and safely. In the first edition of **Basic Clinical Pharmacokinetics**, Part II had nine chapters; the third edition has eighteen. New chapters on cyclosporine and the tricyclic antidepressants have been added as well as updates on other chapters. These updates include new information on the clinical use of serum drug concentrations. New cases and examples have also been added to further expand and exemplify the use of pharmacokinetics in clinical practice.

For each of the drugs, examples of the most common pharmacokinetic manipulations such as calculation of a loading dose and maintenance dose are presented. An example of the process used to interpret a reported plasma concentration is also given. In addition, pathophysiologic factors that influence the pharmacokinetics of these drugs and their significance are considered. Examples of the most common problems encountered in clinical practice are also given to help the reader recognize when caution should be used in making patient care decisions based upon serum drug concentrations and pharmacokinetic principles. Ultimately, it is hoped that the reader will be able to recognize the fundamental principles which are being applied to each of the drugs. As you develop confidence and skill in using pharmacokinetics as a clinical tool, you will be able to apply these same principles to new drugs.

Although plasma drug concentrations are useful in evaluating drug therapy, they constitute only one source of information. They should not, therefore, be used as the sole criterion on which treatment is based. Pharmacokinetic calculations should be considered only as a guide to the determination of dosing regimens.

If a calculated dosing regimen seems unreasonable, re-evaluation is essential since mathematical error is always a possibility. Another problem inherent in these calculations is that the pharmacokinetic parameters utilized may be inappropriate for the patient under consideration. Many of the pharmacokinetic parameters available in the literature are based upon small numbers of patients or normal volunteers. Therefore, values obtained from these experimental data are, at best, estimates for any given patient. If the basic underlying pharmacokinetic assumptions are not applicable to the particular patient, even the most elegant calculation is invalid.

Review articles commonly list pharmacokinetic parameters for a number of drugs, however, the reader is encouraged to seek out the original literature to evaluate the methodology and data from which this information was derived. Some factors that should be considered in scrutinizing these studies include the number and type of subjects, type and specificity of drug assay, degree of inter- and intra-subject variability, statistical analysis of the data, and whether the drug was studied prospectively or retrospectively. The third edition of **Applied Pharmacokinetics: Principles of Therapeutic Drug Monitoring** provides the clinician with an excellent literature review of the pharmacokinetic parameters for many of the most commonly monitored drugs. The potential problems associated with using literature data to predict disposition of a drug within a specific patient emphasize the need to obtain accurate plasma level measurements. Only with appropriate drug sampling, accurate and specific assay procedures and logical pharmacokinetic analysis can patient-specific parameters be derived that will be a useful adjunct to providing optimal patient care and improving clinical outcomes.

Part One _____

Basic Principles

Bioavailability (F)

Definition

Bioavailability is the percentage or fraction of the administered dose which reaches the systemic circulation of the patient. Examples of factors which can alter bioavailability include: the inherent dissolution and absorption characteristics of the administered chemical form (e.g., salt, ester), the dosage form (e.g., tablet, capsule), the route of administration, the stability of the active ingredient in the gastrointestinal tract, and, the extent of drug metabolism before reaching the systemic circulation. Drugs can be metabolized by gastrointestinal bacteria, by the gastrointestinal mucosa, and by the liver before reaching the systemic circulation.

To calculate the amount of drug absorbed, the administered dose should be multiplied by a bioavailability factor, which is usually represented by the letter "F." For example, the bioavailability of digoxin (Lanoxin) is estimated to be 0.7 for orally administered tablets.[1,2] This means that if 250 μg (0.25 mg) of digoxin is given orally, the effective or absorbed dose can be calculated by multiplying the administered dose by F:

$$\text{Amount of Drug Absorbed or Reaching Systemic Circulation} = (F)(\text{Dose})$$

Eq. 1

$$= (0.7)(250 \ \mu g)$$
$$= 175 \ \mu g$$

It should be emphasized that this factor does not take into consideration the *rate* of drug absorption; it only estimates the *extent* of absorption. Although the rate of absorption can be important when rapid onset of pharmacological effects is required, it is not usually important when a drug is administered chronically. The rate of absorption is important only when it is so slow that it limits the absolute bioavailability of the drug, or when it is so rapid that too much drug is absorbed. The former occasionally occurs with some sustained-release preparations.[3,4]

Dosage Form

As noted earlier, bioavailability can vary among different formulations and dosage forms of a drug. For example, digoxin elixir has a bioavailability of approximately 77% (F = 0.77) while the soft gelatin capsules have a bioavailability of 100% (F = 1.0). This is in contrast to the tablets which have a bioavailability of 70% (F = 0.7).[2,5,6] When drugs are administered parenterally, the bioavailability is usually considered to be 100% (F = 1.0). By rearranging Equation 1, this principle can be used to calculate equivalent doses of a drug when a patient is to receive a different dosage form of the same drug.

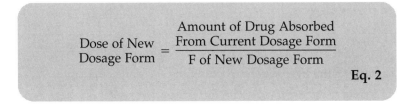

$$\frac{\text{Dose of New}}{\text{Dosage Form}} = \frac{\begin{array}{c}\text{Amount of Drug Absorbed}\\ \text{From Current Dosage Form}\end{array}}{\text{F of New Dosage Form}}$$

Eq. 2

For example, if a patient who has been receiving digoxin 250 µg (0.25 mg) in the tablet dosage form, needs to receive digoxin elixir instead, an equivalent dose of the elixir would be calculated as follows:

$$\text{Dose of Elixir} = \frac{175\ \mu g}{0.77}$$

$$= 227\ \mu g$$

If the soft gelatin capsules of digoxin were to be administered, the bioavailability or F of the new dosage form would have been 1.0 and the equivalent dose would have been 175 µg.

The bioavailability of parenterally-administered drugs usually is considered to be 1.0. Drugs which are administered as inactive precursors that must then be converted to an active product are an exception to this rule. If some of the inactive precursor is excreted or eliminated from the body *before* it can be converted to the active compound, the bioavailability will be <1.0. For example, parenteral chloramphenicol is given as the succinate ester, and this chloramphenicol ester must be hydrolyzed to the active compound. The bioavailability of the parenterally-administered chloramphenicol succinate ranges from 55% to 95%, because from 5% to 45% of the chloramphenicol ester is eliminated renally before it can be converted to the active compound.[7]

Chemical Form (S)

The chemical form of a drug must also be considered when evaluating bioavailability. For example, when a salt or ester of a drug is administered, the bioavailability factor (F) should be multiplied by the fraction of the total molecular weight which the active drug represents. If "S" represents the fraction of the administered dose which is the active drug, then the amount of drug absorbed from a salt or ester form can be calculated as follows:

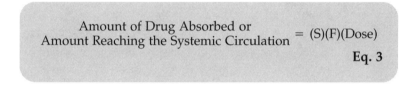

$$\text{Amount of Drug Absorbed or Amount Reaching the Systemic Circulation} = (S)(F)(Dose)$$

Eq. 3

The "S" factor should be included in all bioavailability equations as a constant reminder of its importance in assessing bioavailability of the active drug form. When a drug is administered in its parent or active form, the "S" for that drug is 1.0.

Equation 2 can now be expanded to consider the salt factor as well as the bioavailability when calculating the dose of a new dosage form:

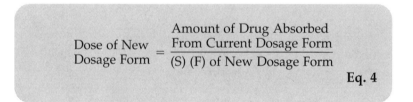

$$\frac{\text{Dose of New}}{\text{Dosage Form}} = \frac{\text{Amount of Drug Absorbed From Current Dosage Form}}{(S)\ (F)\ \text{of New Dosage Form}}$$

Eq. 4

Aminophylline is an excellent example of this principle. (See Figure 1.) Aminophylline is the ethylenediamine salt of the pharmacologically-active moiety, theophylline. Eighty to eighty-five percent (by weight) of this salt is theophylline, so that the "S" for aminophylline is approximately 0.8. Uncoated aminophylline tablets are considered to be completely (100%) bioavailable; the bioavailability factor (F) for this dosage form is, therefore, 1.0. It is important to consider the salt form in determining the amount of theophylline absorbed from an aminophylline tablet. When Equation 3 is applied to this situation, it can be demonstrated that 160 mg of theophylline is absorbed from a 200 mg aminophylline tablet:

$$\text{Amount of Drug Absorbed or Reaching the Systemic Circulation} = \text{(S)(F)(Dose)}$$

$$= (0.8)(1.0)(200 \text{ mg Aminophylline})$$

$$= 160 \text{ mg Theophylline}$$

First-Pass Effect

Since drugs are absorbed from the gastrointestinal tract into the portal circulation, some drugs may be extensively metabolized in the liver before reaching the systemic circulation. This "first-pass effect" can substantially decrease the amount of active drug reaching the systemic circulation and thus, its bioavailability. (See Figure 2.)

Lidocaine is an example of a drug with a first-pass effect that is so great that oral administration is not practical.[8] In the case of propranolol

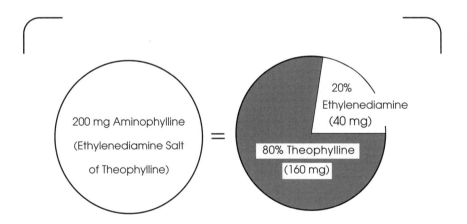

Figure 1. The Effect of the Chemical-Drug Form on Bioavailability. The example above emphasizes the importance of considering the chemical form administered when calculating the amount of active drug actually administered. The amount of active drug administered may represent only a fraction of the salt, ester, or other chemical form of the drug contained in formulation. The bioavailability of the dosage form itself must also be considered when drugs are administered by the oral route.

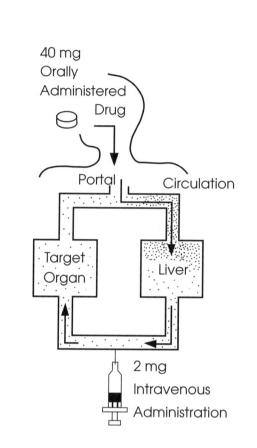

Figure 2. First-Pass Effect. When drugs with a high "first-pass effect" are administered orally, a large amount of the absorbed drug is metabolized before it reaches the systemic circulation. If the drug is administered intravenously, the liver is bypassed and the fraction of the administered dose that reaches the circulation is increased. Parenteral doses of drugs with a "high first-pass" are much smaller than oral doses which produce equivalent pharmacologic effects.

(Inderal), a significant portion of the orally administered dose is metabolized through a first-pass effect; therefore, a much larger oral dose is required to achieve the same pharmacologic response as that obtained from a dose administered intravenously. However, the propranolol issue is further complicated by the fact that one of the metabolites, 4-hydroxy-propranolol, is pharmacologically active.[9]

Administration Rate (R$_A$)

The administration rate is the average rate at which absorbed drug reaches the systemic circulation. This is usually calculated by dividing the amount of drug absorbed (see Equation 3) by the time over which the drug was administered (dosing interval). The dosing interval is usually represented by the symbol, tau (τ).

$$\text{Administration Rate (R}_A) = \frac{(S)(F)(Dose)}{\tau}$$

Eq. 5

When drugs are administered as a continuous infusion, the dosing interval can be expressed in any convenient time unit. For example, the theophylline administration rate resulting from aminophylline infused at a rate of 75 mg/hr is calculated from Equation 5 as follows:

$$R_A = \frac{(S)(F)(Dose)}{\tau}$$

$$= \frac{(0.8)(1.0)(75 \text{ mg})}{1 \text{ hr}}$$

$$= 60 \text{ mg/hr}$$

or

$$= \frac{(0.8)(1.0)(75 \text{ mg})}{60 \text{ min}}$$

$$= 1 \text{ mg/min}$$

When drugs are administered at fixed dosing intervals, the calculated administration rate is an average value. For example, the average administration rate of theophylline in mg/hr resulting from an oral dose of 300 mg aminophylline given every six hours would be calculated using Equation 5 as follows:

$$
\begin{aligned}
R_A &= \frac{(S)(F)(Dose)}{\tau} \\
&= \frac{(0.8)(1.0)(300 \text{ mg})}{6 \text{ hr}} \\
&= 40 \text{ mg/hr}
\end{aligned}
$$

Desired Plasma Concentration (Cp)

Protein Binding

Clinical laboratory reports of drug concentrations in plasma (Cp) represent drug that is bound to plasma protein plus drug that is unbound or free. It is the free or unbound drug which is in equilibrium with the receptor site and is, therefore, the pharmacologically active moiety. Thus, the reported plasma drug concentration indirectly reflects the concentration of free or active drug. (See Figure 3.)

Some disease states are associated with decreased plasma proteins or with decreased binding of drugs to plasma proteins.[10,11] In these situations, drugs which are usually highly protein bound have a larger percent of free or unbound drug present in plasma. Therefore, a greater pharmacological effect can be expected for any given drug concentration in plasma (Cp). Clinicians must always consider altered protein binding and whether the fraction of free drug concentration (alpha or "α") is altered when interpreting or establishing desired plasma drug concentrations.

$$\alpha = \frac{\text{Free Drug Concentration}}{\text{Total Drug Concentration}}$$

$$\alpha = \frac{\text{Cp free}}{\text{Cp bound + Cp free}}$$

Eq. 6

The fraction of drug that is free (α) does not vary with the drug concentration for most drugs that are bound primarily to albumin because the number of protein binding sites far exceeds the number of drug molecules available for binding. When the plasma concentrations for drugs bound to albumin exceed 25 to 50 mg/L, however, albumin binding sites can be saturated. As a result, alpha, or the fraction of drug which is free, will change with the plasma drug concentration. For example, salicylates and valproic acid (Depakene) can saturate plasma protein binding sites and both of these drugs frequently have plasma concentrations exceeding 25 to 50 mg/L. For those drugs that do not reach serum concentrations

Figure 3. Plasma Concentration of a Highly Protein-Bound Drug: Normal Plasma Protein Concentration. The plasma drug concentration reported by the laboratory represents a total of both "bound" and "free" drug. It is the "free" drug that is in equilibrium with the target organs and is the pharmacologically active moiety. In this illustration, alpha (or the fraction of free drug to total drug concentration) is 0.1.

capable of saturating protein-binding sites, the plasma protein concentration (in many cases, this is albumin) and the binding affinity of the drug for the plasma protein are the two major factors which control alpha.

Low Plasma Protein Concentrations

Low plasma protein concentrations decrease the plasma concentration of bound drug (Cp bound); however, the concentration of free drug (Cp free) generally is unaffected. Therefore, the fraction of drug which is free (or alpha) increases as plasma protein concentrations decrease. Free drug concentrations are not significantly increased because the free drug which is released into plasma secondary to low plasma protein concentrations equilibrates with the tissue compartment (See Figure 4 and compare with Figure 3). Therefore, if the volume of distribution (Vd) is relatively large, only a minor increase in Cp free will result. (Also see Volume of Distribution on page 18.)

The relationship between the plasma drug concentration and the plasma protein concentration can be expressed as follows:

$$\frac{Cp'}{Cp_{Normal\ Binding}} = (1 - \alpha)\left[\frac{P'}{P_{NL}}\right] + \alpha$$

Eq. 7

This equation can be used to estimate the degree to which an altered plasma protein concentration will affect the desired therapeutic drug concentration. Cp' represents the patient's plasma drug concentration and P'

Figure 4. Effect of Decreased Plasma Protein Concentration on Plasma Drug Concentration. Compare this figure with Figure 3. The decreased protein concentration decreases the plasma drug concentration reported by the laboratory. In this situation, the concentration of free, or active drug, remains the same because free drug that is released as a result of the lowered plasma protein concentration is taken up by nonspecific tissue binding sites. For this reason, the pharmacologic effect, which can be expected from the reported Cp of 5, will be the same as that produced by the reported Cp of 10 in Figure 3. In this illustration, alpha (or the fraction of free drug to total drug concentration) is increased to 0.2.

the plasma protein concentration. $Cp_{Normal\ Binding}$ is the plasma drug concentration that would be expected if the patient's plasma protein concentration were normal (P_{NL}). Note that α is the free fraction associated with "normal plasma protein binding." The $Cp_{Normal\ Binding}$ for any given drug can be calculated by rearranging Equation 7:

$$Cp_{Normal\ Binding} = \frac{Cp'}{(1 - \alpha)\left[\dfrac{P'}{P_{NL}}\right] + \alpha}$$

Eq. 8

For example, a patient with a low serum albumin of 2.2 gm/dL (normal albumin: 4.4 gm/dL) and an apparently low plasma phenytoin concentration of 5.5 mg/L still has a therapeutically acceptable plasma drug concentration when it is adjusted for the low serum albumin. When the normal alpha (α) for phenytoin (Dilantin) (i.e., 0.1) is substituted into Equation 8, an adjusted phenytoin plasma concentration of 10 mg/L is calculated.

$$
\begin{aligned}
Cp_{Normal\ Binding} &= \frac{Cp'}{(1 - \alpha)\left[\dfrac{P'}{P_{NL}}\right] + \alpha} \\[2ex]
&= \frac{5.5\ \text{mg/L}}{(1 - 0.1)\dfrac{(2.2\ \text{gm/dL})}{(4.4\ \text{gm/dL})} + (0.1)} \\[2ex]
&= \frac{5.5\ \text{mg/L}}{(0.9)(0.5) + 0.1} \\[2ex]
&= \frac{5.5\ \text{mg/L}}{0.55} \\[2ex]
&= 10\ \text{mg/L}
\end{aligned}
$$

The phenytoin concentration that would have been reported from the laboratory if the patient's albumin concentration were "normal" would be approximately 10 mg/L. This calculation is based upon the assumption that phenytoin is primarily bound to albumin and that an average normal albumin concentration is 4.4 gm/dL (range: 3.5 to 5.5 gm/dL). While

Equation 8 could be used to adjust for any drug significantly bound to albumin, the degree to which the drug concentration will be adjusted or "normalized" for the alteration in serum albumin will be minimal and is generally unwarranted as long as the albumin concentrations are within the usual range of 3.5 to 5.5 gm/dL.

Many other drugs are bound primarily to globulin rather than albumin. Adjustments of plasma drug concentrations for these drugs based upon serum albumin concentrations would, therefore, be inappropriate. Unfortunately, adjustments for changes in globulin binding are difficult because drugs usually bind to a specific globulin which is only a small fraction of total globulin concentration. In general, acidic drugs (e.g., phenytoin, most of the anti-epileptic drugs, and some neutral compounds) bind primarily to albumin; basic drugs (e.g., lidocaine and quinidine) bind more extensively to the globulins.[11–15]

Elevated Plasma Protein Concentrations

The alpha value (fraction of total drug concentration which is free) for selected drugs is provided in Table 1. Because increases in serum albumin are uncommon in the clinical setting, the use of Equation 8 for high serum albumin would be rare. Many basic drugs, however, are bound to the acute phase reactive protein,[17,18] alpha$_1$-acid glycoprotein (AAG). This plasma protein has been known to be significantly decreased and increased under certain clinical conditions. (See Part II: Quinidine.) For example, increases in plasma quinidine concentrations have been observed following surgery or trauma.[12,16] The change in the quinidine concentration is the result of increased concentrations of the plasma binding proteins (alpha$_1$-acid glycoproteins) and increased bound concentrations of quinidine. There appears to be little or no change in the free quinidine level because re-equilibration with the larger tissue stores occurs. In this situation, there would be a decrease in alpha (α) and the therapeutic levels of free or unbound drug should correlate with higher-than-usual drug concentration (bound plus free). Unfortunately, alpha$_1$-acid glycoprotein concentrations are seldom assayed in the clinical setting, making it difficult to evaluate the relationship between the total drug concentration and the unbound or free fraction. For this reason, evaluation of plasma levels for basic drugs that are significantly protein bound is often difficult. A careful evaluation of the patient's clinical response to a measured drug level, as well as an evaluation of any concurrent medical problems (such as surgery, trauma, or inflammatory bowel disease) that could influence plasma protein concentrations and drug binding is required.

Patients with cirrhosis vary considerably in their plasma protein binding characteristics. Some patients have markedly elevated binding capa-

Table 1   Drugs and Alpha Values for Plasma Protein Binding

Drug	*Alpha Value*
Amitriptyline	0.04[a]
Carbamazepine	0.2
Chlordiazepoxide	0.05
Chlorpropamide	0.04
Chlorpromazine	0.04[a]
Cyclosporine	<0.1[c]
Diazepam	0.01
Diazoxide	0.09
Digoxin	0.70
Digitoxin	0.10
Ethosuximide	1.0
Imipramine	0.04[a]
Lidocaine	0.30[a]
Lithium	1.0
Methadone	0.13[a]
Methotrexate	0.5
Nafcillin	0.10
Nortriptyline	0.05[a]
Phenylbutazone	0.01
Phenytoin	0.10
Propranolol	0.06[a]
Quinidine	0.20[a]
Salicylic Acid	0.16[b]
Thiopental	0.13
Valproic Acid	0.15[b]
Vancomycin	0.9
Warfarin	0.03

[a] Basic drugs that are bound significantly to plasma proteins other than albumin. From references 10, 12, 13, 90.

[b] Concentration-dependent plasma protein binding (see Salicylate and Valproic Acid chapters).

[c] Bound to lipoproteins and other blood elements. [91, 92]

bilities, while others have markedly decreased binding capabilities. This variation probably reflects the fact that some cirrhotic patients have a strong stimulus for the production of alpha$_1$-acid glycoproteins, while others with more serious hepatic disease are unable to manufacture these binding proteins.[16,17,19]

Binding Affinity

The binding affinity of plasma protein for a drug can also alter the fraction of drug which is free (alpha). (See Figure 5 and compare with Figure 3.) For example, the plasma proteins in patients with uremia (severe end-stage renal failure) have less affinity for phenytoin than do proteins present in nonuremic individuals. As a result, the alpha for pheny-

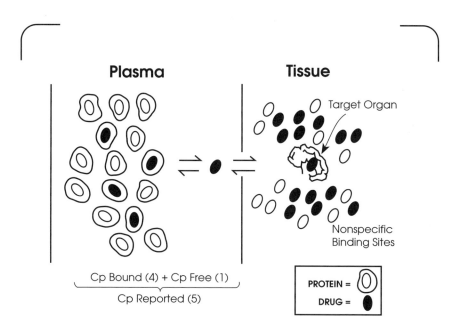

Figure 5. The Effect of Decreased Binding Affinity on Plasma Drug Concentration. Compare this figure with Figure 3. Although the protein concentration is normal, the decreased binding affinity of the drug for protein has decreased the reported drug concentration. The concentration of free or active drug remains the same because free drug that is released as a result of this decreased affinity is taken up by nonspecific binding sites in the tissue. Thus, the pharmacologic effect which can be expected from the reported Cp of 5 will be the same as that produced by the reported Cp of 10 in Figure 3. In this illustration, alpha (or the fraction of free drug to total drug concentration) is increased to 0.2.

toin in uremic patients is estimated to be in the range of 0.2 to 0.3 in contrast to the normal value of 0.1.[15,20] The "effective" or free drug concentration can be calculated by rearranging Equation 6:

$$\alpha = \frac{Cp\ free}{Cp\ bound\ +\ Cp\ free}$$

$$\alpha = \frac{Cp\ free}{Cp\ total}$$

$$Cp\ free = (\alpha)(Cp\ total)$$

Eq. 9

According to Equation 9, the concentration of free phenytoin in uremic patients is comparable to that in nonuremic patients—in spite of lower phenytoin plasma concentrations (Cp total)—because the alpha for phenytoin is increased in uremic patients. The uremic patient with an alpha of 0.2 and a reported phenytoin concentration of 5 mg/L would have the same free drug concentration (and same pharmacologic effect) as a patient with normal renal function who has a reported phenytoin concentration of 10 mg/L (using Equation 9):

$$Cp\ free = (\alpha)(Cp\ total)$$

$$Cp\ free_{(in\ Uremic\ Patient)} = (0.2)(5\ mg/L)$$

$$= 1.0\ mg/L$$

$$Cp\ free_{(in\ Patient\ with\ Normal\ Renal\ Function)} = (0.1)(10\ mg/L)$$

$$= 1.0\ mg/L$$

In summary, any factor which alters protein binding becomes clinically important when a drug is highly protein bound (i.e., if alpha is <0.1 or 10% free). For these drugs, small changes in the fraction bound can substantially increase or decrease the amount of free drug available to pharmacologically active sites for any given drug level. For example, if alpha is increased from 0.1 (10% free) to 0.2 (20% free) because of decreased amounts of protein, the concentration of free, active drug available for any given value of Cp (total or bound + free) would be double the usual values. If, on the other hand, the alpha for a drug is ≥0.5 (50% free), it is unlikely that changes in plasma protein binding will be of clinical consequence. As an illustration, if the alpha for a drug is increased from a normal value 0.5 (50% free) to 0.6 (60% free) because of decreased protein concentrations, the concentration of free active drug (assuming the same total concentration) would actually be increased by only 20%.

As a general rule, if alpha is increased in any given situation, the clinician should reduce the desired Cp by the same proportion.[21] That is, if alpha is increased twofold, the desired Cp or "therapeutic range" should be reduced to one-half the usual value.

Monitoring Free or Unbound Plasma Concentrations.

While many clinicians believe that monitoring free or unbound plasma concentrations is desirable, it is not common in general clinical practice. The reasons are several and include the fact that assay procedures for free or unbound drug are not commercially available for most compounds. Furthermore, the assay procedures available for free drug concentrations are more expensive and increase the cost of providing patient care. Also, most patients exhibit reasonably normal binding characteristics; therefore, monitoring unbound drug concentrations would not add significantly to the evaluation of their clinical status. There is little evidence demonstrating that monitoring unbound drug levels improves the correlation between the plasma concentration and the pharmacologic effect or therapeutic outcome.

If unbound drug concentrations are to be used in clinical practice, the clinician must be aware of factors that can alter the relationship between *in vitro* to *in vivo* plasma binding characteristics. For example, the method used to determine the free drug level (equilibrium dialysis, ultra filtration, saliva sampling, etc.) as well as the conditions under which the sample is obtained can alter the *in vitro* assay results. This in turn can result in an inaccurate estimate of the *in vivo* binding characteristics.[22,23,88] For these reasons, the use of unbound or free plasma level monitoring is still in the developmental stage and used routinely in only a limited number of clinical settings. If unbound serum drug concentrations are used infrequently, the results should be carefully evaluated and compared to both the expected free drug level as well as the clinical response of the patient.

Volume of Distribution (Vd)

The volume of distribution for a drug or the "apparent volume of distribution" does not necessarily refer to any identifiable compartment in the body.[1,24] It is simply the size of a compartment necessary to account for the total amount of drug in the body if it were present throughout the body at the same concentration found in the plasma. (See Figure 6A.) The equation for the volume of distribution is expressed as follows:

$$Vd = \frac{Ab}{Cp}$$

Eq. 10

where Vd is the apparent volume of distribution, Ab is the total amount of drug in the body, and Cp is the plasma concentration of drug.

Apparent volumes of distribution which are larger than the plasma compartment (>3 L) only indicate that the drug is also present in tissues or fluids outside that compartment. The actual sites of distribution cannot be determined from the Vd value. For example, drugs with a volume of distribution similar to total body water (0.65 L/kg) may or may not be extensively bound in certain tissues. Without additional specific information, the actual sites of a drug's distribution are only speculative.

The apparent volume of distribution is a function of the lipid versus water solubilities and of the plasma and tissue protein binding properties of the drug. Factors which tend to keep the drug in the plasma or increase Cp (such as low lipid solubility, increased plasma protein binding, or decreased tissue binding), reduce the apparent volume of distribution. It follows, then, that factors which decrease Cp (such as decreased plasma protein binding, increased tissue binding, and increased lipid solubility), increase the apparent volume of distribution.

Loading Dose

Since the volume of distribution is the factor which accounts for all of the drug in the body, it is an important variable in estimating the loading dose necessary to rapidly achieve a desired plasma concentration:

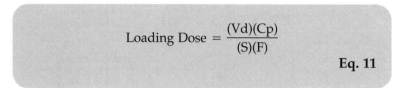

$$\text{Loading Dose} = \frac{(Vd)(Cp)}{(S)(F)}$$

Eq. 11

where Vd is the volume of distribution, Cp is the desired plasma level, and (S)(F) represents the fraction of the dose administered that will reach the systemic circulation. (See Figure 7.)

For example, if one wishes to calculate an oral loading dose of digoxin (i.e., using digoxin tablets) for a 70 kg man that will produce a plasma

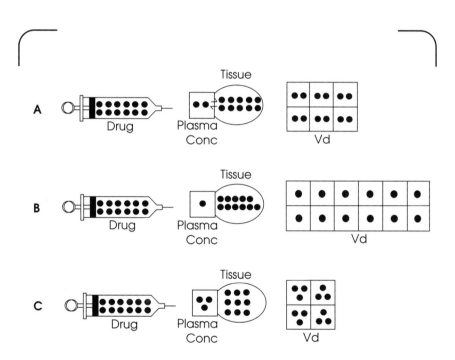

Figure 6. Volume of Distribution (A) The administration of a drug into the body produces a specific plasma concentration. The apparent volume of distribution (Vd) is the volume that accounts for the total dose administered based upon the observed plasma concentration. (B) Any factor that decreases the drug plasma concentration (e.g., decreased plasma protein binding) will increase the apparent volume of distribution. (C) Conversely, any factor that increases the plasma concentration (e.g., decreased tissue binding) will decrease the apparent volume of distribution.

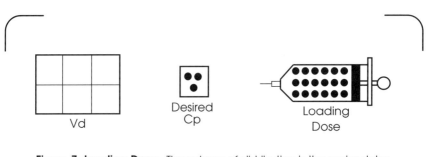

Figure 7. Loading Dose. The volume of distribution is the major determinant of the loading dose. If the Vd for a drug is known, the loading dose that will produce a specific concentration can be easily calculated. (See Equation 11.)

concentration of 1.5 µg/L, Equation 11 can be used. If S is assumed to be 1.0, F to be 0.7, and the Vd to be 7.3 L/kg,[1,25] the loading dose will be 1095 µg or 1.095 mg based upon the following calculation:

$$\text{Loading Dose} = \frac{(Vd)(Cp)}{(S)(F)}$$

$$= \frac{(7.3 \text{ L/kg})(70 \text{ kg})(1.5 \text{ µg/L})}{(1.0)(0.7)}$$

$$= 1095 \text{ µg } or \text{ } 1.095 \text{ mg}$$

A reasonable approximation of this dose would be 1 mg given orally as tablets. The usual clinical approach is to give the loading dose in divided doses (0.25 to 0.5 mg per dose every six hours). The patient is observed and evaluated for therapeutic response and digoxin toxicity before each successive dose is administered. In addition, clinicians frequently use a bioavailability factor >0.7 (e.g., 0.75 or 0.8) to guard against "overshooting" the desired level.

Equation 11 can also be used to estimate the loading dose that will be required to achieve a higher plasma concentration than the present concentration. (See Figure 8.) This new formula is derived by replacing the Cp in Equation 11 with an expression which represents the increment in plasma concentration which is desired.

$$\frac{\text{Incremental}}{\text{Loading Dose}} = \frac{(Vd)(Cp\ desired - Cp\ initial)}{(S)(F)}$$

Eq. 12

For example, if the previous patient had a digoxin level of 0.5 µg/L and the desired concentration was 1.5 µg/L, the loading dose would have been:

$$\begin{aligned}\frac{\text{Incremental}}{\text{Loading Dose}} &= \frac{(Vd)(Cp\ desired - Cp\ initial)}{(S)(F)} \\ &= \frac{(7.3\ L/kg)(70\ kg)(1.5\ µg/L - 0.5\ µg/L)}{(1.0)(0.7)} \\ &= 730\ µg\ or\ 0.73\ mg\end{aligned}$$

A reasonable incremental loading dose in this case would be about 0.75 mg.

Factors Which Alter Volume of Distribution (Vd) and Loading Dose

In analyzing Equation 11, it becomes clear that any factor which alters the volume of distribution will theoretically influence the loading dose.

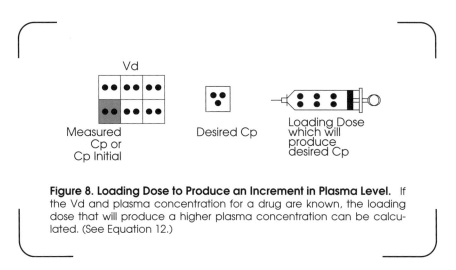

Figure 8. Loading Dose to Produce an Increment in Plasma Level. If the Vd and plasma concentration for a drug are known, the loading dose that will produce a higher plasma concentration can be calculated. (See Equation 12.)

Decreased tissue binding of drugs in uremic patients is a common cause of a reduced apparent volume of distribution for several agents.[26] (See Figure 6C on page 19.) Decreased tissue binding will increase the Cp by allowing more of the drug to remain in the plasma. Therefore, if the desired plasma level remains unchanged, a smaller loading dose will be required. Digoxin is an example of a drug whose loading dose should be altered in uremic patients. This is discussed in Part II: Digoxin.

Decreased plasma protein binding, on the other hand, tends to increase the apparent volume of distribution because more drug is available for tissue binding sites. (See Figure 6B on page 19.) Decreased plasma protein binding, however, also increases the fraction of free or active drug so that the desired Cp which produces a given therapeutic response decreases. To summarize, diminished plasma protein binding increases Vd and decreases Cp in Equation 11, resulting in no net effect on the loading dose. This is based upon the assumption that the majority of drug in the body is actually outside the plasma compartment and that the amount of drug bound to plasma protein comprises only a small percentage of the total amount in the body.

This principle is illustrated by the pharmacokinetic behavior of phenytoin in uremic patients. Plasma phenytoin concentrations in uremic patients are frequently one half of those observed in normal patients given the same dose. The lower plasma levels, however, produce the same free or pharmacologically-active phenytoin concentration as levels twice as high in non-uremic patients because the free fraction (alpha) is increased from 0.1 to 0.2 in these individuals. Furthermore, a loading dose of phenytoin which produces a normal therapeutic effect is the same for both uremic and non-uremic patients because the volume of distribution increases by approximately twofold (0.65 L/kg to 1.44 L/kg) in uremic individuals.[20] This statement assumes there is no change in bioavailability:

$$(2 \times Vd)(\tfrac{1}{2} \times Cp \text{ desired}) = \text{No Change in LD}$$

Two-Compartment Models

Pharmacokinetic Parameters. If one thinks of the body as a single compartment, pharmacokinetic calculations are relatively simple. However, there are some situations when it is more appropriate to conceptualize the body as two, and occasionally, more than two compartments when thinking about drug distribution, elimination, and pharmacologic effect. The first compartment can be thought of as a rapidly-equilibrating volume, usually made up of blood and those organs or tissues that have high blood flow. This first compartment has a volume referred to as Vi or initial volume. The second compartment equilibrates with the drug over a somewhat longer time period. This volume is referred to as Vt or tissue volume.[24] The half-time for the distribution phase is referred to as the alpha (α) half-life, and the half-time for drug elimination from the body is referred to as the beta (β) half-life. The sum of Vi and Vt is the apparent volume of distribution (Vd). Drugs are assumed to enter into and be eliminated from Vi. That is, any drug that distributes into the tissue compartment (Vt) must re-equilibrate into Vi before it can be eliminated. (See Figure 9.)

Effects of a Two-Compartment Model on the Loading Dose and Plasma Concentration (Cp). Since some time is required for a drug to distribute into Vt, a rapidly-administered loading dose calculated on the basis of Vd (Vi + Vt) would result in an initial Cp that is larger than predicted because of the smaller initial volume of distribution (Vi). The consequences of such an inaccurate prediction depend upon whether the target organ behaves as though it were located in Vi or Vt.

Drugs such as lidocaine, quinidine, and procainamide exert therapeutic and toxic effects on target organs which behave as though they are located in Vi. In these instances, the concentration of drug delivered to the target organs could be much higher than expected and produce toxicity if the loading dose is not adjusted appropriately. This problem can be circumvented by calculating the total loading dose based on the total volume of distribution (Vd). Then, the loading dose should be administered at a rate slow enough to allow for drug distribution into Vt, or the total loading dose should be given in sufficiently small bolus doses such that the Cp in Vi does not exceed some predetermined critical concentration.[27,28]

When the drug's target organ is in the second or tissue compartment, Vt (e.g., digoxin), the rather high Cp which may be observed before distribution occurs is not dangerous. Plasma concentrations which are obtained before distribution is complete, however, will not reflect the tissue concentration at equilibrium; therefore, these plasma samples cannot be used to predict the therapeutic or toxic effects of these drugs.[29,30] For example, clinicians usually wait one to three hours after an intravenous bolus dose before evaluating the effect of digoxin. This delay allows the digoxin to distribute to the site of action (myocardium) so that the full therapeutic or toxic effects of a dose can be observed. (See Part II: Digoxin and Figure 4.1.)

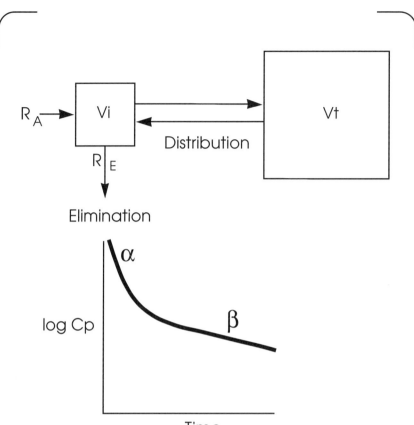

Figure 9. Two-Compartment Model. Volumes of distribution for a two-compartment model. Vi is the initial volume of distribution. Drug administration (R_A) and elimination (R_E) are assumed to occur in Vi. The lower graph shows how a drug administered into Vi follows a biphasic decay pattern. The initial decay half-life ($\alpha t\frac{1}{2}$) is usually due to drug distribution into Vt. The second decay half-life ($\beta t\frac{1}{2}$) is usually due to drug elimination from the body.

Slow drug distribution into the tissue compartment can pose problems in the accurate interpretation of Cp when a drug is given by the intravenous route. It is not generally a problem when a drug is given orally because the rate of absorption is usually slower than the rate of distribution from Vi into Vt. Nevertheless, digoxin and lithium are exceptions to this rule. Even when these drugs are given orally, several hours are required for complete absorption and distribution.

Plasma samples obtained <6 hours after an oral dose of digoxin or <12 hours after an oral dose of lithium are of questionable value. For these two drugs, the end-organs behave as though they are located in the more slowly-equilibrating tissue compartment or Vt. Plasma concentrations obtained during the distribution phase (before equilibrium with the deep tissue compartment is complete) will be increased, and the pharmacologic response will be much less than the plasma concentration would indicate.

Drugs with Significant and Non-Significant Two-Compartment Modeling. As illustrated in Figure 9, the alpha phase for most drugs represents distribution of drug from Vi into Vt; relatively little drug is eliminated during the distribution phase. Drugs which behave in this way are generally referred to as "non-significant" two-compartmental drugs. It is important to recognize that for some drugs, increased drug plasma concentrations during the alpha phase can be clinically significant because the patient may experience serious toxicity if the end-organ behaves as though it lies within the initial volume of distribution (Vi). These drugs are considered to exhibit "non-significant" two-compartmental modeling only after the alpha phase has been completed. That is, plasma samples are obtained for pharmacokinetic modeling only during the beta or elimination phase.

Drugs with "significant" two-compartment modeling are those which are eliminated to a significant extent during the initial alpha phase. For these drugs, the alpha phase cannot be thought of simply as a distribution phase, since significant elimination occurs as well. Two drugs which border on having significant two-compartment modeling are lithium and lidocaine. Some clinicians have suggested that these drugs could be more successfully monitored by use of two-compartmental model pharmacokinetics. The complexity of these models, however, as well as the number of plasma samples required for patient-specific dose adjustments, usually limits the use of two-compartmental modeling techniques. When a one-compartment model is used for drugs that exhibit significant two-compartment modeling, the actual trough concentrations will be lower than those predicted by the one-compartment model because a significant amount of drug is eliminated during the distribution phase. (See Interpretation of Plasma Drug Concentrations on page 73.)

Clearance (Cl)

Clearance can be thought of as the intrinsic ability of the body or its organs of elimination (usually the kidneys and the liver) to remove drug from the blood or plasma. Clearance is expressed as a volume per unit of time. It is important to emphasize that clearance is not an indicator of how much drug is being removed; it only represents the theoretical volume of blood or plasma which is completely cleared of drug in a given period of time. The amount of drug removed depends on the plasma concentration of drug as well as the clearance. (See Figure 10.)

At steady state, the rate of drug administration (R_A) and rate of drug elimination (R_E) must be equal. (Also see Elimination Rate Constant (Kd) on page 37.)

$$R_A = R_E$$

Eq. 13

Clearance (Cl) can best be thought of as the proportionality constant that makes the average steady-state plasma drug level equal to the rate of drug administration (R_A):

$$R_A = (Cl)(Cpss\ ave)$$

Eq. 14

where R_A is $(S)(F)(Dose)/\tau$ (see Equation 5) and Cpss ave is the average steady-state drug concentration.

If an average steady-state plasma concentration and the rate of drug administration are known, the clearance can be calculated by rearranging Equation 14:

$$Cl = \frac{(S)(F)(Dose/\tau)}{Cpss\ ave}$$

Eq. 15

STEADY STATE

Rate In (R$_A$) Rate Out (R$_E$)

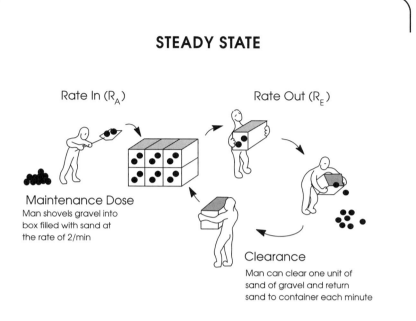

Maintenance Dose
Man shovels gravel into
box filled with sand at
the rate of 2/min

Clearance
Man can clear one unit of
sand of gravel and return
sand to container each minute

Figure 10. Steady State, Maintenance Dose, Clearance, Elimination Rate Constant. At steady state, the rate of drug administration (R$_A$) is equal to the rate of drug elimination (R$_E$), and the concentration of drug remains constant. In this example, the man on the left is able to shovel gravel or ``drug'' into a container of sand at the rate of 2/min. The man on the right is able to remove one unit of sand containing gravel or ``drug'' from the container, dump the gravel, and return the sand to the container each minute. The *amount* of gravel or drug removed per unit of time (rate of elimination) will be determined by the concentration of gravel per unit of sand as well as the clearance (volume of sand cleared of gravel). The elimination rate constant (Kd) can be thought of as the fraction of the total volume cleared per unit of time. In this case, Kd would be equal to ⅙ or 0.17^{-1}.

For example, if intravenous lidocaine is infused continuously at a rate of 2 mg/min and if the concentration of lidocaine at steady state is 3 mg/L, the calculated lidocaine clearance using Equation 15 would be 0.667 L/min:

$$Cl = \frac{(S)(F)(Dose/\tau)}{Cpss\ ave}$$

$$= \frac{(1.0)(1.0)(2\ mg/min)}{3\ mg/L}$$

$$= 0.667\ L/min$$

F is considered to be 1.0 because the drug is being administered intravenously. S is also assumed to be 1.0 because the hydrochloride salt represents only a small fraction of the total molecular weight for lidocaine and correction for the salt form is unnecessary.

Maintenance Dose

If an estimate for clearance is obtained from the literature, the clearance formula (Equation 15) can be rearranged slightly and used to calculate the rate of administration or maintenance dose which will produce a desired average plasma concentration at steady state:

$$\text{Maintenance Dose} = \frac{(Cl)(Cpss\ ave)(\tau)}{(S)(F)}$$

Eq. 16

For example, using the literature estimate for theophylline clearance of 2.8 L/hr, the rate of intravenous administration for aminophylline that will produce a steady-state plasma theophylline concentration of 15 mg/L is illustrated below:

$$\text{Maintenance Dose} = \frac{(Cl)(Cpss\ ave)(\tau)}{(S)(F)}$$

$$= \frac{(2.8\ L/hr)(15\ mg/L)(1\ hr)}{(0.8)(1.0)}$$

$$= 52.5\ mg$$

Since τ is one hour, the rate of administration is 52.5 mg/hr. If the aminophylline were to be given every six hours, the dose would be 315 mg or six times the hourly administration rate.

$$\text{Maintenance Dose} = \frac{(Cl)(Cpss\ ave)(\tau)}{(S)(F)}$$

$$= \frac{(2.84\ hr)(15\ mg/L)(6\ hr)}{(0.8)(1.0)}$$

$$= 315\ mg$$

Factors Which Alter Clearance (Cl) *(See Table 2)*

Body Surface Area (BSA). Most literature values for clearance are expressed as volume/kg/time or as volume/70 kg/time. There is some evidence, however, that drug clearance is best adjusted on the basis of body surface area rather than weight.[31-34] Body surface area can be calculated using Equation 17 or it can be obtained from various charts and nomograms.[35,36] (See Appendix I.)

$$\text{BSA in m}^2 = \left(\frac{\text{Patient's Weight in kg}}{70 \text{ kg}}\right)^{0.73} (1.73 \text{ m}^2)$$

Eq. 17

The following formulas can be used to adjust the clearance values reported in the literature for specific patients.

$$\text{Patient's Cl} = (\text{Literature Cl per m}^2)(\text{Patient's BSA})$$

Eq. 18

$$\text{Patient's Cl} = (\text{Literature Cl per 70 kg})\left(\frac{\text{Patient's BSA}}{1.73 \text{ m}^2}\right)$$

Eq. 19

$$\text{Patient's Cl} = (\text{Literature Cl per 70 kg})\left(\frac{\text{Patient's Weight in kg}}{70 \text{ kg}}\right)$$

Eq. 20

$$\text{Patient's Cl} = (\text{Literature Cl per kg})(\text{Patient's Weight in kg})$$

Eq. 21

Equations 20 and 21 adjust clearance in proportion to weight, whereas Equations 18 and 19 adjust clearance in proportion to body surface area.

The underlying assumption in using weight or surface area to adjust clearance values is that the patient's liver and kidney size (and hopefully function) vary in proportion to these physical measurements. If the patient's weight is reasonably close to 70 kg (BSA = 1.73 m²), the patient's

Table 2	Factors Which Alter Clearance (Cl)
	Body weight
	Body surface area
	Plasma protein binding
	Extraction ratio
	Renal function
	Hepatic function
	Cardiac output

calculated clearance will be similar whether weight or body surface area are used to calculate clearance. If, however, the patient's weight differs significantly from 70 kg, then the use of weight or surface area is likely to generate substantially different estimates of the patient's clearance. When a patient's size is substantially greater or less than the standard 70 kg, or 1.73 m², a careful assessment should be made to determine if the patient's body stature is normal, obese, or emaciated. In obese and emaciated patients, neither weight nor surface area is likely to be helpful in predicting clearance, since the patient's body size will not reflect the size or function of the liver and kidney.

Plasma Protein Binding. For highly protein-bound drugs, diminished plasma protein binding is associated with a decrease in reported steady-state plasma drug concentrations (total of unbound plus free drug) for any given dose which is administered. (See Figure 5 on page 15 and Desired Plasma Concentration (Cp) on page 9.) According to Equation 15, a decrease in the denominator, Cpss ave, increases the calculated clearance.

$$Cl = \frac{(S)(F)(Dose/\tau)}{Cpss\ ave}$$

It would be misleading, however, to assume that because the calculated clearance is increased, the *amount* eliminated per unit of time has increased. Equation 15 assumes that when Cpss ave (total of bound plus free drug) changes, the free drug concentration which is available for metabolism and renal elimination changes proportionately. In actuality, the free or unbound *fraction* of drug in the plasma[11,37] generally increases (even though Cpss ave decreases) with diminished plasma protein binding. As a result, the *amount* of free drug eliminated per unit of time remains unchanged. This should be apparent if one considers that at steady state, the amount of drug administered per unit of time (R_A) must equal the amount eliminated per unit of time (R_E). If R_A has not changed, R_E must remain the same.

In summary, when the same daily dose of a drug is given in the presence of diminished protein binding, an amount equal to that dose will be eliminated from the body each day at steady state despite a diminished steady-state plasma concentration and an increase in the calculated clearance. This lower plasma concentration (Cp bound + Cp free) is associated with an increased *fraction* of free drug (α) but the same free concentration (Cp free) as that observed under normal binding conditions.

$$\uparrow\alpha = \frac{\text{Cp free}}{\downarrow \text{Cp bound} + \text{Cp free}}$$

Eq. 22

Therefore, the pharmacologic effect achieved will be similar to that produced by the higher serum concentration observed under normal protein binding conditions. This example re-emphasizes the principle that clearance alone is not a good indicator of the *amount* of drug eliminated per unit of time (R_E). (See Figures 11 and 12.)

This principle is illustrated by comparing the calculated phenytoin clearances for a uremic and non-uremic patient at steady state. As noted previously in the discussion of desired plasma concentration on page 16, the steady-state plasma phenytoin concentration in the uremic individual receiving 300 mg/day will be lower ($\approx$5 mg/L) than that of the non-uremic patient ($\approx$10 mg/L) who is receiving the same dose due to decreased protein binding. Nevertheless, the concentration of free or active drug will be approximately the same for both patients because the alpha or free fraction is equal to 0.2 in the uremic individual and 0.1 in the non-uremic individual. Consequently, even though the calculated clearance (Equation 15) for the uremic patient is higher than the non-uremic patient (60 L/day versus 30 L/day), the amount of drug cleared per day (300 mg) is the same, because at steady state the rate of drug administration (R_A) is equal to the rate of drug elimination (R_E) for both the uremic and non-uremic patient. (See Equation 15.)

$$Cl = \frac{(S)(F)(Dose/\tau)}{Cpss\ ave}$$

Uremic

$$Cl = \frac{(1)(1)(300\ mg/day)}{5\ mg/L}$$

$$= 60\ L/day$$

Non-Uremic

$$Cl = \frac{(1)(1)(300\ mg/day)}{10\ mg/L}$$

$$= 30\ L/day$$

$$R_A = R_E$$
$$300\ mg/day = 300\ mg/day$$

When protein binding is decreased, the increase in calculated clearance is generally proportional to the change in alpha. Although the calculated clearance may be used to estimate a maintenance dose, careful

STEADY STATE

PROTEIN ◎
FREE DRUG ●

Rate In (R_A)

Rate Out (R_E)

Maintenance Dose

$\alpha = 0.25$

Clearance (Cl = 0.25)

Figure 11. Clearance (Cl) of a Highly Protein-Bound Drug with a Low Extraction Ratio. The free drug fraction α is available for clearance. Protein-bound drug is returned to the container so that the actual volume cleared of drug is ½ of the volume removed by the man on the right each minute. (Compare with Figure 10.)

STEADY STATE

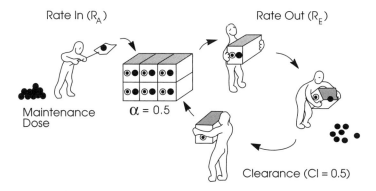

Rate In (R$_A$)   Rate Out (R$_E$)

Maintenance Dose α = 0.5

Clearance (CI = 0.5)

Figure 12. Effect of Diminished Protein Binding on Clearance (CI) of a Highly Protein-Bound Drug Which Has a Low Extraction Ratio. Compare this figure with Figure 11. The plasma concentration of drug has decreased, but the free concentration remains the same (α is increased). (See Figure 4.) The volume actually cleared of drug has increased compared to that cleared in Figure 11, even though the *amount* of drug cleared per unit of time has remained unchanged. This illustrates the principle that the amount of a highly protein-bound drug cleared per unit of time (R$_E$) remains the same if the increase in clearance is proportional to the increase in fraction free when protein binding is decreased.

selection of the plasma level that will produce the desired pharmacologic effect is critical to the determination of a therapeutically-correct maintenance dose.

Extraction Ratio. The direct proportionality between calculated clearance and alpha does not apply to drugs that are so efficiently metabolized or excreted that some (perhaps all) of the drug bound to plasma protein is removed as it passes through the eliminating organ.[33,38] In this situation the plasma protein acts as a "transport system" for the drug, carrying it to the eliminating organs, and clearance becomes dependent upon the blood or plasma flow to the eliminating organ. To determine whether the clearance for a drug with significant plasma binding will be influenced primarily by blood flow or plasma protein binding, its extraction ratio is estimated and compared to its alpha value.

The extraction ratio is the fraction of the drug presented to the eliminating organ that is cleared after a single pass through that organ. It can be estimated by dividing the blood or plasma clearance of a drug by the blood or plasma flow to the eliminating organ. If the extraction ratio exceeds alpha, then the plasma proteins are acting as a transport system and clearance will not change in proportion to alpha. If, however, the extraction ratio is less than alpha, clearance is likely to increase by the same proportion that alpha changes. This approach does not take into account other factors that may affect clearance such as red blood cell binding, elimination from red blood cells, or changes in metabolic function.

Renal and Hepatic Function. Drugs can be eliminated or cleared as unchanged drug through the kidney (renal clearance) and by metabolism in the liver (metabolic clearance). These two routes of clearance are assumed to be independent of one another and additive.[24,39]

$$Cl_t = Cl_m + Cl_r$$

Eq. 23

Where Cl_t is total clearance, Cl_m is metabolic clearance or the fraction cleared by metabolism, and Cl_r is renal clearance or the fraction cleared by the renal route. Since the kidneys and liver function independently, it is assumed that a change in one does not affect the other. Thus, Cl_t can be estimated in the presence of renal or hepatic failure or both. Since metabolic function is difficult to quantitate, Cl_t is most commonly adjusted when there is decreased renal function:

$$Cl \text{ Adjusted} = [Cl_m] + [Cl_r]\left[\frac{\text{Fraction of Normal Renal}}{\text{Function Remaining}}\right]$$

Eq. 24

A clearance that has been adjusted for renal function can be used to estimate the maintenance dose for a patient with diminished renal function. (See Equation 16 on page 28.) This adjusted clearance equation, however, is only valid if the drug's metabolites are inactive and if the metabolic clearance is indeed unaffected by renal dysfunction as assumed.

A decrease in the function of an organ of elimination is most significant when that organ serves as the primary route of drug elimination. However, as the major elimination pathway becomes increasingly compromised, the "minor" pathway becomes more significant because it assumes a greater proportion of the total clearance. For example, a drug that is usually 67% eliminated by the renal route and 33% by the metabolic route will be 100% metabolized in the event of complete renal failure; the total clearance, however, will only be one-third of the normal value.

Most pharmacokinetic adjustments for drug elimination are based upon renal function because hepatic function is usually more difficult to quantitate. Hepatic function can be evaluated using the prothrombin time, serum albumin concentration, and serum bilirubin concentration. Unfortunately, each of these laboratory tests is affected by variables other than altered hepatic function. For example, the serum albumin may be low due to decreased protein intake or increased renal or gastrointestinal loss, as well as to decreased hepatic function. Although liver function tests do not provide quantitative data, pharmacokinetic adjustments must still take into consideration liver function because this route of elimination is important for a significant number of drugs.

Cardiac output also affects drug metabolism. Hepatic or metabolic clearances for some drugs can be decreased by 25% to 50% in patients with congestive heart failure. For example, the metabolic clearances of theophylline[40] and digoxin[31] are reduced by about one-half in patients with congestive heart failure. Since the metabolic clearance for both of these drugs is much lower than the hepatic blood or plasma flow (low extraction ratio), it would not have been predicted that their clearances would have been influenced by cardiac output or hepatic blood flow to this extent. The decreased cardiac output and resultant hepatic congestion must, in some way, decrease the intrinsic metabolic capacity of the liver. The effect of diminished clearance on plasma drug concentrations is illustrated in Figure 13 (compare with Figure 10 on page 27).

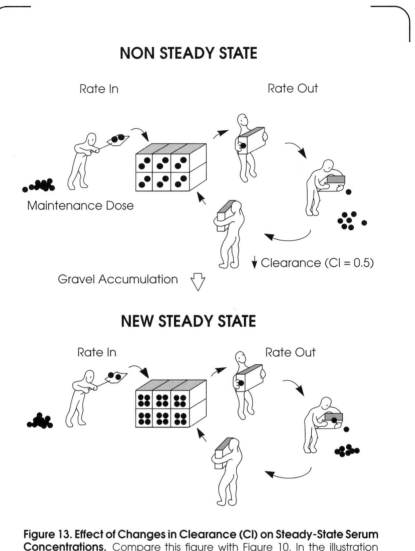

NON STEADY STATE

Rate In   Rate Out

Maintenance Dose

Gravel Accumulation

↓ Clearance (Cl = 0.5)

NEW STEADY STATE

Rate In   Rate Out

Figure 13. Effect of Changes in Clearance (Cl) on Steady-State Serum Concentrations. Compare this figure with Figure 10. In the illustration above, the maintenance dose or amount of gravel added to the container per unit of time remains the same; however, the volume of sand cleared of gravel (clearance) has been halved. Initially, the amount of gravel or "drug" cleared per unit of time is less than the maintenance dose; the concentration of gravel in the container increases until a new steady state is reached. At this point, the rate at which gravel is added to the container again equals the rate at which gravel is eliminated from the container. If clearance had increased, the concentration of gravel would have decreased until the amount removed per unit of time (R_E) again equaled the rate of administration (R_A).

Elimination Rate Constant (Kd) and Half-Life (t½)

It is often desirable to predict how drug plasma levels will change with time. For drugs which are eliminated by first-order pharmacokinetics, these predictions are based on the elimination rate constant (Kd).

First-Order Pharmacokinetics

First-order elimination pharmacokinetics refers to a process in which the amount or concentration of drug in the body diminishes logarithmically over time. (See Figure 14.)

The rate of elimination (R_E) is proportional to the drug concentration; therefore, the *amount* of drug removed per unit of time (R_E) will vary proportionately with drug concentration. The *fraction or percentage* of the total amount of drug present in the body (Ab) that is removed at any instant in time, however, will remain constant and independent of dose. That fraction or percentage is expressed by the elimination rate constant, Kd. The equations which describe first-order elimination of a drug from the body are as follows:

$$Ab = (Ab^\circ)(e^{-Kdt})$$

Eq. 25

or

$$Cp = (Cp^\circ)(e^{-Kdt})$$

Eq. 26

where Ab° and Ab represent the total amount of drug in the body at the beginning and end of the time interval, t, respectively; and e^{-Kdt} is the fraction of Ab° remaining at time t. Cp° and Cp are the plasma concentrations at the beginning and end of the time interval, respectively. Since the drug concentration diminishes logarithmically, a graphic plot of the logarithm of the plasma level versus time yields a straight line. (See Figure 15.)

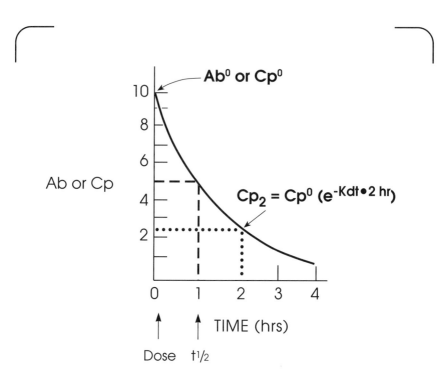

Figure 14. First-Order Elimination. The amount or concentration of drug diminishes logarithmically over time. The initial amount of plasma concentration produced by a loading dose is Ab^0 or Cp^0. The half-life (t½) is the time required to eliminate one-half of the drug. The concentration at the end of a given time interval (in this example, 2 hr) is equal to the initial concentration times the fraction of drug remaining at the end of that time interval ($e^{-Kd \times 2 hr}$). The amount or concentration of drug lost in each 1-hour interval diminishes over time (5, 2.5, 1.25); however, the fraction of drug which is lost each unit of time remains constant (0.5). For example, over the first hour, one-half of the total amount of drug in the body (10) was lost (5). In the next time interval (1–2 hr), one half of the amount of drug which remained (5) was lost (2.5).

This type of graphical analysis of declining plasma drug concentrations is often used to determine if a drug is eliminated by a first-order process.

Another important characteristic of first-order elimination is that both clearance and volume of distribution remain constant and do not vary with dose or concentration. Therefore, concentrations can be adjusted by altering the drug dosage in proportion to the desired change in concentration. (See Figure 16.)

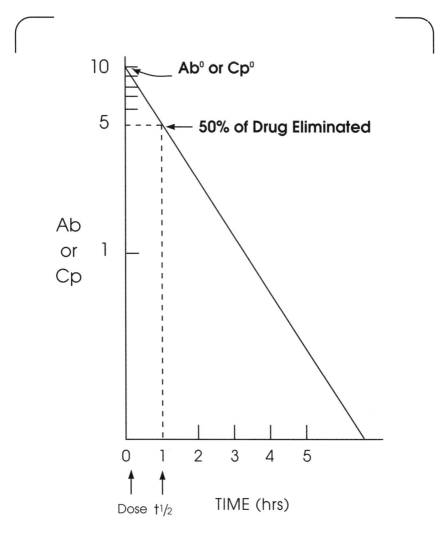

Figure 15. First-Order Elimination. A graph of the log of Ab or Cp versus time yields a straight line. The half-life is the time required for Ab or Cp to decline to one-half the original value.

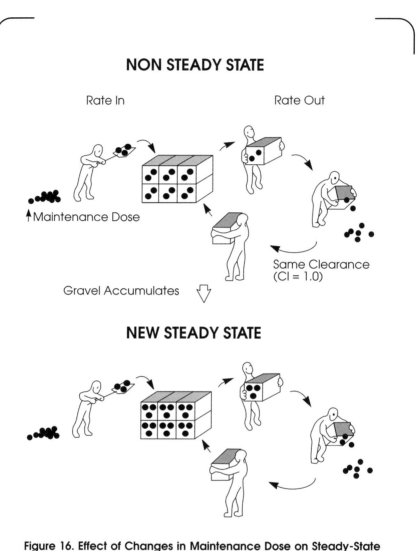

NON STEADY STATE

Rate In   Rate Out

↑Maintenance Dose

Same Clearance
(Cl = 1.0)

Gravel Accumulates

NEW STEADY STATE

Figure 16. Effect of Changes in Maintenance Dose on Steady-State Plasma Concentrations. Compare this figure with Figure 10. In the illustration above, the clearance or volume of sand cleared of gravel remains the same; however, the maintenance dose or the amount of gravel added to the container per unit of time has been increased from 2/min to 3/min. Therefore, the concentration of gravel or "drug" increases until a new steady state is reached. At this point, the rate at which gravel is added to the container again equals the rate at which gravel is eliminated from the container. If the maintenance dose decreased, the concentration of gravel would have gradually decreased until a new steady state had been achieved.

Elimination Rate Constant (Kd)

The elimination rate constant, Kd, is the fraction or percentage of the total amount of drug in the body removed per unit of time and it is a function of clearance and volume of distribution:

$$Kd = \frac{Cl}{Vd}$$

Eq. 27

As Equation 27 illustrates, Kd can also be thought of as the fraction of the volume of distribution which will be effectively cleared of drug per unit of time. (See Figure 10 on page 26.) For example, a drug with a clearance of 10 L/day and a Vd of 100 L would have an elimination rate constant of 0.1 days^{-1}.

Since the drug elimination rate constant is the slope of the ln Cp versus time plot, two plasma concentrations measured during the decay or elimination phase (i.e., between doses or following a single dose) can be used to calculate the Kd for a specific patient:

$$Kd = \frac{\ln\left(\frac{Cp_1}{Cp_2}\right)}{t}$$

Eq. 28

where Cp_1 is the first or higher plasma concentration, Cp_2 is the second or lower plasma concentration, and t is the time interval between the plasma samples. For example, if Cp_1 is 5 mg/L and Cp_2 is 2 mg/L, and the time interval between the samples is eight hours, the elimination rate constant (Kd) will be 0.115 hr^{-1}.

$$Kd = \frac{\ln\left(\frac{5 \text{ mg/L}}{2 \text{ mg/L}}\right)}{8 \text{ hr}}$$

$$= 0.115 \text{ hr}^{-1}$$

To estimate Kd accurately, the time which elapses between samples should span at least one half-life. [See Half-Life (t½) on page 43.] Although Kd is dependent upon the volume of distribution and clearance, some authors have suggested that Kd be adjusted for renal failure in a manner similar to that for clearance (Equation 24 on page 34), and that the adjusted Kd be used to estimate a clearance value in renal failure by use of Equation 30.[41,42] [See Clearance (Cl): Factors Which Alter Clearance on page 29.]

$$Kd_{adjusted} = \left[K_{metabolic} \right] + \left[(K_{renal}) \left(\begin{array}{c} \text{Fraction of Normal} \\ \text{Renal Function} \\ \text{Remaining} \end{array} \right) \right]$$

Eq. 29

$$Cl_{adjusted} = (Kd_{adjusted})(Vd_{normal})$$

Eq. 30

This adjusted clearance is then used to calculate a maintenance dose for the patient in renal failure using Equation 16 on page 28:

$$\text{Maintenance Dose} = \frac{(Cl)(Cpss\ ave)(\tau)}{(S)(F)}$$

This method of adjusting the maintenance dose in a patient with renal failure is based on the assumption that changes in clearance are proportional to changes in Kd if the volume of distribution does not change in renal failure. However, this often is not the case. Protein binding changes that occur in renal failure can change Vd. (See Figure 6 on page 19.) Nevertheless, one may have to resort to this indirect method of determining clearance on occasion because elimination rate constants for drugs are more readily available in the literature than clearance values. While the adjusted Kd calculated by this approach can be used to estimate an adjusted clearance in renal failure, it *cannot* be reliably used to estimate the half-life of a drug in a patient with renal failure if the Vd is altered.[42,43] If Vd is altered in renal failure and if the indirect method of determining clearance is being utilized, the normal value for Vd must still be used in Equation 30 because Kd was adjusted on the assumption that Vd had *not* changed in renal failure. A more direct approach is to first estimate the independent parameters, clearance and volume of distribution. From these, the elimination rate constant, which is the dependent variable, can be calculated.

Half-Life (t½)

The elimination rate constant is often expressed in terms of a drug's half-life, a value which is more conveniently applied to the clinical setting. The half-life (t½) of a drug is the amount of time required for the total amount of drug in the body or the plasma drug concentration to decrease by one-half. (See Figure 15 on page 39.) It sometimes is referred to as the βt½ to distinguish it from the half-life for distribution (αt½) in a two-compartment model and it is a function of the elimination rate constant, Kd:

$$t\tfrac{1}{2} = \frac{0.693}{Kd}$$

Eq. 31

If the Kd used in Equation 31 is derived from plasma concentrations obtained during the decay phase, then the time interval in which the samples are drawn should span at least one half-life. (See discussion of Equation 28 on page 41.) Shorter time periods can be used, but small errors in the assayed concentrations can alter the calculated half-life considerably.

This rule makes it impractical to obtain peak and trough levels within a dosing interval to determine the half-life because the dosing interval is frequently equal to, or shorter than, the usual half-life for most drugs (e.g., theophylline, quinidine, procainamide, digoxin, phenobarbital).

If the volume of distribution and clearance for a drug are known, the half-life can be estimated by using Equation 32 below. The half-life, like Kd, is dependent upon and determined by Cl and Vd. This relationship is illustrated in Equation 32 which was obtained by substituting Equation 27 into Equation 31:

$$t\tfrac{1}{2} = \frac{(0.693)(Vd)}{Cl}$$

Eq. 32

The dependence of t½ or Kd on Vd and Cl is emphasized because the volume of distribution and clearance for a drug can change *independently*

Table 3	Clinical Application of the Elimination Rate Constant (Kd) and Half-Life (t½)

1. Estimating the time to reach steady-state plasma concentrations after initiation of change in the maintenance dose.

2. Estimating the time required to eliminate all or a portion of the drug from the body once it is discontinued.

3. Predicting nonsteady-state plasma levels following the initiation of an infusion.

4. Predicting a steady-state plasma level from a nonsteady-state plasma level obtained at a specific time following the initiation of an infusion.

5. Given the degree of fluctuation in plasma concentration desired within a dosing interval, determine that interval. Given the interval, determine the fluctuation in the plasma concentration.

of one another and thus, affect the half-life or elimination constant in the same or opposite directions.

Another caution is appropriate at this point. It is a common misconception that because Equation 27 can be rearranged to:

$$Cl = (Kd)(Vd)$$

Eq. 33

that clearance is determined by Kd (or t½) and Vd; however, this is incorrect. Instead, Kd and t½ are dependent upon clearance and the volume of distribution; it is therefore invalid to make any assumptions about the volume of distribution or clearance of a drug based solely upon knowledge of its half-life. For example, if the half-life of a drug is prolonged, the clearance may be increased, decreased, or unchanged depending upon corresponding changes in the volume of distribution.

Clinical Application of Elimination Rate Constant (Kd) and Half-Life (t½) (See Table 3)

Time to Reach Steady State. Half-life is an important variable to consider when answering questions concerning time such as: "How long will it take a drug concentration to reach steady state on a constant dosage regimen?" or "How long will it take for the drug concentration to reach steady state if the dosage regimen is changed?" When drugs are given chronically, they accumulate in the body until the amount administered in a given time period (maintenance dose) is equal to the amount eliminated in that same period. When this occurs, drug concentrations in the plasma will plateau and will have reached "steady state." (See Figures 10 and 16 on pages 27 and 40, respectively.) The time required for a drug concentration to reach steady state is determined by the drug's half-life. It takes one half-life to reach 50%, two half-lives to reach 75%, three half-lives to reach 87.5%, and four half-lives to reach 93.75% of steady state. With each additional half-life the residual fraction away from steady state diminishes, and at some point (usually ≤10%) this residual is considered negligible and steady state is assumed to have been achieved. *In most clinical situations, the attainment of steady state can be assumed after three to four half-lives.* (See Figure 17.)

Time for Drug Elimination. The half-life can also be used to determine how long it will take to effectively eliminate all of the drug from the body after the drug has been discontinued. It takes one half-life to eliminate 50%, two half-lives to eliminate 75%, three half-lives to eliminate 87.5%, and four half-lives to eliminate 93.75% of the total amount of drug in the body. Again, in *most* clinical situations it can be assumed that all of the drug has been effectively eliminated after three to four half-lives. (See Figure 18.)

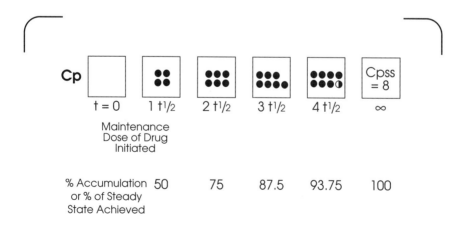

Figure 17. First-Order Accumulation. When a maintenance dose is initiated, it takes 4 or more half-lives to reach steady-state plasma levels. This example assumes that the maintenance dose administered will produce an average steady-state level (Cpss ave or Cpss) of 8.

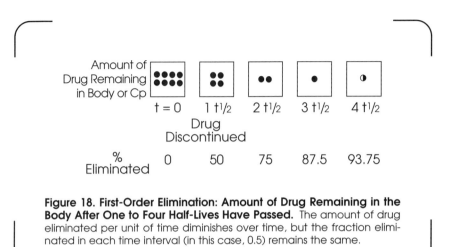

Figure 18. First-Order Elimination: Amount of Drug Remaining in the Body After One to Four Half-Lives Have Passed. The amount of drug eliminated per unit of time diminishes over time, but the fraction eliminated in each time interval (in this case, 0.5) remains the same.

Prediction of Plasma Levels Following Initiation of an Infusion. Often, when drugs are given by constant infusion, it is useful to predict the plasma concentrations that will be achieved at a specific period of time. (See Figure 19.) The rate at which a drug approaches steady state is also governed by the elimination rate constant; therefore, this parameter can be used to calculate the fraction of steady state which is achieved at any time after the initiation of the infusion (t_1):

$$\text{Fraction of Steady State Achieved at } t_1 = (1 - e^{-Kdt_1})$$

Eq. 34

The average plasma concentration at steady state (Cpss ave) can be calculated by rearranging the clearance formula (Equation 15 on page 26):

$$Cl = \frac{(S)(F)(Dose/\tau)}{Cpss\ ave}$$

$$Cpss\ ave = \frac{(S)(F)(Dose/\tau)}{Cl}$$

Eq. 35

$$Cp_1 = \frac{(S)(F)(Dose/\tau)}{Cl}(1 - e^{-Kdt_1}) \qquad \text{(Eq. 37)}$$

$$Cp_2 = \frac{(S)(F)(Dose/\tau)}{Cl}(1 - e^{-Kdt_1})(e^{-Kdt_2}) \qquad \text{(Eq. 41)}$$

Figure 19. Graphic Representation of an Infusion That Is Discontinued Before Steady State. Cp_1 is a concentration which is achieved any time (t_1) after the infusion is initiated, and Cp_2 is a concentration that results any interval of time (t_2) after the infusion has been discontinued.

The plasma concentration which can be expected at a specific time after initiation of the infusion (Cp_1) can be calculated by multiplying the average steady-state concentration by the fraction of steady state achieved at t_1.

$$Cp_1 = \left(Cpss\ ave\right)\left(\begin{array}{c}\text{Fraction of Steady State} \\ \text{Achieved at } t_1\end{array}\right)$$

Eq. 36

If Equation 34 for "fraction of steady state achieved at t_1" and Equation 35 for Cpss ave are substituted into Equation 36 above, a new equation for plasma concentration at t_1 (Cp$_1$) is derived:

$$Cp_1 = \frac{(S)(F)(Dose/\tau)}{Cl}(1 - e^{-Kdt_1})$$

Eq. 37

All of the time units (i.e., days, hours, or minutes) used in Equation 37 (τ, Cl, t_1) should be the same. According to Equation 36, as the duration of the infusion (t_1) approaches four or more half-lives, the fraction of steady state achieved approaches one, and for all practical purposes steady state has been achieved. Conversely, if a drug plasma concentration was obtained before steady-state concentration was attained (Cp$_1$), the approximate steady-state concentration which should be achieved can be estimated through rearrangement of Equation 37:

$$Cpss\ ave = \frac{Cp_1}{(1 - e^{-Kdt_1})}$$

Eq. 38

If the predicted steady-state concentration is too high, side effects or toxicities might be avoided by reducing the maintenance infusion before the achievement of steady state.

Prediction of Plasma Levels Following Discontinuation of an Infusion. (See Figure 19 on page 47.) The plasma concentration any time after an infusion is discontinued (Cp$_2$), can be estimated by multiplying the measured or predicted plasma concentration at the time the infusion is discontinued by the fraction of drug remaining at t_2.

$$\text{Fraction of Drug Remaining at } t_2 = (e^{-Kdt_2})$$

Eq. 39

$$Cp_2 = (Cp_1)(e^{-Kdt_2})$$

Eq. 40

If Equation 37 for Cp_1 is substituted into Equation 40, the plasma concentration (Cp_2) at any time (t_2) after an infusion is discontinued is as follows:

$$Cp_2 = \frac{(S)(F)(Dose/\tau)}{Cl}\left(1 - e^{-Kdt_1}\right)\left(e^{-Kdt_2}\right)$$

Eq. 41

While Equation 41 looks complicated, it is only a variation of Equation 26 on page 37, the first-order equation which describes elimination:

$$Cp = (Cp^\circ)(e^{-Kdt})$$

where Cp° is the concentration at the beginning of the time interval (t) which, in this case, is the point at which the infusion was discontinued. (See Figure 19 on page 47.)

Calculation of a theophylline concentration, which will be expected 8 hours after an aminophylline infusion of 100 mg/hr is discontinued, can be used to illustrate this principle. Assume that aminophylline has been administered for 16 hours to a patient with a theophylline clearance of 2.8 L/hr and a half-life of 8 hours (Kd of 0.087 hr^{-1}). The calculations can be accomplished step by step as follows:

1) The expected steady-state theophylline concentration resulting from an aminophylline infusion of 100 mg/hr to a patient with a theophylline clearance of 2.8 L/hr can be calculated using Equation 35:

$$Cpss\ ave = \frac{(0.8)(1.0)(100\ mg/hr)}{2.8\ L/hr}$$
$$= 28.6\ mg/L$$

2) The expected concentration after 16 hours of infusion (t_1) can be calculated using Equation 37:

$$
\begin{aligned}
Cp_1 &= (28.6 \text{ mg/L})(1 - e^{(-0.087 \text{ hr}^{-1})(16 \text{ hr})}) \\
&= (28.6 \text{ mg/L})(1 - e^{-1.392}) \\
&= (28.6 \text{ mg/L})(1 - 0.25) \\
&= 21.45 \text{ mg/L}
\end{aligned}
$$

3) The expected concentration 8 hours after the end of the infusion can be calculated using Equation 40:

$$
\begin{aligned}
Cp_2 &= (21.45 \text{ mg/L})(e^{(-0.087 \text{ hr}^{-1})(8 \text{ hr})}) \\
&= (21.45 \text{ mg/L})(e^{-0.693}) \\
&= (21.45 \text{ mg/L})(0.5) \\
&= 10.7 \text{ mg/L}
\end{aligned}
$$

Dosing Interval (τ). The half-life can also be used to estimate the appropriate dosing interval or tau (τ) for maintenance therapy. For example, if the goal of therapy is to minimize plasma fluctuations to no more than 50% between doses, the dosing interval (τ) should be less than or equal to the half-life. The maintenance dose can be calculated using Equation 16 on page 28:

$$
\text{Maintenance Dose} = \frac{(Cl)(Cpss \text{ ave})(\tau)}{(S)(F)}
$$

If tau is less than or equal to the half-life of a drug, the calculated maintenance dose will produce plasma concentrations which will fluctuate by ≤50% during that dosing interval. The plasma levels will be above the average steady-state plasma level for the first half of the dosing interval and below the average steady-state plasma level during the second half of the dosing interval. (See Figure 20.)

If the approximate half-life and dosing interval are known, the degree of change in plasma drug concentration which will occur over a dosing

$$\text{Cpss ave} = \frac{(S)(F)(Dose/\tau)}{Cl} \qquad\qquad \text{(Eq. 35)}$$

$$\text{Cpss max} = \frac{\dfrac{(S)(F)(Dose)}{Vd}}{(1 - e^{-Kd\tau})} \qquad\qquad \text{(Eq. 43)}$$

$$\text{Cpss min} = \frac{\dfrac{(S)(F)(Dose)}{Vd}}{(1 - e^{-Kd\tau})}(e^{-Kd\tau}) \qquad\qquad \text{(Eq. 47)}$$

$$\text{Cpss}_1 = \frac{\dfrac{(S)(F)(Dose)}{Vd}}{(1 - e^{-Kd\tau})}(e^{-Kdt_1}) \qquad\qquad \text{(Eq. 48)}$$

Figure 20. Plasma Level-Time Curve for Intermittent Dosing at Steady State. When the dosing interval is equal to the half-life, plasma concentrations are above the average steady-state plasma concentration (Cpss ave) approximately 50% of the time. Oral administration dampens the curve considerably and the maximum concentration at steady state (Cpss max) occurs later and is lower than that produced by IV bolus. The minimum concentration at steady state (Cpss min) is greater than that produced by IV bolus doses because of the effect of absorption. In the equations above, τ is the interval between doses and t_1 is the time from the theoretical peak concentration following a dose to the time of sampling.

interval can be determined. Once the degree of fluctuation is known, one can then determine whether the primary determinant of plasma levels between dosing intervals is the volume of distribution or the clearance.

In certain situations, the *dosing interval is much longer than the half-life* and, for practical purposes, all of the drug is eliminated before the next dose. Therefore, each new dose is essentially a new loading dose. In this situation the peak concentration will be determined primarily by the volume of distribution because almost no drug remains from the previous dose.

Antibiotics are commonly dosed in this manner. The therapeutic index for antibiotics is usually so large that wide fluctuations in plasma level are acceptable and perhaps even desirable.[44] Furthermore, the therapeutic effect may require a plasma level that is above the minimal bactericidal or inhibitory concentration for only a brief period of time relative to the dosing interval.[89]

When the *dosing interval is much shorter than the half-life*, the plasma concentration fluctuates very little throughout the dosing interval. In this case, the plasma concentration will be primarily determined by clearance. Digoxin and phenobarbital given orally and any drug administered by a constant infusion are good examples of such a situation. (Also see Maximum and Minimum Plasma Concentrations on page 53.)

Determining the parameter which primarily affects plasma concentration for any given dosage regimen (when τ is longer or shorter than t½) is important because one then knows which parameters can be calculated reliably from the reported steady-state plasma concentrations. For example, if a patient who has been taking a dose of 0.375 mg of digoxin daily has a reported steady-state trough plasma concentration of 3.8 µg/L, one can reliably calculate the digoxin clearance for this patient using Equation 15 on page 26. Since the dosing interval is much shorter than the half-life, clearance is the major determinant of the patient's plasma concentration. One cannot reliably use the reported plasma concentration to calculate Vd and Kd (see Maximum and Minimum Plasma Concentrations on page 53) because Vd is not the major determinant of plasma concentration when τ is much shorter than the half-life. With a new clearance value, one can estimate a new maintenance dose for the patient described. Loading doses, however, which require knowledge of volume of distribution would require a literature estimate as no patient-specific information on Vd can be determined from this drug level.

Maximum and Minimum Plasma Concentrations

It is often important to estimate the maximum (Cpss max or peak) and minimum (Cpss min or trough) plasma drug concentrations produced by a given dose of drug during the dosing interval at steady state. (See Figure 20 on page 51.) For example, while it is critical in gentamicin therapy to achieve an acceptable peak concentration for efficacy, it is also important that the trough level be below a specified concentration to minimize concentration-related toxicity.

For drugs with a narrow therapeutic index (e.g., theophylline), it is useful to determine the degree of fluctuation in plasma drug concentration that will occur between doses. This can be particularly important if the dosing interval is longer than the half-life (i.e., fluctuations will be large) and Cpss min levels are being used to monitor therapy.

Most frequently, plasma specimens for drug assays are drawn just before the next dose because Cpss min levels are the most reproducible. Although the reported plasma drug concentrations for these specimens are often considered to be average steady-state concentrations (Cpss ave), a patient's pharmacokinetic parameters can be more accurately estimated by using an equation which describes Cpss min for drugs that are administered at dosing intervals which equal or exceed their half-lives. [See Minimum Plasma Drug Concentration (Cpss min) on page 55.]

Maximum Plasma Drug Concentration (Cpss max)

The maximum plasma drug concentration can be calculated from Equation 43 if the dose, salt form (S), bioavailability (F), volume of distribution (Vd), and elimination rate constant (Kd) are known:

$$\text{Cpss max} = \frac{\Delta Cp}{\text{Fraction of Drug Lost in } \tau}$$

Eq. 42

or

$$\text{Cpss max} = \frac{\dfrac{(S)(F)(\text{Dose})}{Vd}}{(1 - e^{-Kd\tau})}$$

Eq. 43

where ΔCp and $(S)(F)(Dose)/Vd$ represent the change in drug concentration that occurs over the dosing interval and $(1 - e^{-Kd\tau})$ represents the fraction of drug that is lost in the dosing interval.

Some pharmacokineticists have chosen to describe the fraction lost in a dosing interval $(1 - e^{-Kd\tau})$ as the *accumulation factor* and express it as:

$$\frac{1}{1 - e^{-Kd\tau}}$$

and the Cpss max equation as:

$$\text{Cpss max} = \left(\frac{(S)(F)(Dose)}{Vd}\right)\left(\frac{1}{1 - e^{-Kd\tau}}\right)$$

This equation is essentially the same as Equation 43 expressed in a slightly different format.

Equation 43 assumes drug absorption and distribution rates are rapid in relation to the drug half-life and dosing interval. This assumption is valid as long as drug concentrations are not sampled during the absorption and distribution phase. Following intravenous injection, the absorption and distribution phases are relatively short compared to the dosing interval and half-life for most drugs. When drugs are administered orally, the primary concern is with the absorption phase because the distribution component associated with two-compartment modeling is usually negligible. Digoxin and lithium are two notable exceptions in that a distribution phase continues for several hours following oral administration.

For *digoxin*, the observed peak concentration will be greater than that predicted by Equation 43 for Cpss max because drug distribution into tissue requires a minimum of six hours. When procainamide is dosed every three or four hours, the observed peak concentration will be lower than that predicted on the basis of Equation 43 for Cpss max because absorption is slow relative to the short dosing interval and the half-life of the drug. This tends to blunt or dampen the peak and trough levels of procainamide because elimination begins before all of the drug enters the body. For most drugs, the time required to reach peak concentrations after oral administration is between one and two hours.

Minimum Plasma Drug Concentration (Cpss min)

The minimum plasma drug concentration can be estimated by subtracting ΔCp or the magnitude of change in plasma concentration in one dosing interval from the maximum plasma concentration:

$$\text{Cpss min} = \text{Cpss max} - \Delta Cp \qquad \text{Eq. 44}$$

or

$$\text{Cpss min} = \text{Cpss max} - \frac{(S)(F)(Dose)}{Vd} \qquad \text{Eq. 45}$$

Alternatively, Cpss min can be calculated by multiplying Cpss max by the fraction of drug which remains at the end of the dosing interval $(e^{-Kd\tau})$.

$$\text{Cpss min} = (\text{Cpss max})(e^{-Kd\tau}) \qquad \text{Eq. 46}$$

Substituting Equation 43 for Cpss max into Equation 46 enables one to calculate Cpss min if the dose, elimination rate constant (Kd), volume of distribution (Vd), salt form (S), and bioavailability (F) are known:

$$\text{Cpss min} = \frac{\dfrac{(S)(F)(Dose)}{Vd}}{(1 - e^{-Kd\tau})}(e^{-Kd\tau}) \qquad \text{Eq. 47}$$

If a steady-state sample is obtained at some time other than the true peak or trough, the concentration can be calculated by the following equation:

$$Cpss_1 = \frac{\dfrac{(S)(F)(Dose)}{Vd}}{(1 - e^{-Kd\tau})} (e^{-Kdt_1})$$

Eq. 48

where t_1 is the number of hours since the last dose and $Cpss_1$ is the steady-state plasma concentration "t_1" hours after the last dose or Cpss max, which is "assumed" to occur at the time of dose administration. Note that although steady state has been achieved, not all plasma concentrations within the dosing interval represent the average concentration or Cpss ave. If the dosing interval (τ) is short compared to the half-life, however, the plasma concentration changes very little within the dosing interval and all concentrations are a close approximation of Cpss ave. (See Figure 20 on page 51.)

One note of caution: When a slow absorption rate significantly dampens the plasma drug concentration-versus-time curve (as for procainamide or sustained release dosage forms), the Cpss min can be assumed to be in close approximation of the average steady-state concentration (Cpss ave) and Equation 15 on page 26 is used to calculate the patient's pharmacokinetic parameters (i.e., clearance). (See Figure 20 on page 51.) This assumption also is applicable when the dosing interval is short relative to the half-life. The Kd and Vd values which can be calculated from the Cpss min equation may be misleading. When the dosing interval is much shorter than the half-life or there is a substantial blunting of the plasma drug concentration-versus-time curve, peak and trough plasma levels are about equal to the average concentration and are, therefore, primarily determined by clearance. Although the product of the Vd and Kd obtained by this method may closely approximate clearance, there can be no confidence in the Vd and Kd values *per se* because Vd and, therefore, Kd may vary independently of the clearance. [Also see Elimination Rate Constant (Kd) and Half-Life (t½) on page 37.]

Selecting the Appropriate Equation

It is often difficult to determine which of the many equations should be used to solve specific clinical problems. A technique used by this author to avoid the use of inappropriate equations is to draw a graphical representation of the plasma drug concentration-versus-time curve which would be expected on the basis of the dosage regimen the patient is receiving. Once the graph is drawn and the plasma concentration visualized, mathematical equations which describe the drug's pharmacokinetic behavior are selected. To facilitate this process, a series of typical plasma level-time curves and their corresponding formulas is presented in Figures 21 through 27.

Loading Dose or Bolus Dose

When a loading dose or a bolus of drug has been administered (see Figure 21), the initial plasma concentration (Cp°) can be determined by rearranging the "loading dose" equation (See Equation 11 on page 19):

$$Cp^\circ = \frac{(S)(F)(\text{Loading Dose})}{Vd}$$

Eq. 49

A subsequent plasma level (Cp_1) any time (t_1) after the dose has been administered can be calculated by using a variation of the equation that describes first-order elimination (Equation 26):

$$Cp = (Cp^\circ)(e^{-Kdt})$$

or

$$Cp_1 = \frac{(S)(F)(\text{Loading Dose})}{Vd}(e^{-Kdt_1})$$

Eq. 50

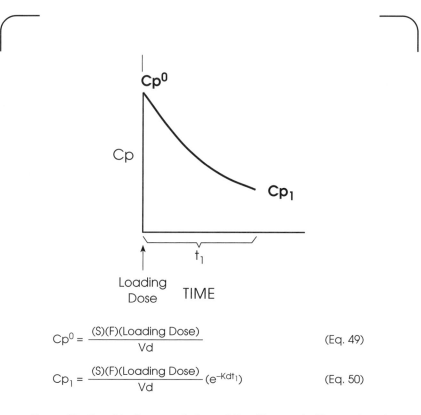

$$Cp^0 = \frac{(S)(F)(\text{Loading Dose})}{Vd} \qquad \text{(Eq. 49)}$$

$$Cp_1 = \frac{(S)(F)(\text{Loading Dose})}{Vd}(e^{-Kdt_1}) \qquad \text{(Eq. 50)}$$

Figure 21. Graphic Representation of the Change in Plasma Level that Occurs Over Time Following a Loading Dose. Cp° represents the initial concentration and Cp_1 represents the concentration at any interval of time (t_1) after the dose has been administered. Assume a one-compartment model and rapid absorption if the drug is given orally.

Continuous Infusion to Steady State

The plasma concentration-versus-time curve produced by a continuous infusion which has been administered until steady state has been achieved is represented by Figure 22. The average steady-state concentration (Cpss ave) that will be produced by the infusion can be calculated using Equation 35:

$$\text{Cpss ave} = \frac{(S)(F)(\text{Dose}/\tau)}{Cl}$$

Discontinuation of Infusion After Steady State

The curve which represents a change in the plasma concentration after the infusion has been discontinued is also represented in Figure 22. The concentration (Cp_2) produced any time (t_2) after the infusion has been discontinued can be calculated using a variation of the first-order elimination equation (Equation 26). (Also see discussion of Equations 35–41 on pages 46–49):

$$Cp_2 = (Cpss\ ave)(e^{-Kdt_2})$$

or

$$Cp_2 = \frac{(S)(F)(Dose/\tau)}{Cl}(e^{-Kdt_2})$$

Eq. 51

Initiation and Discontinuation of Infusion Before Steady State

When an infusion is initiated and discontinued *before* steady state is achieved ($<4\ t\frac{1}{2}$) the plasma concentration time curve can be described as depicted in Figure 19 on page 47. In this situation, the concentration (Cp_1) which occurs at any time (t_1) after the infusion has been initiated and the concentration (Cp_2) which occurs any time (t_2) after the infusion was discontinued can be approximated by Equations 37 and 41. (Also see earlier discussion of Equations 37–41 on pages 48–49.)

Whether a bolus or infusion model is used depends upon the relationship between the duration of drug input versus the drug's half-life. For example, if a drug is administered as an intravenous bolus, or if a drug administered orally is absorbed rapidly relative to the drug's half-life, very little drug will be cleared or eliminated during the absorption or administration process; therefore, the bolus model can be used. If, however, a drug is absorbed over a long time period relative to its half-life, a significant amount of drug will be eliminated during the input or absorption period and the plasma level concentrations resulting from oral administration would resemble those resulting from an infusion model. As a general rule, if the drug input time is less than one-tenth its half-life, then it can be successfully modeled as a bolus dose; however, if the drug input time is greater than one-half its half-life, it is more appropriate to use an infusion model. When the duration of drug input falls between one-tenth and one-half of its half-life, an arbitrary choice can be made between a bolus dose and an infusion model.

As a clinical guideline, the author uses one-sixth of a drug half-life as an arbitrary break point. That is, for those drugs that are absorbed over a time period equal to one-sixth of a half-life or less, the bolus model is used; for those drugs absorbed over a time period that is greater than one-sixth of the half-life, the infusion model is used. While the one-sixth of a half-life "rule" is arbitrary, it was selected because the difference in the calculated plasma concentrations when using the bolus or short infusion model is <10%. (See Figure 24.)

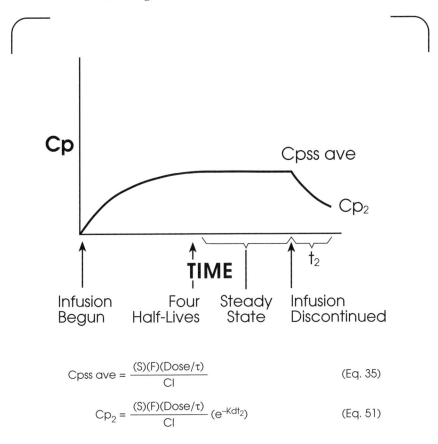

$$Cpss\ ave = \frac{(S)(F)(Dose/\tau)}{Cl} \qquad (Eq.\ 35)$$

$$Cp_2 = \frac{(S)(F)(Dose/\tau)}{Cl} (e^{-Kdt_2}) \qquad (Eq.\ 51)$$

Figure 22. Graphic Representation of the Plasma Concentration-Versus-Time Curve that Results When an Infusion Is Continued Until Steady State Is Reached and Then Discontinued. Cpss ave is the steady-state concentration and Cp_2 is the concentration at any interval of time (t_2) after the infusion has been discontinued.

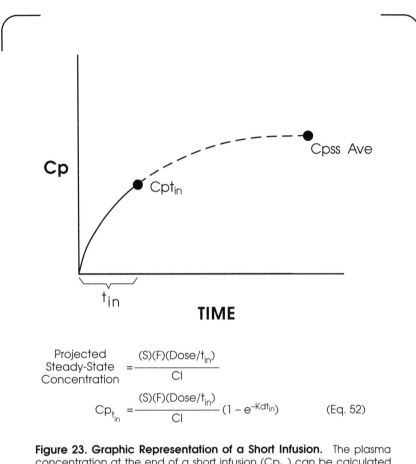

$$\text{Projected Steady-State Concentration} = \frac{(S)(F)(Dose/t_{in})}{Cl}$$

$$Cp_{t_{in}} = \frac{(S)(F)(Dose/t_{in})}{Cl}(1 - e^{-Kdt_{in}}) \qquad \text{(Eq. 52)}$$

Figure 23. Graphic Representation of a Short Infusion. The plasma concentration at the end of a short infusion ($Cp_{t_{in}}$) can be calculated by multiplying the "projected steady-state concentration" (-----) by the fraction of steady state achieved ($1 - e^{-Kdt_{in}}$) during the infusion period (t_{in}).

If there is any uncertainty about which model is more appropriate, the infusion model should be used because it more closely approximates the actual absorption and plasma concentration curve during drug absorption and elimination. Figure 23 represents the plasma concentration obtained at the end of a short infusion, as calculated by Equation 52.

$$Cp_{t_{in}} = \frac{(S)(F)(Dose/t_{in})}{Cl}(1 - e^{-Kdt_{in}})$$

Eq. 52

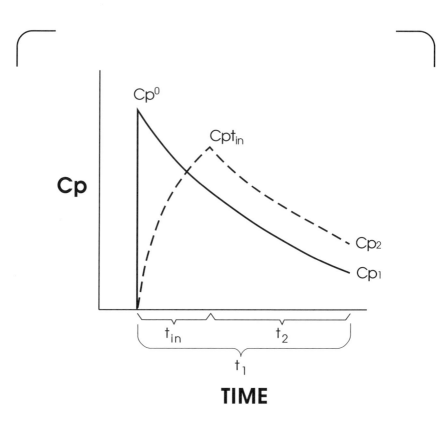

$$Cp^0 = \frac{(S)(F)(\text{Loading Dose})}{Vd} \qquad\qquad (\text{Eq. 49})$$

$$Cp_1 = \frac{(S)(F)(\text{Loading Dose})}{Vd}\,(e^{-Kdt_1}) \qquad\qquad (\text{Eq. 50})$$

$$Cp_{t_{in}} = \frac{(S)(F)(\text{Dose}/t_{in})}{Cl}\,(1 - e^{-Kdt_{in}}) \qquad\qquad (\text{Eq. 52})$$

$$Cp_2 = \frac{(S)(F)(\text{Dose}/t_{in})}{Cl}\,(1 - e^{-Kdt_{in}})(e^{-Kdt_2}) \qquad\qquad (\text{Eq. 53})$$

Figure 24. Graphic Representation of a Drug Administered as a Bolus (—) or as a Short Infusion (---). The bolus dose model assumes that drug input or absorption is instantaneous. The decay interval, t_1 (i.e., t_{in} + t_2), is therefore assumed to begin at the start of the infusion. In contrast, the infusion model assumes that the decay interval (t_2) begins at the conclusion of the infusion period (t_{in}).

Note in the above equation that t_{in} represents the duration of drug input and that $(1 - e^{-Kdt_{in}})$ represents the fraction of steady state that would be achieved during the infusion time. This concentration ($Cp_{t_{in}}$) therefore, represents the peak level at the end of the infusion.

Conceptually, it is useful to compare Equation 52 to Equation 37 on page 48. Both equations represent the process of multiplying a steady-state average concentration by the fraction of steady state achieved. In Equation 37 the dosing interval (τ) and duration of infusion (t_1) are replaced in Equation 52 with the duration of drug input (t_{in}). Although both equations represent the same basic process, Equation 37 is most commonly used when a continuous infusion (e.g., theophylline) is discontinued before steady state is achieved, and Equation 52 is used when a dose is to be administered over a relatively short time period (e.g., aminoglycoside antibiotics).

Once the infusion has been concluded, any subsequent drug concentration (Cp_2) can be calculated by multiplying the concentration at the end of the infusion ($Cp_{t_{in}}$) by the fraction remaining at any time interval since the end of the infusion (t_2).

$$Cp_2 = \frac{(S)(F)(Dose/t_{in})}{Cl}(1 - e^{-Kdt_{in}})(e^{-Kdt_2})$$

Eq. 53

The relationship between plasma concentrations predicted by the bolus dose equation (Equations 49 and 50) and the short infusion equation (Equations 52 and 53) is depicted in Figure 24. Note that the bolus dose is assumed to be instantaneously absorbed at the beginning of the infusion; therefore, the initial peak concentrations are higher than would be predicted by the short infusion model. However, plasma concentrations corresponding to the conclusion of the short infusion model (t_{in} hours after starting the infusion) and all subsequent plasma levels are lower for the bolus-dose model than for the infusion model. If the infusion time t_{in} is less than one-sixth of a drug's half-life, then the difference between the plasma concentrations predicted by the bolus dose and the short infusion

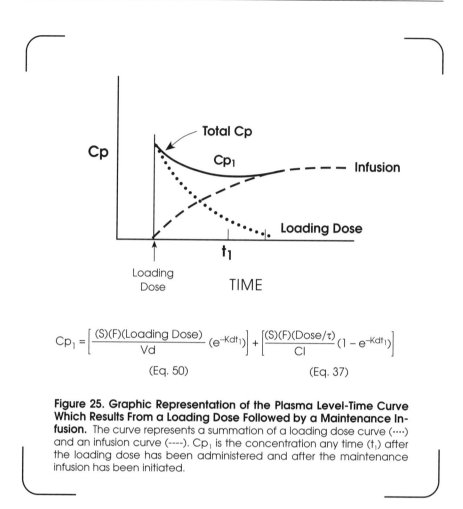

$$Cp_1 = \left[\frac{(S)(F)(\text{Loading Dose})}{Vd} (e^{-Kdt_1}) \right] + \left[\frac{(S)(F)(\text{Dose}/\tau)}{Cl} (1 - e^{-Kdt_1}) \right]$$

(Eq. 50)   (Eq. 37)

Figure 25. Graphic Representation of the Plasma Level-Time Curve Which Results From a Loading Dose Followed by a Maintenance Infusion. The curve represents a summation of a loading dose curve (·····) and an infusion curve (----). Cp_1 is the concentration any time (t_1) after the loading dose has been administered and after the maintenance infusion has been initiated.

model will be minimal. Although either equation can be used, the bolus dose model is much simpler.

Loading Dose Followed By Infusion

When a patient is given a loading dose followed by an infusion, the plasma concentration (Cp_1) at any time (t_1) can be calculated by summing the equations which describe the concentration produced by the loading dose at t_1 (Equation 50 on page 57) and the concentration produced by the infusion at t_1 (Equation 37 on page 48). Refer to Cp_1 in Figure 21 on page 58 and Cp_1 in Figure 19 on page 47.

$$Cp_1 = \begin{array}{c} \text{Concentration} \\ \text{Produced By the} \\ \text{Loading Dose At } t_1 \text{ (Eq. 50)} \end{array} + \begin{array}{c} \text{Concentration} \\ \text{Produced By the} \\ \text{Infusion At } t_1 \text{ (Eq. 37)} \end{array}$$

$$Cp_1 = \frac{(S)(F)(\text{Loading Dose})}{Vd}(e^{-Kdt_1}) + \frac{(S)(F)(\text{Dose}/\tau)}{Cl}(1 - e^{-Kdt_1})$$

Note that $(S)(F)(\text{Dose}/\tau)$ in the second portion of the above equation represents the infusion rate. It is important to recall in this situation that the loading dose is eliminated according to first-order pharmacokinetics as described in Figure 21 even when a maintenance infusion is initiated. This must be taken into account when predicting a plasma concentration. In other words, the maintenance infusion is accumulating while the concentration resulting from the loading dose is diminishing. (See Figure 25.)

Intermittent Administration at Regular Intervals to Steady State

When a drug is administered intermittently at regular dosing intervals until steady state (at least three to five half-lives) is achieved, the average concentration, the maximum concentration, and the minimum concentration between dosing intervals can be approximated using Equations 35, 43, and 47, respectively. Prediction of the plasma concentration at any time (t_1) following the peak can be accomplished by using Equation 48. Figure 26 depicts the plasma concentration-versus-time curve which occurs with this type of dosing regimen. (Also see Maximum and Minimum Plasma Concentrations on page 53.)

$$\text{Cpss ave} = \frac{(S)(F)(\text{Dose}/\tau)}{Cl}$$

$$\text{Cpss max} = \frac{\dfrac{(S)(F)(\text{Dose})}{Vd}}{(1 - e^{-Kd\tau})}$$

$$\text{Cpss min} = \frac{\dfrac{(S)(F)(\text{Dose})}{Vd}}{(1 - e^{-Kd\tau})}(e^{-Kd\tau})$$

$$\text{Cpss}_1 = \frac{\dfrac{(S)(F)(\text{Dose})}{Vd}}{(1 - e^{-Kd\tau})}(e^{-Kdt_1})$$

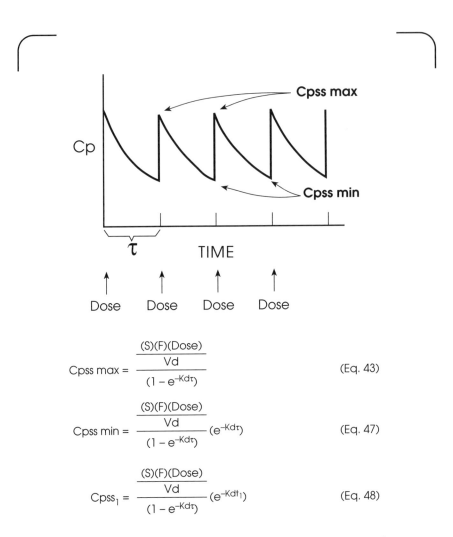

$$Cpss\ max = \frac{\dfrac{(S)(F)(Dose)}{Vd}}{(1 - e^{-Kd\tau})} \qquad (Eq.\ 43)$$

$$Cpss\ min = \frac{\dfrac{(S)(F)(Dose)}{Vd}}{(1 - e^{-Kd\tau})}\ (e^{-Kd\tau}) \qquad (Eq.\ 47)$$

$$Cpss_1 = \frac{\dfrac{(S)(F)(Dose)}{Vd}}{(1 - e^{-Kd\tau})}\ (e^{-Kdt_1}) \qquad (Eq.\ 48)$$

Figure 26. Graphic Representation of the Steady-State Plasma Concentration Versus Time Curve Which Occurs When Drugs Are Given Intermittently At Regular Dosing Intervals. Any maximum concentration (Cpss max) is interchangeable with any other maximum concentration and any minimum concentration (Cpss min) is interchangeable with any other minimum concentration.

Series of Individual Doses

When a series of individual doses is administered and a concentration before steady state must be calculated, there are several approaches that can be taken. One approach is to sum the contributions of each individual dose. This is done by decaying the peak concentration of each dose to the time at which the plasma concentration needs to be predicted. Figure 27 represents a series of three doses whose individual contributions were calculated and then summed to estimate the total plasma concentration existing at some time point after the third dose. Note that this is simply the sum of three individual doses as modeled by Equation 50. This approach is most practical when the interval between doses or the amount of drug administered with each dose varies.

If each dose and the intervals between doses are the same, it may be simpler to multiply Cpss max or the peak concentration that would be

$$Cp_{sum} = \left[\frac{(S)(F)(D_1)}{Vd}(e^{-Kdt_1}) \right] + \left[\frac{(S)(F)(D_2)}{Vd}(e^{-Kdt_2}) \right] + \left[\frac{(S)(F)(D_3)}{Vd}(e^{-Kdt_3}) \right]$$

Figure 27. Graphic Representation of Nonsteady-State Summation of Individual Doses. The solid line represents a plasma concentration which is the total or sum of the individual doses (D_1, D_2, D_3). The dashed line represents the contribution of each of the individual doses to the total. The t_1, t_2, and t_3 represent the time interval between the time of administration of each of the doses and the time at which the plasma concentration is to be calculated.

achieved at steady state (Equation 43 on page 53) by the fraction of steady state achieved after N doses (Equation 54):

$$\text{Cpss max} = \frac{\dfrac{(S)(F)(Dose)}{Vd}}{(1 - e^{-Kd\tau})}$$

$$\text{Fraction of Steady State Achieved After (N) Doses} = (1 - e^{-Kd(N)\tau})$$

Eq. 54

In Equation 54, τ is the interval between each dose and N represents the number of doses that have been administered. The peak concentration following N doses can be calculated by combining Equations 43 and 54. Any concentration (Cp_2) following the Nth dose can be calculated by multiplying the peak concentration following N doses by (e^{-Kdt_2}), where t_2 is the number of hours since the last dose.

$$Cp_2 = \frac{\dfrac{(S)(F)(Dose)}{Vd}}{(1 - e^{-Kd\tau})}(1 - e^{-Kd(N)\tau})(e^{-Kdt_2})$$

Eq. 55

Note that if the doses and dosing intervals were the same in Figure 27, the concentration (Cp_{sum}) could be calculated using Equation 55 where N would be 3 and t_2 would be the number of hours after the third dose. Equation 55 is most useful when a number of doses have been administered with a consistent τ but steady state has not yet been achieved. Equation 55 represents the concentration of drug produced by a series of consistently administered bolus doses that have not yet achieved steady state. This equation can be further expanded to represent a series of doses that are absorbed over a significant fraction of the drug's half-life (i.e., $t_{in} > \frac{1}{6}t\frac{1}{2}$).

$$Cp = \frac{\dfrac{(S)(F)(Dose/t_{in})}{Cl}(1 - e^{-Kdt_{in}})}{(1 - e^{-Kd\tau})}(1 - e^{-Kd(N)\tau})(e^{-Kdt_2})$$

Eq. 56

Equation 56 is similar to Equation 55 except that the bolus dose input model is now replaced with the short infusion input model. In clinical practice, Equation 56 is seldom used. This is because the half-life of the drug which requires the use of a short infusion input model is likely to be sufficiently brief that steady state will be achieved after two to three doses have been administered.

Sustained-Release Dosage Forms

Most sustained-release dosage forms are designed to produce concentrations that fluctuate little within the dosage interval. In most cases, therefore, concentrations produced by these sustained-release products can be estimated by use of the equation that describes the average steady-state concentration (Equation 35):

$$\text{Cpss ave} = \frac{(S)(F)(Dose/\tau)}{Cl}$$

As illustrated below, the use of the Cpss ave formula for sustained release products is based on the assumption that the time required for absorption (t_{in}) is approximately equal to the dosing interval (τ).

$$Cpss_2 = \frac{\dfrac{(S)(F)(Dose/t_{in})}{Cl}(1 - e^{-Kdt_{in}})}{(1 - e^{-Kd\tau})}(e^{-Kdt_2})$$

Eq. 57

$$Cpss_2 = \frac{\dfrac{(S)(F)(Dose/\tau)}{Cl}(1 - e^{-Kd\tau})}{(1 - e^{-Kd\tau})}(e^{-Kdt_2})$$

As can be seen from this example, Equation 35

$$\text{Cpss ave} = \frac{(S)(F)(Dose/\tau)}{Cl}$$

is the result of having t_{in} exactly equal to τ, as each of the short infusions would last for exacly one dosing interval and stop at the same time the next dose begins its infusion process, resulting in an average steady-state concentration with no rise or fall within the dosing interval. In practice, absorption times are not exactly equal to the dosing interval, but for most sustained-release drug products, they are reasonably close and, therefore, plasma concentrations can be considered as an average steady-state value. It should be emphasized, however, that the use of Equation 35 is not universal and depends upon not only the absorption of the drug product, but also the dosing interval selected and half-life of the drug in the specific patient. As a general rule, absorption times which exceed the dosing interval are not a problem. However, if absorption time (t_{in}) is substantially less than the dosing interval, then there will be some fluctuation of the plasma concentrations. A useful approach is to consider the duration over which the plasma concentrations will decay following the end of absorption. This can be approximated by subtracting the absorption time from the dosing interval.

$$\tau - t_{in} = \frac{\text{Time Within the Dosing}}{\text{Interval With No Drug Absorption}}$$

If this time within the dosing interval is short compared to the drug half-life, it suggests that there will be little fluctuation of the plasma concentration within the dosing interval. As a clinical guideline, if $\tau - t_{in}$ is $\leq \frac{1}{3}t\frac{1}{2}$, the average steady-state equation (Equation 35) can be used. Note that this guideline is very similar to the guidelines used for substituting the average steady-state equation (Equation 35) for the intermittent bolus dose equation (Equation 48). (See Figure 31.) Note, however, in Figure 31 the time of decay is considered to be the entire dosing interval as the absorption is assumed to be instantaneous and t_{in} is zero.

Algorithm for Choosing the Appropriate Equation

Selecting the appropriate equation to use in a specific clinical situation can be a complex process. The algorithm that appears on the following pages offers a step-wise approach to this process. The rules follow those outlined in the text. First, one must consider whether steady state has been achieved; then, the appropriate model is chosen to predict or calculate drug concentrations.

Algorithm for Choosing the Appropriate Pharmacokinetic Model

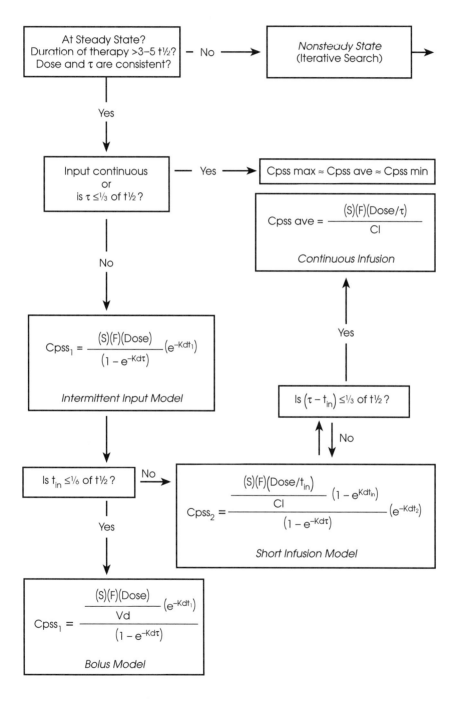

At Steady State?
Duration of therapy >3–5 t½?
Dose and τ are consistent? — No ⟶ *Nonsteady State (Iterative Search)* ⟶

Yes ↓

Input continuous
or
is τ ≤⅓ of t½? — Yes ⟶ Cpss max ≈ Cpss ave ≈ Cpss min

$$Cpss\ ave = \frac{(S)(F)(Dose/\tau)}{Cl}$$

Continuous Infusion

No ↓

$$Cpss_1 = \frac{(S)(F)(Dose)}{(1 - e^{-Kd\tau})}(e^{-Kdt_1})$$

Intermittent Input Model

Yes ↑

$$Is\ (\tau - t_{in}) \leq \tfrac{1}{3}\ of\ t½?$$

↑ No ↓

Is $t_{in} \leq \tfrac{1}{6}$ of t½? — No ⟶

$$Cpss_2 = \frac{\dfrac{(S)(F)(Dose/t_{in})}{Cl}(1 - e^{Kdt_{in}})}{(1 - e^{-Kd\tau})}(e^{-Kdt_2})$$

Short Infusion Model

Yes ↓

$$Cpss_1 = \frac{\dfrac{(S)(F)(Dose)}{Vd}(e^{-Kdt_1})}{(1 - e^{-Kd\tau})}$$

Bolus Model

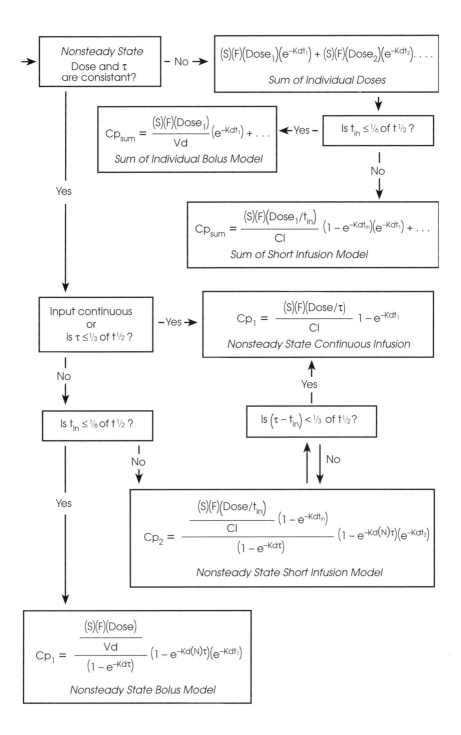

Interpretation of Plasma Drug Concentrations

Plasma drug concentrations are measured in the clinical setting to determine whether a therapeutic or toxic concentration has been produced by a given dosage regimen. This process is based on the assumption that plasma drug concentrations reflect drug concentrations at the receptor and, therefore, can be correlated with pharmacologic response. This assumption is not always valid, however, when plasma samples are obtained at inappropriate times or when other factors (such as delayed absorption) confound the usual pharmacokinetic behavior of a drug. These factors are discussed below.

Plasma Sampling Time

To properly interpret a plasma concentration, it is essential to know when a plasma sample was obtained in relation to the last dose administered and when the drug regimen was initiated. If a plasma sample is obtained before distribution of the drug into tissue is complete (e.g., digoxin), the plasma concentration will be higher than predicted on the basis of dose and response. Peak (Cpss max) plasma levels are helpful in evaluating the dose of antibiotics used to treat severe, life-threatening infections. Although serum concentrations for many antibiotics peak one to two hours after the dose is administered, factors such as slow or delayed absorption can significantly delay the time at which peak serum concentrations are attained. Large errors in the estimation of Cpss max can occur if the plasma sample is obtained at the wrong time. (See Figure 29.) Therefore, with few exceptions, plasma samples should be drawn just before the next dose (Cpss min) when determining routine drug concentrations in plasma. These trough levels are less likely to be influenced by absorption and distribution problems.

When the full therapeutic response of a given drug dosage regimen is to be assessed, plasma samples should not be obtained until steady-state concentrations of the drug have been achieved. If drug doses are increased or decreased on the basis of drug concentrations that have been measured while the drug is still accumulating, disastrous consequences can occur. Nevertheless, in some clinical situations it *is* appropriate to measure drug levels before steady state. For example, pharmacokinetic parameters for a drug administered to a severely ill patient may change so rapidly that extrapolations from a reported plasma concentration may

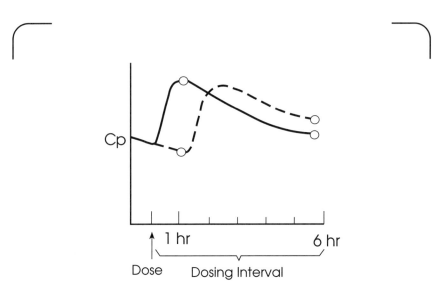

Figure 29. Schematic Representation of the Effect of Delayed Absorption (-----) on Plasma Level Measurements. Note the magnitude of error at one hour (theoretical time to reach Cpss max) as compared to six hours (Cpss min).

not be valid from one day to the next. Similarly, if there is reason to suspect that the pharmacokinetic parameters in a given patient are likely to differ substantially from those reported in the literature (e.g., lidocaine in a patient with congestive heart failure),[45] it may be reasonable to obtain plasma samples before steady state to avoid toxic or subtherapeutic levels from the current dose. If possible, plasma samples should be drawn after a minimum of two half-lives because clearance values calculated from drug levels obtained less than one half-life after a regimen has been initiated are very sensitive to small differences in the volume of distribution and minor assay errors. (See Figure 30.)

Revising Pharmacokinetic Parameters

The process of using a patient's plasma drug concentrations and dosing history to determine patient-specific pharmacokinetic parameters can be complex and difficult. If the relationship between pharmacokinetic equations, the specific parameters, and the resultant plasma levels is understood, however, this process can be simplified. Depending on the dosing history, a single plasma sample obtained at the appropriate time can yield information to revise either the volume of distribution or clearance, but not both. Drug concentrations measured from poorly-timed samples may prove to be useless in estimating a patient's Vd or clearance values. Thus, the goal is to obtain plasma samples at times that are likely to yield data that can be used with confidence to estimate pharmacokinetic parameters. In the alternative, one can evaluate available plasma concentration data to determine whether they can be used to estimate, with some degree of confidence, Vd or clearance. Which pharmacokinetic parameter is revised has much to do with the timing of the sample and the drug's pharmacokinetic profile. The goal in pharmacokinetic revisions is not only to

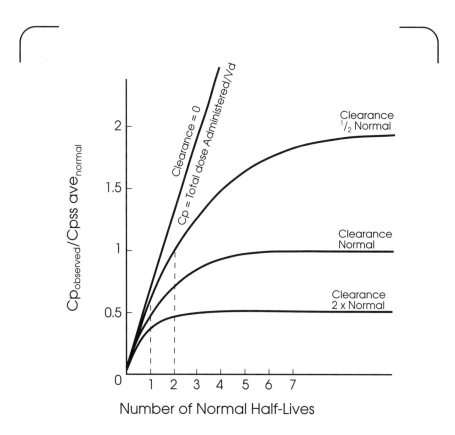

Figure 30. Relationship Between Observed Plasma Concentrations (Cp$_{Observed}$) and the Normal Steady-State Concentration (Cpss ave$_{normal}$). Following the Initiation of a Maintenance Regimen at Various Clearance Values. At steady state, the plasma concentrations are inversely proportional to clearance. Plasma concentrations obtained at or before one normal half-life are all very similar regardless of clearance. After two half-lives, alterations in a patient's clearance and ultimately steady-state concentrations can be detected by unexpectedly high or low plasma drug concentrations. After three half-lives, more confident predictions of steady-state concentrations can be made.

recognize which pharmacokinetic parameter can be revised, but also the accuracy or confidence one has in the revised or patient-specific pharmacokinetic parameter.

Volume of Distribution. A plasma level that has been obtained soon after a bolus dose has been administered is primarily determined by the dose administered and the volume of distribution. This assumes that both the absorption and distribution phases have been avoided. This is illustrated by Equation 50 on page 57:

$$Cp_1 = \frac{(S)(F)(\text{Loading Dose})}{Vd} (e^{-Kdt_1})$$

The plasma concentration at time t_1 (Cp_1) is primarily a function of the administered dose and the apparent volume of distribution when e^{-Kdt_1} approaches unity (i.e., when $t_1 \ll t\frac{1}{2}$). At this point, very little drug has been eliminated from the body. As a clinical guideline, a patient's volume of distribution can be estimated when t_1, or the interval between the administration and sampling time, is less than or equal to one-third of the drug's half-life. As t_1 exceeds one-third of a half-life, the measured concentration is increasingly influenced by clearance. At this point it is difficult to estimate the patient's Vd with any certainty. The specific application of this clinical guideline depends upon the confidence with which one knows clearance. If clearance is extremely variable and uncertain, a time interval of less than one-third of a half-life might be appropriate. On the other hand, if a patient-specific value for clearance has already been determined, then t_1 could exceed one-third of a half-life and a reasonably accurate estimate of volume of distribution could be obtained. It is important to recognize that the pharmacokinetic parameter which most influences the drug concentration is not determined by the model chosen to represent the drug level. For example, even if the dose is modeled as a short infusion (Equation 53 on page 63), the volume of distribution can still be the important parameter controlling the plasma concentration. Vd is not clearly defined in the equation; nevertheless, it is incorporated into the elimination rate constant (Kd):

$$Cp_2 = \frac{(S)(F)(\text{Dose}/t_{in})}{Cl} (1 - e^{-Kdt_{in}})(e^{-Kdt_2})$$

Although one would not usually select Equation 53 to demonstrate that drug concentration is primarily a function of volume of distribution, it is important to recognize that the relationship between the observed drug concentration and volume is not altered as long as the total elapsed time $[t_{in} + t_2]$ does not exceed one-third of a half-life.

Clearance. A plasma drug concentration that has been obtained at steady state in a patient who is receiving a constant drug infusion is determined by clearance. This is illustrated by Equation 35 on page 46:

$$\text{Cpss ave} = \frac{(S)(F)(Dose/\tau)}{Cl}$$

Note that the average steady-state plasma concentration is *not* influenced by the apparent volume of distribution. Therefore, plasma concentrations which represent the average steady-state level can be used to estimate a patient's clearance value, but they cannot be used to estimate a patient's volume of distribution. As illustrated in Figure 31, all steady-state plasma concentrations within a dosing interval that is short relative to a drug's half-life ($\tau \leq \frac{1}{3}t\frac{1}{2}$) approximate the average concentration. Therefore, these concentrations are also primarily a function of clearance. If the average drug concentration is assumed to occur approximately in the middle of the dosing interval, the trough concentration will have decayed from the average for only half of the dosing interval or by one-sixth of a drug half-life. Under these conditions, the trough concentration is approximately 90% of the average drug level, an error which is usually acceptable in clinical practice. Thus, in this circumstance, the equation for Cpss ave (Equation 35 on page 46) or the equation which represents a steady-state plasma concentration sampled any time within the dosing interval (Equation 48 on page 56) can be used to estimate a patient-specific clearance.

$$\text{Cpss}_1 = \frac{\dfrac{(S)(F)(Dose)}{Vd}}{(1 - e^{-Kd\tau})} (e^{-Kdt_1})$$

If Equation 48 is used, the expected volume of distribution should be retained and the elimination rate constant adjusted such that Cpss at t_1

$$\text{Cpss ave} = \frac{(S)(F)(Dose/\tau)}{Cl} \qquad\qquad \text{(Eq. 35)}$$

$$Cpss_1 = \frac{\dfrac{(S)(F)(Dose)}{Vd}}{(1 - e^{-Kd\tau})} (e^{-Kdt_1}) \qquad\qquad \text{(Eq. 48)}$$

Figure 31. Plasma Concentrations Relative to Cpss Ave (—) when τ is Much Less Than (····) and Greater Than (----) the Half-Life. When τ is much less than the t½ (···), all plasma concentrations approximate the average concentration (Cpss ave) and are therefore primarily a function of clearance. When τ is much greater than t½ (----), the plasma concentrations fluctuate significantly. The degree to which plasma concentrations are determined by clearance and/or volume of distribution is a function of when the plasma level is obtained within the dosing interval.

equals the observed drug plasma concentration. Clearance could then be calculated using Equation 33 on page 44:

$$Cl = (Kd)(Vd)$$

Sensitivity Analysis. Whether a measured drug concentration is a function of clearance or volume of distribution is not always apparent.

When this is difficult to ascertain, one can examine the sensitivity or responsiveness of the predicted plasma concentration to a parameter by changing one parameter while holding the other constant. For example, Equation 37 on page 48 represents a plasma concentration (Cp_1) at some time interval (t_1) after a maintenance infusion has been started.

$$Cp_1 = \frac{(S)(F)(Dose/\tau)}{Cl}(1 - e^{-Kdt_1})$$

When the fraction of steady state which has been reached $(1 - e^{-Kdt_1})$ is small, large changes in clearance are frequently required to adjust a predicted plasma concentration to the appropriate value. If a large percentage change in the clearance value results in a disproportionately small change in the predicted drug level, then the volume of distribution and the amount of drug administered are the primary determinants of the observed concentration. This concept is illustrated graphically in Figure 30 on page 75. Note that plasma concentrations within the first two half-lives are all very similar, while the steady-state concentrations are quite different. Within the first two half-lives of initiating a maintenance regimen, very large changes in clearance are required to account for small changes in plasma levels.

This type of sensitivity analysis is useful to reinforce the concept that the most reliable revisions in pharmacokinetic parameters are made when the predicted drug concentration changes by approximately the same percentage as the pharmacokinetic parameter undergoing revision. To illustrate this principle, let us examine the relationship between a theophylline drug concentration obtained 6.93 hours after starting a theophylline infusion of 30 mg/hr in a patient with the following expected parameters for theophylline: Cl 3 L/hr, Vd 30 L, Kd 0.1 hr^{-1}, t½ 6.93 hr. Because the drug being administered is theophylline, S and F are assumed to be 1.0. Using Equation 37, the expected plasma concentration [Cp_1] is calculated to be 5 mg/L:

$$Cp_1 = \frac{(S)(F)(Dose/\tau)}{Cl}(1 - e^{-Kdt_1})$$

$$= \frac{(1)(1)(30 \text{ mg/hr})}{3 \text{ L/hr}}(1 - e^{-(0.1)(6.93 \text{ hr})})$$

$$= 10 \text{ mg/L} (1 - 0.5)$$

$$= 5 \text{ mg/L}$$

As can be seen from the calculations, the expected steady-state concentration is 10 mg/L and the fraction of steady state achieved $(1-e^{-Kdt_1})$ is 0.5 since the time of sampling is at one drug half-life and 50% of the steady-state plasma concentration has been achieved. If the observed plasma concentration was 6 mg/L, only slightly higher than the calculated or expected value of 5 mg/L, one might expect the patient's clearance on revision to be only slightly less than the expected 3 L/hr. This relationship, however, is deceiving because, in order to calculate a plasma concentration of 6 mg/L at 6.93 hr with a volume of 30 L, a clearance of approximately 1.32 L/hr with a corresponding Kd and t½ of 0.044 hr^{-1} and 15.7 hr, respectively, is required.

$$Cp_1 = \frac{(S)(F)(Dose/\tau)}{Cl}(1 - e^{-Kdt_1})$$

$$= \frac{(1)(1)(30 \text{ mg/hr})}{1.32 \text{ L/hr}}(1 - e^{-(0.044)(6.93)})$$

$$= 22.7 \text{ mg/L }(1 - 0.737)$$

$$= 22.7 \text{ mg/L }(0.263)$$

$$= 5.97 \text{ mg/L } or \approx 6 \text{ mg/L}$$

As can be seen from this illustration, the clearance value of 3 L/hr had to be reduced by more than one-half (1.32 L/hr) in order to increase the predicted drug concentration by $\approx$20%. This poor response of the calculated drug concentration to a change in clearance suggests that clearance is not the primary pharmacokinetic parameter responsible for the drug concentration. Therefore, any estimates of clearance based upon these calculations would be tenuous at best.

When a predicted drug concentration changes in direct proportion to an alteration in only one of the pharmacokinetic parameters, it is likely that a measured drug concentration can be used to estimate that patient-specific parameter. When both clearance and volume of distribution have a significant influence on the prediction of a measured drug concentration, however, revision of a patient's pharmacokinetic parameters will be less certain since there are an infinite number of combinations for clearance and volume of distribution values that could be used to predict the observed drug concentration. When this occurs, the patient's specific pharmacokinetic characteristics can be estimated by adjusting one or both of the pharmacokinetic parameters. Nevertheless, in most cases such as this, additional plasma level sampling will be needed to accurately predict the patient's clearance or volume of distribution so that subsequent dosing regimens can be adjusted.

If a plasma drug concentration calculated from a specific equation is similar to the reported value, the pharmacokinetic parameters used in that equation may not necessarily be the most important determinants of the drug concentration. Equation 48 on page 56 and Figure 31 on page 77 can be used to demonstrate this principle.

$$Cpss_1 = \frac{\frac{(S)(F)(Dose)}{Vd}}{(1 - e^{-Kd\tau})} (e^{-Kdt_1})$$

When the dosing interval is much shorter than the drug's half-life, the changes in concentration within a dosing interval are relatively small, and any drug concentration obtained within a dosing interval can be used as an approximation of the average steady-state concentration. Even though Equations 43 on page 53 and 47 on page 55 could be used to predict peak and trough concentrations, a reasonable approximation could also be achieved by using Equation 35 on page 46 for Cpss ave:

$$Cpss \ ave = \frac{(S)(F)(Dose/\tau)}{Cl}$$

This suggests that even though Equations 43 and 47 do not contain the parameter clearance *per se*, the elimination rate constant functions in such a way that the clearance derived from Equations 43 or 47 and 35 would all be essentially the same.

Even though the elimination rate constant and volume of distribution might be manipulated in Equations 43 and 47, it is only the product of those two numbers (i.e., clearance) that can be known with any certainty so long as the dosing interval is less than the drug half-life. See Equation 33 on page 44:

$$Cl = (Kd)(Vd)$$

Conversely, if a drug is administered at a dosing interval that is much longer than the apparent half-life (see Figure 31 on page 77), peak concentrations may be primarily a function of volume of distribution. Since most of the dose is eliminated within a dosing interval, each dose can be treated like a new loading dose. At some point within the dosing interval, the plasma concentration is primarily determined by clearance. Trough plasma concentrations in this situation are a function of both clearance and volume of distribution. Since clearance and volume of distribution are critical to the prediction of peak and trough concentrations in this situation, a minimum of two plasma concentrations is needed to accurately establish a dosing regimen that will achieve desired peak and trough concentrations. Aminoglycosides are examples of drugs that are administered at dosing intervals that exceed their apparent half-life; therefore, at least two plasma concentrations are measured within a dosing interval for these agents. (See Part II: Aminoglycoside Antibiotics.)

When an observed drug concentration correlates with the level that was predicted based upon pharmacokinetic parameters from the literature, the particular pharmacokinetic parameter that is the primary determinant of the observed drug concentration should be determined before making future predictions. Successful prediction of an appropriate loading dose to achieve specific plasma levels, for example, does not guarantee that the maintenance dose is correct. Therefore, critical evaluation of the parameters affecting a patient's measured drug concentration will minimize incorrect assumptions about the applicability of literature-based pharmacokinetic parameters to a specific patient's situation or about the predictability of future plasma concentrations.

Choosing a Model to Revise or Estimate a Patient's Clearance at Steady State

As previously discussed, a drug's half-life often determines the pharmacokinetic model that should be used to estimate a pharmacokinetic parameter that is specific for the patient under treatment. A common problem encountered clinically, however, is that the half-life observed in the patient often differs from the expected value. Since a change in either clearance or volume of distribution or both may account for this unexpected value, the pharmacokinetic model is often unclear. One way to approach this dilemma is to compare the expected change in plasma drug concentration associated with each dose to the steady-state trough concentration measured in the patient.

$$\frac{\text{(S)(F)(Dose)}}{\text{Vd}} \text{ versus Cpss min}$$

or

$$\Delta Cp \text{ versus Cpss min}$$

Note in Figure 31 on page 77 that when the dosing interval (τ) is much less than the drug half-life that ΔCp will be small when compared to Cpss min. As the dosing interval increases relative to τ, ΔCp will increase relative to Cpss min. Therefore, a comparison of ΔCp or (S)(F)(Dose)/Vd to Cpss min can serve as a guide to estimating the drug t½ and the most appropriate pharmacokinetic model or technique to use for revision. With few exceptions, drugs are most often dosed at intervals which equal or exceed their half-lives. Therefore, clearance is the pharmacokinetic parameter most often revised or calculated for the patient in question. The following guidelines can be used to select the pharmacokinetic model that is the least complex and therefore the most appropriate to estimate a patient-specific pharmacokinetic parameter.

Condition 1

➤ When:
$$\frac{\text{(S)(F)(Dose)}}{\text{Vd}} \leq \tfrac{1}{4} \text{ Cpss min}$$

➤ Then:
$$\tau \leq \tfrac{1}{3}t½$$

➤ Under these conditions:
Cpss min ≈ Cpss ave

➤ And Cl can be estimated by Equation 15:
$$Cl = \frac{\text{(S)(F)(Dose}/\tau)}{\text{Cpss ave}}$$

➤ Rules/Conditions: Must be at steady state.

Condition 2

➤ When:
$$\frac{\text{(S)(F)(Dose)}}{\text{Vd}} \leq \text{Cpss min}$$

➤ Then:
$$\tau \leq t½$$

➤ Under these conditions:

$$\text{Cpss min} + (\tfrac{1}{2})\frac{(S)(F)(Dose)}{Vd} \approx \text{Cpss ave}$$

➤ And clearance can be estimated by:

$$Cl = \frac{(S)(F)(Dose/\tau)}{\text{Cpss ave}}$$

➤ Rules/Conditions: Must be at steady state.
  Cp is Cpss min.
  Bolus model acceptable.
    Dosage form is not sustained release.
    Short infusion model does not apply.
    $t_{in} \leq \tfrac{1}{6}t\tfrac{1}{2}$

Condition 3

➤ When:

$$\frac{(S)(F)(Dose)}{Vd} > \text{Cpss min}$$

➤ Then:

$$\tau > t\tfrac{1}{2}$$

➤ Under these conditions:

$$\text{Cpss min} + \frac{(S)(F)(Dose)}{Vd} = \text{Cpss max}$$

➤ And clearance can be estimated by first revising Kd:

$$\text{Kd Revised} = \frac{\ln\left(\dfrac{\text{Cpss min} + \dfrac{(S)(F)(Dose)}{Vd}}{\text{Cpss min}}\right)}{\tau} = \frac{\ln\left(\dfrac{\text{Cpss max}}{\text{Cpss min}}\right)}{\tau}$$

$$Cl = \text{Kd Revised} \times Vd$$

➤ Rules/Conditions: Must be at steady state.
  Cp is Cpss min.
  Bolus model acceptable.
    Dosage form is not sustained release.
    Short infusion model does not apply.
    $t_{in} \leq \tfrac{1}{6}t\tfrac{1}{2}$

Note that the approaches used become more complex as the dosing interval increases relative to the drug half-life. If a drug is administered at a dosing interval less than or equal to one-third of its half-life and the technique in Condition 3 is used to revise clearance, the clearance value derived would be essentially correct. However, if a drug is administered at a dosing interval that exceeds one half-life and the technique in Condition 1 is used to revise clearance, the revised clearance value would be inaccurate because Cpss min cannot be assumed to be equal to Cpss ave. While it could be argued that the technique used in Condition 3 would suffice for all the previous conditions, it is more cumbersome and tends to focus on the intermediate parameters, elimination rate constant and volume of distribution. One should also be aware that, as the dosing interval increases, the confidence in a revised clearance diminishes because the volume of distribution begins to influence the revised clearance to a greater degree.

Nonsteady-State Revision of Clearance (Iterative Search)

The techniques described in the previous section allow one to calculate a revised clearance directly. However, there are a number of situations when revision of the clearance value is possible, but there are no explicit solutions. These situations require an iterative search technique. The first situation is when the parameter being revised appears in both the exponential and nonexponential portions of the equations, as illustrated by Equation 37 on page 48.

$$Cp_1 = \frac{(S)(F)(Dose/\tau)}{Cl}(1 - e^{-Kdt_1})$$

While it may not be obvious that clearance appears in both the exponential and nonexponential portions of the equation, the elimination rate constant consists of both clearance and Vd. Therefore, if Vd is held constant, the revision process would be associated with a changing clearance (and the corresponding elimination rate constant) to match the observed plasma concentration [Cp_1]. The clearance that "fits" Cp_1 will be the revised clearance. As stated earlier, there is no direct solution and the clearance value (which when placed in Equation 37 calculates the specific Cp_1) can only be found by trial and error.

The second situation which requires an iterative search is anytime there are multiple exponential terms (e^{-Kdt}) where t differs. This might occur when there are multiple bolus doses being administered and the plasma concentration is the sum of the residual of each of these doses. (See Figure 27 on page 67.) Another example is the short infusion model or Equation 57.

$$Cpss_2 = \frac{\dfrac{(S)(F)(Dose/t_{in})}{Cl}(1 - e^{-Kdt_{in}})}{1 - e^{-Kd\tau}}(e^{-Kdt_2})$$

In Equation 57, clearance is expressed in both the exponential (as Kd) and nonexponential portions. In addition, each of the exponential terms has a different value for t, which in itself requires an iterative search. While an iterative search process can be cumbersome, in most cases approximate values for the revised clearance can be arrived at within one to three tries. Most pharmacokineticists, however, use programmed calculators or computers to facilitate these repetitive trial and error calculations. While use of computers is to be encouraged as a labor saving device, the user must understand the fundamental process and the limits of the method.

Nonsteady-State Revision of Clearance (Mass Balance)

The mass balance technique has been suggested as a more direct alternative to the iterative approach.[46,47] The mass balance technique is relatively simple and can be best visualized by examining the relationship between the rate of drug administration and the rate of drug elimination. At steady state, the rate of drug elimination (R_E) is equal to the rate of administration (R_A) and the change in the amount of the drug in the body with time is zero.

$$R_A - R_E = \frac{\text{Change in Amount of}}{\text{Drug in the Body with Time}} = 0$$

Under nonsteady-state conditions, however, there will be a change in the amount of drug in the body with time. This change can be estimated by multiplying the difference in the plasma concentration (ΔCp) by the volume of distribution and dividing by the time interval between the two drug concentrations.

$$R_A - R_E = \frac{(\Delta Cp)(Vd)}{t}$$

By substituting the appropriate values in the above equation, an estimate of clearance can be derived as follows:

$$R_A - R_E = \frac{(\Delta Cp)(Vd)}{t}$$

$$(S)(F)(Dose/\tau) - R_E = \frac{(Cp_2 - Cp_1)Vd}{t}$$

$$(S)(F)(Dose/\tau) - \frac{(Cp_2 - Cp_1)Vd}{t} = R_E$$

$$(S)(F)(Dose/\tau) - \frac{(Cp_2 - Cp_1)Vd}{t} = Cl \times Cp\ ave$$

$$\frac{(S)(F)(Dose/\tau) - \dfrac{(Cp_2 - Cp_1)Vd}{t}}{Cp\ ave} = Cl$$

Eq. 58

Note that the average plasma concentration [Cp ave] is generally assumed to be the average of Cp_1 and Cp_2.

$$Cp\ ave = \frac{Cp_1 + Cp_2}{2}$$

While this Cp ave is not the steady-state average, it is assumed to be the average concentration which results in the loss of drug as it proceeds towards steady state. Equation 58 is an accurate method for estimating clearance if the following conditions are met:

1) t, or time interval between the first and second plasma concentration, should be equal to at least one but no longer than two, of the revised drug half-lives.

2) The plasma concentration values should be reasonably close to one another. If the drug concentrations are increasing, C_2

should be less than two times C_1; if the plasma concentrations are declining, C_2 should be more than one-half of C_1 (i.e., $0.5 < Cp_2/Cp_1 < 2.0$).

3) The rate of drug administration $[(S)(F)(Dose/\tau)]$ should be regular and result in a reasonably smooth progression from Cp_1 to Cp_2 such that the value of Cp ave $((Cp_1 + Cp_2)/2)$ is approximately equal to the true average drug concentration between Cp_1 and Cp_2.

The mass balance approach is a useful technique if the above conditions are met. It is relatively simple and allows for the calculation of clearance under nonsteady-state conditions by a direct process. There are certain situations where the above conditions are not met, but the mass balance technique still works relatively well. For example, if the time interval between Cp_1 and Cp_2 is substantially greater than two half-lives and the value of Cp_2 is very close to Cp_1, then Equation 58 approximates Equation 15 on page 26 because the average plasma concentration approximates the average steady-state value.

$$\frac{(S)(F)(Dose/\tau) - \dfrac{(Cp_2 - Cp_1)Vd}{t}}{Cp \text{ ave}} = Cl$$

$$\frac{(S)(F)(Dose/\tau) - (\approx 0)}{Cp \text{ ave}} = Cl$$

$$\frac{(S)(F)(Dose/\tau)}{Cp \text{ ave}} = Cl$$

The mass balance approach is most commonly applicable for drugs that are given as a continuous intravenous infusion, as a sustained-release product, or for drugs that are administered at a dosing interval that is much shorter than the half-life.

Single-Point Determination of Clearance. A drug concentration that is obtained approximately 1.44 half-lives after a single bolus dose is primarily a function of clearance. This concept is represented in Figure 32 on page 89. The ability to predict clearance using this principle is based upon a complex relationship between volume of distribution, clearance, and half-life. As can be seen from Equations 49 on page 57 for Cp° and 32 on page 43 for $t\frac{1}{2}$, if clearance is held constant, and volume of distribution is decreased, the initial plasma levels will be higher and the elim-

$$Cp = \frac{(S)(F)\, Dose}{Vd_1}$$

$$Cp = \frac{(S)(F)\, Dose}{Vd}$$

$$Cp = \frac{(S)(F)\, Dose}{Vd_2}$$

Cp

Dose

≈1.44 t½'s

TIME

Figure 32. Single-Point Determination of Clearance. The plasma concentrations following a single bolus dose when clearance is held constant and volume of distribution is altered tend to pivot around a single point which occurs at approximately 1.44 half-lives after the dose. When the volume of distribution is small (--- Vd_1), the concentrations before the 1.44 half-life points are elevated, relative to the concentrations found in patients with larger volumes of distribution (···· Vd_2). The opposite is true after the 1.44 half-life point.

ination half-life will be decreased. However, if volume of distribution is increased, the initial plasma concentrations will be lower and the elimination half-life will be longer.

$$Cp^\circ = \frac{(S)(F)(Loading\ Dose)}{Vd}$$

$$t^{1}\!/_{2} = \frac{(0.693)(Vd)}{Cl}$$

By examining Figure 32 it can be seen that over a range of volume of distribution values, there is a locus or point about which the decaying plasma concentration versus time curves appears to pivot. This pivot point is at 1.44 half-lives. For this reason, a single plasma concentration obtained at 1.44 half-lives following an initial bolus dose[48,49,50] can be used with Equation 50 on page 57 for Cp_1 to predict a patient-specific clearance:

$$Cp_1 = \frac{(S)(F)(\text{Loading Dose})}{Vd}(e^{-Kdt_1})$$

It is important to recognize that if the patient's clearance or volume of distribution values differ substantially from those assumed in Equation 50, a sampling time based upon a literature-derived half-life may not represent 1.44 half-lives for the patient. In this instance, accurate patient-specific clearance values would not be derived from this method. For example, if a patient has a very low clearance and a longer-than-expected elimination half-life, plasma samples obtained at 1.44 times the drug's reported half-life will represent a sampling time that is sooner than 1.44 times the patient's elimination half-life for this drug. Plasma samples obtained at this time are primarily a function of volume of distribution and would be influenced minimally by clearance.

It is often difficult to accurately plan a sampling time which can be used for the single-point method. However, if sensitivity testing reveals that clearance is the primary determinant of a concentration obtained approximately 1.44 half-lives after a bolus dose, this concentration may be used to ascertain a patient-specific clearance.

Assay Specificity

The accuracy and specificity of assays used by the clinical laboratory to measure serum drug concentrations are critical. Historically, laboratories developed their assay procedures using a variety of analytical methods ranging from radio-immunoassays to high performance liquid chromatography (HPLC) assay procedures. Currently, however, the vast majority of drug assays performed in the clinical setting are some variant of commercially available immuno-binding assay procedures. The most commonly used procedures are the fluorescence polarization immunoassay, or TDX by Abbott Laboratories, and the enzyme-multiplied immunoassay, or EMIT System by Syva. In general, these assays are accurate, relatively inexpensive, and require little technical expertise to perform. These assays are generally specific for the parent compound; however, in isolated instances, metabolites or other drug-like substances are also recognized by the antibody.[51,52,53]

Since plasma concentrations that are measured by more specific assays will result in lower values, the pharmacokinetic parameters derived from these concentrations (volume of distribution and clearance) will be higher than those derived from less specific assay measurements. (See Equations 10 and 15 on pages 18 and 26, respectively.) While the current literature usually is associated with relatively specific drug assays, use caution when the older literature is employed since pharmacokinetic parameters that have been derived from assays with differing specificities are not interchangeable. The usual therapeutic range will also be altered when less specific assays are used. To illustrate, the therapeutic range for quinidine derived from nonspecific assays was 4 to 8 mg/L.[54,55] In contrast, the therapeutic range for levels measured by the more specific HPLC is 1 to 4 mg/L.[56,57]

For assays that measure the parent compound only, it is important to determine the pharmacologic activity and pharmacokinetic behavior of the metabolites. Many drugs have *active metabolites* that may affect a patient's pharmacologic response (see Table 4); the pharmacokinetic behavior of these metabolites cannot be predicted by an assay that measures only the parent compound. Procainamide has an active metabolite, N-acetyl-procainamide (NAPA), which accumulates to rather high concentrations in patients with renal failure.[58] For this drug, therefore, an assay that measures only procainamide could underestimate the pharmacologic response of the patient.

Whenever possible, one should evaluate the patient's clinical response directly. If drug levels and clinical response do not correlate as predicted, it may be due to a laboratory error. Similarly, factors unique to the patient such as concurrent disease states or antagonist drug therapy may alter one's interpretation of the plasma drug concentration. For example, it is

Table 4	Examples of Drugs with Active Metabolites[59]	
	Amitriptyline	Lidocaine
	Carbamazepine	Primidone
	Chlordiazepoxide	Procainamide
	Chlorpromazine	Propranolol
	Chlorpropamide	Warfarin
	Diazepam	

a common clinical observation that higher-than-usual plasma concentrations of digoxin are required to achieve a clinical response in patients with atrial fibrillation and in patients receiving propranolol. Furthermore, for drugs that have high plasma protein binding, the same therapeutic effect will be achieved with a lower plasma concentration when plasma protein binding is decreased. This is because both bound and free drug levels are measured, and decreased binding lowers the bound concentration but not the free, pharmacologically active concentration. [See Desired Plasma Concentration (Cp) on page 9.] The formation of aberrant metabolites and tachyphylaxis are other reasons why plasma drug concentrations fail to correlate with an expected therapeutic response.

Creatinine Clearance (Cl$_{Cr}$)

Since many drugs are partially or totally eliminated by the kidney, an accurate estimation of renal function is crucial to the application of pharmacokinetics to drug therapy. The creatinine clearance is considered by most clinicians to be the most accurate test of renal function. In the actual clinical setting, however, an accurate Cl$_{Cr}$ may be difficult to obtain because it is based on a 24-hour collection of urine. Frequently, the urine collection is inaccurate because a portion is accidentally discarded, or the time of collection is shorter or longer than requested. An incomplete collection will result in a gross underestimation of renal function.[60] Furthermore, the method is expensive and time-consuming. Because decisions with regard to drug dosing must often be made quickly, several authors have suggested a variety of methods by which Cl$_{Cr}$ can be estimated using a serum creatinine value.

Creatinine Pharmacokinetics

The pharmacokinetics of creatinine are presented in far more detail elsewhere,[60–62] but a brief overview is necessary. Creatinine is a metabolic by-product of muscle and its rate of formation (R$_A$) is primarily determined by an individual's muscle mass or lean body weight. It varies, therefore, with age (lower in the elderly) and gender (lower in the females).[63–65] For any given individual, the rate of creatinine production is assumed to be constant. Once creatinine is released from muscle into plasma, it is eliminated almost exclusively by renal glomerular filtration. Any decrease in the glomerular filtration rate ultimately results in a rise in the serum creatinine level until a new steady state is reached and the *amount* of creatinine cleared per day equals the rate of production. In other words, at steady state, the rate in must equal the rate out. Since the rate of creatinine production *remains* constant even when renal clearance diminishes, the serum creatinine must rise until the product of the clearance and the serum creatinine again equals the rate of production. This concept is represented by Equation 14 on page 26 which has been discussed earlier in the section on clearance:

$$R_A = (Cl)(Cpss\ ave)$$

where R$_A$ is the rate of creatinine production, Cl is creatinine clearance, and Cpss ave is a steady-state serum creatinine level or SrCr$_{ss}$.

Estimating Creatinine Clearance from Steady-State Serum Creatinine Concentrations

The degree to which a *steady-state* serum creatinine rises is *inversely* proportional to the fall in creatinine clearance. Therefore, the new creatinine clearance can be estimated by multiplying a normal Cl$_{Cr}$ value by the fraction increase in the serum creatinine: Normal SrCr/patient's SrCr$_{ss}$. For the 70 kg man, it can be assumed that the normal SrCr is 1.0 mg/dL and that the corresponding Cl$_{Cr}$ is 120 mL/min:

$$\text{New Cl}_{Cr} = (120 \text{ mL/min})\left[\frac{1.0 \text{ mg/dL}}{\text{SrCr}_{ss}}\right]$$

Eq. 59

On the basis of this concept, one can see that each time the serum creatinine doubles, the creatinine clearance falls by one-half and that small changes in the serum creatinine at low levels are of much greater consequence than equal changes in the serum creatinine at high levels. To illustrate, if a patient whose normal serum creatinine is 1.0 mg/dL is reported to have a new steady-state serum creatinine of 2 mg/dL, the creatinine clearance has dropped from 120 mL/min to 60 mL/min. However, if a patient with chronic renal failure has a usual serum creatinine of 8 mg/dL (Cl$_{Cr}$ = 15 mL/min), a similar 1.0 mg/dL increase in the serum creatinine to 9 mg/dL would result in a small drop in the Cl$_{Cr}$ (1.7 mL/min) and a new clearance value of 13.3 mL/min.

The estimation of Cl$_{Cr}$ from SrCr$_{ss}$ is reasonably satisfactory as long as the patient's daily creatinine production is average (i.e., 20 mg/kg/day); the serum creatinine is at steady state (i.e., not rising or falling); and the patient weighs approximately 70 kg.

Adjusting to Body Size and Weight. To account for any changes in creatinine production and clearance which may result from a difference in body size, Equation 59 can be modified to compensate for any deviation in body surface area (BSA) from the 70 kg patient (1.73 m^2):

$$\text{New Cl}_{Cr} = (120 \text{ mL/min})\left(\frac{1.0 \text{ mg/dL}}{\text{SrCr}_{ss}}\right)\left(\frac{\text{Patient's BSA}}{1.73 \text{ m}^2}\right)$$

Eq. 60

The patient's BSA can be obtained from a nomogram (See Appendix I) or estimated from Equation 17 on page 29:

$$\text{BSA in m}^2 = \left(\frac{\text{Patient's Weight in kg}}{70 \text{ kg}}\right)^{0.73} (1.73 \text{ m}^2)$$

A disadvantage of this method is that elderly and emaciated patients who have a reduced muscle mass do not have a "normal" creatinine clearance of 120 mL/min/1.73m^2 with a serum creatinine value of 1.0 mg/dL. For this reason, it may be erroneous to assume that a SrCr of 1.0 mg/dL is indicative of a creatinine clearance of 120 mL/min/1.73 m^2 in these individuals.

As patients grow older, their muscle mass represents a smaller proportion of their total weight and creatinine production is decreased. (See Table 5.) The following methods for estimating creatinine clearance from a steady-state serum creatinine concentration consider age and gender-related alterations in creatinine production.[64,66,67]

$$\frac{\text{Cl}_{\text{Cr}} \text{ for Males}}{(\text{mL/min/70 kg})} = \frac{98 - [(0.8)(\text{Age} - 20)]}{\text{SrCr}_{\text{ss}}}$$

Eq. 61

$$\frac{\text{Cl}_{\text{Cr}} \text{ for Females}}{(\text{mL/min/70 kg})} = (0.9) \frac{98 - [(0.8)(\text{Age} - 20)]}{\text{SrCr}_{\text{ss}}}$$

Eq. 62

$$\frac{\text{Cl}_{\text{Cr}} \text{ for Males}}{(\text{mL/min})} = \frac{(140 - \text{Age})(\text{Weight})}{(72)(\text{SrCr}_{\text{ss}})}$$

Eq. 63

$$\frac{\text{Cl}_{\text{Cr}} \text{ for Females}}{(\text{mL/min})} = (0.85) \frac{(140 - \text{Age})(\text{Weight})}{(72)(\text{SrCr}_{\text{ss}})}$$

Eq. 64

Where age is in years, weight is in kg, and serum creatinine is in mg/dL. In Equations 61 and 62, the creatinine clearance is calculated for the average 70 kg or 1.73 m^2 person. In contrast, Equations 63 and 64 calculate a creatinine clearance for the size or weight of the patient entered

Table 5   Expected Daily Creatinine Production for Males[65,a]

Age (yr)	Daily Creatinine Production (mg/kg/day)
20–29	24
30–39	22
40–49	20
50–59	19
60–69	17
70–79	14
80–89	12
90–99	9

[a] Daily creatinine production for females would be expected to be 85% of the above values.

in the equation. There are numerous other ways to calculate creatinine clearance based on age, weight, and gender; however, all of these result in similar creatinine clearance values.

The two most critical factors to consider when using the above equations are the assumptions that 1) the serum creatinine is at steady state and 2) the weight used in Equations 63 and 64 reflects normal muscle mass. For example, when estimating a creatinine clearance for an obese patient, the nonobese or ideal body weight should be used in Equations 63 and 64. This estimate can be based upon ideal body weight tables or the following equations:

$$\text{Ideal Body Weight for Males in kg} = 50 + (2.3)(\text{Height in Inches} < 60)$$

Eq. 65

$$\text{Ideal Body Weight for Females in kg} = 45 + (2.3)(\text{Height in Inches} < 60)$$

Eq. 66

It should be pointed out, however, that an ideal body weight derived from one's height, as in Equations 65 and 66, may not represent the actual nonobese weight of a patient. Although there are some potential flaws in estimating the nonobese weight from height, the use of any estimated lean body weight is usually preferable to the use of actual weight when a patient is markedly obese. As a clinical guideline, adjustment for ideal body weight is necessary if the patient's actual weight is >120% of their ideal body weight. A number of studies indicate that total body weight overestimates renal function in markedly obese subjects, and ideal body weight underestimates renal function. It has been suggested that an adjusted body weight between ideal and total body weight be used to estimate renal function in obese individuals. While this adjustment factor is extremely variable, 40% of the excess weight is commonly used:[68,69]

$$\text{Adjusted Body Weight} = \text{IBW} + 0.4(\text{TBW} - \text{IBW})$$

$$\textbf{Eq. 67}$$

where IBW is the patient's ideal body weight in kg as calculated from Equation 65 or 66, and TBW is the total body weight in kg.

While it may seem counter-intuitive, a creatinine clearance calculated from an emaciated subject also tends to over-predict the patient's creatinine clearance. This is because patients who are emaciated tend to have a proportionally greater loss in their muscle mass. Consequently, their serum creatinine in the denominator of Equations 63 and 64 decreases more than the numerator, resulting in an over-estimate of creatinine clearance. For this reason, the actual rather than ideal body weight should be used when calculating creatinine clearance in emaciated subjects. Even then, creatinine clearance is likely to be overestimated.

In addition, it has been suggested that when serum creatinine values are <1.0 mg/dL, more accurate predictions of creatinine clearance can be obtained if these levels are upwardly adjusted to a value of at least 1.0 mg/dL. This suggestion is based on the assumption that low serum creatinine values are related to small muscle mass rather than to an unusually large creatinine clearance. Because it is difficult to estimate muscle mass and appropriate serum creatinine values for obese or emaciated patients, the adjustment techniques discussed above are subject to considerable error. While it is a common practice for clinicians to normalize serum creatinine values <1 mg/dL to 1 mg/dL, there is evidence suggesting that using the actual rather than the normalized serum creatinine is more appropriate.[70,71] Because of this continuing controversy and the difficulty in estimating creatinine clearance accurately, it is important to use clinical judgment in estimating the risk versus the benefit of drug therapy. A decision to take a more conservative approach by using a normalized versus actual serum creatinine for patients with measured values of <1.0 mg/dL should be dictated by clinical judgment rather than a specific rule.

Pediatric Patients. Estimation of creatinine clearance in children is difficult. The most commonly used equation follows:[72]

$$\frac{Cl_{Cr} \text{ for Children}}{(mL/min/1.73 \text{ m}^2)} = \frac{(0.48)(\text{Height in cm})}{SrCr_{ss}}$$

Eq. 68

The above equation is limited to patients between the ages of 1 to 18 years and calculates the creatinine clearance for the standard 1.73 m² or 70 kg patient. To calculate the actual creatinine clearance for the child, the creatinine clearance value calculated in Equation 68 should be adjusted for the patient's body size:

$$\frac{Cl_{Cr} \text{ for Children}}{(mL/min)} = (Cl_{Cr} \text{ mL/min/1.73 m}^2)\left(\frac{BSA}{1.73 \text{ m}^2}\right)$$

Eq. 69

where the body surface area is in m² as calculated from the nomogram in Appendix I. Although Equation 68 was designed to be used for children between the ages of 1 to 18 years, it appears to be less accurate in children <100 cm tall.[67]

The use of Equation 68 does not require a patient's weight in order to calculate creatinine clearance. As noted from the equation, the creatinine clearance calculated is not for the patient; rather, it is a value that has been normalized to a body surface area of 1.73 m². It should be pointed out that while no weight is used in Equation 68, the muscle mass for the child is assumed to be normal for the child's height. For example, a child with an unusually low muscle mass for his height would produce less creatinine. Therefore, for any given degree of renal function, the average serum creatinine would be lower than that of a child with normal muscle mass. For this reason, Equations 68 or 69 need to be used carefully to calculate a child's creatinine clearance in children whose muscle mass is not average. As with adults, if the actual weight is used for either an obese or an emaciated child, it is likely that the creatinine clearance calculated by Equations 68 and 69 will overestimate the actual value. Caution should be used in the application of pharmacokinetics to calculate doses for these patients. For these reasons, plasma level monitoring as a guide to therapy is even more important for these children than in the average child.

Estimating Time to Reach a Steady-State Serum Creatinine Level

All of the above methods for estimating Cl_{Cr} require a steady-state serum creatinine concentration. When a patient's renal function suddenly changes, some period of time will be required to achieve a new steady-state serum creatinine concentration. In this situation, it is important to be able to estimate how long it will take for the SrCr to reach steady state. If a rising serum creatinine is used in any of the previous equations, the patient's creatinine clearance will be overestimated.

As presented earlier, half-life is a function of both the volume of distribution and clearance. If the Vd for creatinine (0.5 to 0.7 L/kg)[73,74] is assumed to remain constant, the time required to reach 95% of steady state in patients with 50%, 25%, and 10% of normal renal function has been estimated to be 0.92, 1.85, and 4.6 days, respectively.[73,75] It is difficult, however, to estimate the percentage of renal function lost clinically. If two determinations of serum creatinine concentration are obtained at 12-hour intervals, a steady-state condition probably has not been reached if the serum creatinine concentration increases by 0.2 mg/dL or more. As renal function decreases, a longer period of time is needed for the serum creatinine concentration to reach a steady state.

Estimating Creatinine Clearance from Nonsteady-State Serum Creatinine Concentrations

Using nonsteady-state serum creatinine values to estimate creatinine clearance is difficult, and a number of approaches have been proposed.[61,62] The author uses Equation 70 to estimate creatinine clearance when steady-state conditions have not been achieved:

$$Cl_{Cr}\ L/day = \frac{\left[\begin{array}{c}\text{Daily Production}\\\text{of Creatinine in mg}\end{array}\right] - \left[\dfrac{(SrCr_2 - SrCr_1)(Vd_{cr})}{t}\right]}{SrCr_2}$$

Eq. 70

The daily production of creatinine in mg is calculated by multiplying the daily production value in mg/kg/day from Table 5 by the patient's weight. The two serum creatinine values in Equation 70 are expressed in units of mg/L; therefore, the serum creatinine concentrations that are reported as mg/dL should be multiplied by 10. SrCr$_1$ represents the first sample and SrCr$_2$ represents the second sample. The volume of distribution for creatinine (Vd$_{Cr}$) is calculated by multiplying the patient's weight times 0.5 L/kg, and the time between samples (t) is expressed in days. Equation 70 is essentially a modification of Equation 58:

$$\frac{(S)(F)(\text{Dose}/\tau) - \dfrac{(Cp_2 - Cp_1)Vd}{t}}{Cp \text{ ave}} = Cl$$

where the daily production of creatinine in mg has replaced the infusion rate of the drug. In addition, the second serum creatinine value was used rather than the average value, primarily because Equation 70 is most commonly applied when creatinine clearance is decreasing, and using the higher of the two serum creatinine values results in a lower, more conservative estimate of renal function. Some have suggested that the iterative search process, as represented by the combination of Equations 26 on page 37 and 37 on page 48, be used:

$$Cp_2 = (Cp^{\circ})(e^{-Kdt}) + \frac{(S)(F)(\text{Dose}/\tau)}{Cl}(1 - e^{-Kdt})$$

where Cp$_2$ represents SrCr$_2$, and Cp$^{\circ}$ represents SrCr$_1$. (S)(F)(Dose/τ) represents the daily production of creatinine, and t represents the time interval between the first and second serum creatinine concentrations. Cl represents the creatinine clearance with the corresponding elimination rate constant Kd being the creatinine clearance divided by the creatinine volume of distribution. As discussed previously [see Interpretation of Plasma Drug Concentrations: Nonsteady-State Revision of Clearance (Iterative Search) on page 85], the solution would require an iterative search, and the inherent errors in the calculation process probably do not warrant this type of calculation.

The use of Equation 70 can be illustrated by considering a 45-year-old, 70 kg male who has a serum creatinine concentration of 1.0 mg/dL on Day 1 and a concentration of 2.0 mg/dL on Day 2. Using Table 5 on page 96, the expected daily production of creatinine for this patient would be 1400 mg/day (20 mg/kg/day × 70 kg). The volume of distribution for creatinine is 35 L (0.5 L/kg × 70 kg), and the time between samples (t) is 1 day. SrCr$_1$ (sampled on Day 1) is 10 mg/L and SrCr$_2$ (sampled on Day 2) is 20 mg/L. Using these values, Equation 70 estimates a creatinine clearance of 52 L/day, or 36.5 mL/min.

$$\frac{Cl_{Cr}}{(L/day)} = \frac{\left[\begin{array}{c} \text{Daily Production} \\ \text{of Creatinine in mg} \end{array}\right] - \frac{(SrCr_2 - SrCr_1)(Vd_{Cr})}{t}}{SrCr_2}$$

$$= \frac{[1400 \text{ mg/day}] - \frac{(20 \text{ mg/L} - 10 \text{ mg/L})(35 \text{ L})}{1 \text{ day}}}{20 \text{ mg/L}}$$

$$= \frac{1400 \text{ mg/day} - 350 \text{ mg/day}}{20 \text{ mg/L}}$$

$$= 52 \text{ L/day}$$

or

$$\frac{Cl_{Cr}}{(mL/min)} = (52 \text{ L/day}) \frac{1000 \text{ mL/L}}{1440 \text{ min/day}}$$

$$= 36.5 \text{ mL/min}$$

This estimated creatinine clearance of approximately 36 mL/min is less than the 46 mL/min that would have been calculated had Equation 63 been used, assuming the serum creatinine of 2.0 represented a steady-state level.

$$\frac{Cl_{Cr} \text{ for Males}}{(mL/min)} = \frac{(140 - Age)(Weight)}{(72)(SrCr_{ss})}$$

$$= \frac{(140 - 45)(70 \text{ kg})}{(72)(2.0 \text{ mg/dL})}$$

$$= 46.2 \text{ mL/min}$$

While Equation 70 may more closely estimate the creatinine clearance when a patient's serum creatinine is rising or falling, there are potential problems associated with this and all other approaches using nonsteady-state serum creatinine values. First, a rising serum creatinine concentration may represent a continually declining renal function. To help compensate for the latter possibility, the second creatinine ($SrCr_2$) rather than the average is used in the denominator of Equation 70. Furthermore, there are nonrenal routes of creatinine elimination that become significant in patients with markedly diminished renal function.[73] Since as much as 30% of a patient's daily creatinine excretion is the result of dietary intake, the ability to predict a patient's daily creatinine production in the clinical setting is limited.[75] One should also consider the potential errors in the serum creatinine measurements, as well as the uncertainty in the volume of distribution estimate for creatinine.

Evaluating Creatinine Clearance Values

The accuracy of a reported creatinine clearance is dependent upon the complete and accurate collection of urine over a 12- or 24-hour period. Therefore, in the evaluation of a reported creatinine clearance, it is essential to validate the completeness of the urine collection. The predicted amount of creatinine produced or excreted for the patient (considering age, gender, weight, and body stature) should be compared with the amount of creatinine actually collected in the urine sample. At steady state, rate in (creatinine production) equals rate out (creatinine excretion). If the amount collected differs significantly from the patient's predicted production, the reported creatinine clearance is likely to be inaccurate. The patient's age, gender, and muscle mass should be considered when estimating the amount of creatinine produced. Increasing age and smaller muscle mass will reduce the expected amount of creatinine produced. (See Table 5 on page 96.)

This principle will be illustrated using the following example: The data below were reported for a 55-year-old, 50 kg female patient for whom a Cl_{Cr} was ordered.

Total Collection Time : 24 hours

Urine Volume : 1200 mL

Urine Creatinine Concentration : 42 mg/dL

Serum Creatinine : 1.5 mg/dL

Creatinine Clearance : 23 mL/min (Uncorrected)
30 mL/min (Corrected)

To determine whether the collection was complete, the total amount of creatinine collected in the 24-hour period should first be calculated:

$$\text{Amount of Creatinine Excreted per Day} = \frac{(\text{Urine Volume per 24 hr})}{(\text{Urine Creatinine Concentration})}$$

Eq. 71

$$= (1200 \text{ mL}/24 \text{ hr})(42 \text{ mg}/100 \text{ mL})$$
$$= 504 \text{ mg Creatinine}/24 \text{ hr}$$

Since the patient weighs 50 kg, the apparent creatinine production per day can be calculated as follows:

$$\text{Apparent Rate of Creatinine Production mg/kg/day} = \frac{\text{Amount of Creatinine Excreted per Day}}{\text{Patient's Weight}}$$

Eq. 72

$$= \frac{504 \text{ mg Creatinine}/1 \text{ day}}{50 \text{ kg}}$$
$$= 10.08 \text{ mg/kg/day}$$

This apparent production rate of creatinine of approximately 10 mg/kg/day is considerably less than the normal production rate of 16 mg/kg/day (19 mg/kg/day × 0.85) as estimated from Table 5. Therefore, the urine collection was probably incomplete, and the reported value for creatinine clearance was much less than the patient's actual Cl$_{Cr}$. However, if the patient has a small muscle mass, the urine collection may be considered adequate and the reported creatinine clearance of 23 mL/min accurate.

As depicted in the patient's data above, both uncorrected and corrected creatinine clearance values are frequently reported by clinical laboratories. The "uncorrected" value usually represents the patient's actual creatinine clearance and the "corrected" value is what the patient's creatinine clearance would be if he or she were 70 kg or 1.73 m^2.

Dialysis of Drugs

Pharmacokinetic Modeling

The pharmacokinetic model for drugs in patients undergoing intermittent hemodialysis generally follows one of two patterns. In Figure 33, a maintenance drug dose produces plasma concentrations that are relatively constant between dialysis periods. This plasma concentration of drug represents the steady-state condition. The rapid decline in the drug concentration corresponds to periods of hemodialysis, and the rapid return of the plasma drug concentration to steady state reflects the administration of a post-dialysis replacement dose. This pattern can be represented by the following equations,

$$\text{Cpss ave} = \frac{(S)(F)(\text{Dose}/\tau)}{Cl_{pat}}$$

Eq. 73

$$\text{Dose} = \frac{(\text{Cpss ave})(Cl_{pat})(\tau)}{(S)(F)}$$

Eq. 74

where S and F are the salt form and bioavailability, τ is a convenient dosing interval, and Cl_{pat} is the drug clearance exhibited by the patient during nondialysis periods. This equation may be used to predict a steady-state plasma concentration produced by a maintenance drug dose if the dosing interval (τ) is considerably shorter than the patient specific half-life. This maintenance dose replaces the amount of drug lost due to the patient's ability to eliminate drug, both by residual renal function (if present) and by nonrenal or metabolic pathways. In addition to a maintenance dose, the patient may also require additional doses following dialysis to replace the drug lost during the dialysis period.

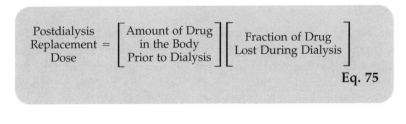

$$\begin{array}{c}\text{Postdialysis} \\ \text{Replacement} = \\ \text{Dose}\end{array} \left[\begin{array}{c}\text{Amount of Drug} \\ \text{in the Body} \\ \text{Prior to Dialysis}\end{array}\right]\left[\begin{array}{c}\text{Fraction of Drug} \\ \text{Lost During Dialysis}\end{array}\right]$$

Eq. 75

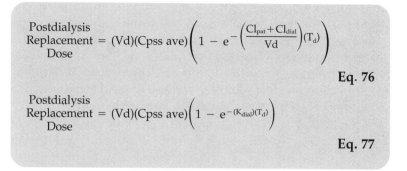

$$\text{Postdialysis Replacement Dose} = (Vd)(Cpss\ ave)\left(1 - e^{-\left(\frac{Cl_{pat} + Cl_{dial}}{Vd}\right)(T_d)}\right)$$

Eq. 76

$$\text{Postdialysis Replacement Dose} = (Vd)(Cpss\ ave)\left(1 - e^{-(K_{dial})(T_d)}\right)$$

Eq. 77

Where (Vd $\times$ Cpss ave) is the amount of drug in the body at the beginning of dialysis and the elimination rate constant during the dialysis (K_{dial}) represents the patient's clearance added to the clearance by dialysis divided by the volume of distribution ($Cl_{pat} + Cl_{dial}$)/Vd). T_d is the duration of dialysis. If the patient's maintenance dose is given once daily, then the patient's dose would be calculated using Equation 74 on nondialysis days. On dialysis days, the patient's daily dose would be the sum of Equations 74 and 76 or 77.

The second pharmacokinetic model for drug dosing in patients undergoing hemodialysis is depicted in Figure 34. In this model, a single dose is given at the conclusion of each dialysis period. Significant amounts of drug are lost between dialysis periods, and additional drug is lost during dialysis. The replacement dose administered at the end of dialysis replaces all of the drug lost by the patient's own clearance, as well as by dialysis clearance and returns the drug level to a critical concentration. This replacement dose can be calculated by use of Equations 78 or 79:

$$\text{Postdialysis Replacement Dose} = (Vd)(Cpss\ peak)\left(1 - \left[\left(e^{-\left(\frac{Cl_{pat}}{Vd}\right)(t_1)}\right)\left(e^{-\left(\frac{Cl_{pat} + Cl_{dial}}{Vd}\right)(T_d)}\right)\right]\right)$$

Eq. 78

$$\text{Postdialysis Replacement Dose} = (Vd)(Cpss\ peak)\left(1 - \left[\left(e^{(-Kd_{pat})(t_1)}\right)\left(e^{(-K_{dial})(T_d)}\right)\right]\right)$$

Eq. 79

where t_1 is the interdialysis period, or the period from the peak concentration to the beginning of dialysis, and T_d is the dialysis period, or the time interval from the beginning to the end of dialysis. Kd_{pat} and K_{dial} are the elimination rate constants during the inter- and intradialysis periods, respectively. In some cases it may be appropriate to calculate the drug concentrations at the beginning and end of the dialysis period. This can be accomplished by use of Equations 80 and 81.

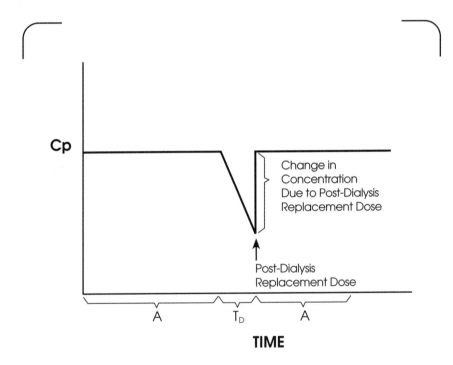

Figure 33. Plasma Concentration Curve Between Dialysis. This figure represents a plasma concentration curve for a patient receiving a maintenance dose of a drug between dialysis procedures at intervals that result in small fluctuations in plasma concentration. The dosing interval during the interdialysis period (A) is arbitrary, but should be less than the half-life of the drug. During the intradialysis period (T_d), the drug is rapidly removed by the dialysis procedure. The subsequent increase in the plasma concentration of drug is due to the postdialysis replacement dose. This model assumes that the drug is significantly removed during dialysis.

$$\begin{array}{c} \text{Predialysis} \\ \text{Drug} \\ \text{Concentration} \end{array} = (\text{Cpss peak})\left(e^{-\frac{Cl_{pat}}{Vd}(t_1)} \right)$$

Eq. 80

$$\begin{array}{c} \text{Postdialysis} \\ \text{Drug} \\ \text{Concentration} \end{array} = \left(\begin{array}{c} \text{Predialysis} \\ \text{Drug} \\ \text{Concentration} \end{array} \right)\left(e^{-\left(\frac{Cl_{pat}+Cl_{dial}}{Vd}\right)(T_d)} \right)$$

Eq. 81

These equations are used when even transient declines in the plasma concentrations might result in therapeutic failures, as with antiarrhythmics or anticonvulsant agents. In the case of aminoglycoside antibiotics, the postdialysis drug concentration should *not* be treated as the "trough concentration" since this level is not at all analogous to the trough concentrations in patients with normal renal function. Because of the unusually long half-life of aminoglycosides in dialysis patients, the targets for the steady-state peak and subsequent predialysis drug concentrations are about 5 mg/L and 2 mg/L, respectively for tobramycin and gentamicin. In some cases, higher drug concentrations may be desired, but it should be recognized that it is not possible to achieve low trough concentrations in dialysis patients in this situation; therefore, the risk of ototoxicity is substantially higher.

Estimating Drug Dialyzability

To calculate dosing requirements for patients undergoing intermittent hemodialysis, the dialysis clearance must be known. Although a number of general references are available,[76–78] it is frequently difficult to find information on specific drugs, especially for drugs that are poorly dialyzable. The doses of these drugs generally do not need to be adjusted following hemodialysis. To determine the dialyzability of a drug, the apparent volume of distribution, plasma protein binding, the patient's clearance, and the drug's half-life should be considered as follows:

1) Divide the volume of distribution by alpha (α) or the usual free fraction to calculate the apparent unbound volume of distribution against which the drug will be dialyzed. If this value exceeds 250 L/70 kg, it is unlikely that the drug will be dialyzable.

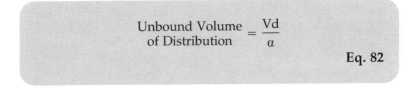

$$\text{Unbound Volume of Distribution} = \frac{Vd}{\alpha}$$

Eq. 82

2) Estimate the patient's clearance. If this value exceeds 500 to 700 mL/70 kg/min, it is unlikely that hemodialysis will add significantly to this clearance value. This is because most drugs have a hemodialysis clearance in the range of 5 to 100 mL/min.

Figure 34. Plasma Profile for a Drug Administered only at the Postdialysis Period for a Patient Receiving Intermittent Hemodialysis. The interdialysis period (t_1) represents the time from the steady-state peak concentration to the beginning of dialysis and may vary according to the number of days between each hemodialysis period. The intradialysis period is represented by T_d. The postdialysis dose represents the amount of drug that is lost from the body due to the patient's clearance during the interdialysis period, as well as the dialysis clearance during the intradialysis period.

3) If the drug's half-life is very short (i.e., <1 to 2 hours), it is unlikely that hemodialysis will significantly alter the dosing regimen. Since most drugs with a very short half-life do not accumulate to a significant extent when dosed intermittently, replacement doses will be required with and without hemodialysis.

If a drug has an unbound volume of <250 L, a clearance value of <500 to 700 mL/min, and a half-life >1 to 2 hours, it is possible that hemodialysis will significantly alter the drug elimination pattern. In these cases it is necessary to review the literature to establish the actual hemodialysis clearance values. If this clearance value adds significantly to the patient's clearance, then additional drug replacement following hemodialysis may be appropriate.

As an additional check, the drug half-life during the dialysis period can be calculated using Equation 83:

$$t\frac{1}{2} \text{ during Hemodialysis} = \frac{(0.693)(Vd)}{(Cl_{pat} + Cl_{dial})}$$

Eq. 83

In order for dialysis to remove a significant amount of drug, the half-life of the drug during the dialysis period should not exceed the duration of dialysis.

While the techniques outlined above can be used to estimate the dialyzability of drugs and thereby model their pharmacokinetic behavior during dialysis, there are a number of potential limitations. For example, relatively little is known about either the activity of metabolites for many drugs or their dialyzability. These guidelines must also be used cautiously in acute overdose situations since plasma and tissue binding saturation as well as possible alterations in the pathways for elimination under these circumstances make the use of standard pharmacokinetic parameters somewhat speculative. Considerable differences in dialysis equipment and the types of membranes used in hemodialysis can result in data that may not be applicable to all dialysis situations.

For example, high-flux hemodialysis utilizes a different type of membrane in the artificial kidney. It is more efficient than the standard dialysis procedure, making the above techniques to estimate dialyzability inaccurate. To illustrate, very little vancomycin is removed during a standard hemodialysis run because of its large molecular weight, but when high-flux dialysis is used, approximately 17% to 30% is removed.[79,80] Another blood purifying technique, continuous arteriovenous hemofiltration (CAVH), utilizes a "large pore" efficient artificial kidney membrane and has been shown to significantly remove vancomycin and other drugs.[81,93] While the clearance values for CAVH are significantly less than for high-flux hemodialysis, significant amounts of drug can be removed because CAVH is a continuous rather than intermittent process. While CAVH is increasing in use, it is available in only a few acute care settings and it is limited to patients who are hemodynamically unstable and therefore unsuitable candidates for intermittent hemodialysis.[82,83,93]

Although it would be ideal to have data derived from the specific dialysis equipment used for the patient in question, this will not be the case in most instances. Instead, one must rely on the data in the literature to estimate the average amount of drug that most likely would be removed during the patient's hemodialysis.

Dialysis procedures also vary in duration and effectiveness. The duration of dialysis can usually be found on the hemodialysis record sheets. When the patient's blood flow during the dialysis period is less than the usual 200 to 350 mL/min, when the patient experiences significant periods of hypotension, or when the dialysis period is cut short, the estimated drug loss during dialysis should be reduced.

The uncertainties and potential problems associated with predictions of drug levels during hemodialysis suggest that plasma drug concentrations guide the approach to therapy. When obtaining plasma samples, the distribution phase associated with IV drug administration, as well as the transient period of disequilibrium between the plasma and tissue compartments associated with the hemodialysis process should be avoided. While this disequilibrium is not documented for most drugs, it would seem reasonable to wait at least 30 to 60 minutes following the end of hemodialysis before obtaining plasma samples.

Peritoneal Dialysis

Peritoneal dialysis, and especially continuous ambulatory peritoneal dialysis (CAPD), is a commonly-used alternative to intermittent hemodialysis. This technique takes advantage of the large intraperitoneal surface area and is performed by instilling dialysate fluid via a catheter into the peritoneal space. The dialysate is allowed to equilibrate with the surrounding tissue fluids, and then is removed. This creates a clearance mechanism for solutes which include both body waste products and drugs. The usual volume instilled into the peritoneal space for an adult is ≈ 2 L, although this can vary somewhat depending on the size of the patient and the intent of dialysis. The efficiency of peritoneal dialysis in removing both drugs and body waste products depends upon a number of factors. Assuming that the solute comes to equilibrium with the dialysate fluid and that there is no plasma protein binding, the maximum expected CAPD clearance would be approximately equal to:

$$\text{Volume Dialysate}/T_D$$

where T_D is the dialysate exchange or dwell time.

If the usual volume of dialysate is ≈ 2000 mL and the usual dwell time or exchange rate (T_D) is ≈ 6 hours, or four times daily, the expected maximum clearance for solute and drugs is approximately 5.5 mL/min.

$$2000 \text{ mL}/6 \text{ hr} = \frac{333.33 \text{ mL/hr}}{60 \text{ min/hr}}$$
$$= 5.5 \text{ mL/min}$$

For this reason, drugs which have a residual Cl_{pat} that is substantially greater than 5.5 mL/min will not be significantly influenced by peritoneal dialysis. As a general guideline, if the dialysis exchange rate is <10% to 20% of the residual patient clearance (Cl_{pat}), one would not anticipate a need to adjust a drug's dose if peritoneal dialysis is initiated or discontinued. Many drugs are significantly bound to plasma protein, however, and this will result in a less efficient peritoneal dialysis clearance because only the unbound drug will readily equilibrate with the dialysate. In addition, large molecules tend to reach equilibrium much more slowly than small molecules; therefore, it is possible that clearance by peritoneal dialysis will be substantially lower than the dialysis exchange rate.

$$Cl_{CAPD} \cong (\alpha)\left(\frac{\text{Volume Dialysate}}{T_D}\right)(1 - e^{(-Keq)(T_D)})$$

In the above equation, Cl_{CAPD} is the clearance by CAPD, alpha is the free fraction in plasma of the compound or drug in question, and $[1 - e^{(-Keq)(T_D)}]$ is the fraction of equilibrium achieved during the dialysate dwell time (T_D). While the free fraction or alpha is available for many drugs, it should be recognized that in renal disease the free fraction is often increased. The time required to achieve equilibrium, or the equilibrium rate constant (Keq), is not generally available. The fraction of equilibrium achieved can be estimated, however, based upon a drug's molecular weight. For example, urea and creatinine, with molecular weights of approximately 60 and 113 daltons, respectively, appear to come to relatively rapid and complete equilibrium within two hours.[84] This suggests that the equilibrium half-time for these compounds is probably less than an hour and may be in the range of one-half an hour. Larger compounds such as the aminoglycosides appear to have a dialysis clearance (Cl_{CAPD}) which approaches the dialysis exchange rate when the dwell (T_D) is ≈ 6 hours.[84,85] This suggests that if equilibrium is approached in six hours, the equilibrium half-time is probably in the range of one to two hours or less. Vancomycin, on the other hand, has a peritoneal dialysis clearance of only 1 to 3 mL/min, suggesting that it does not come to equilibrium within the usual six-hour dwell time. This observation is consistent with the fact that vancomycin is assumed to have relatively little plasma protein binding.[81,86] Therefore, the low peritoneal dialysis clearance can probably be attributed to vancomycin's large molecular weight of ≈ 1500 daltons.

The significance of high plasma protein binding on drug clearance is fairly obvious. Compounds that are extensively bound to plasma proteins and have low free concentrations are not likely to be significantly cleared by peritoneal dialysis unless their residual clearance is exceedingly low. The influence of molecular weight and time to reach equilibrium on a drug's diazability is less well understood because relatively few data are available. However, the clearance of compounds that appear to come to equilibrium rapidly is likely to be altered if the dwell time is changed. For example, if a patient is taking a drug that has low molecular weight, more drug will be removed if the peritoneal dialysate fluid is exchanged more frequently. As a result, replacement doses of a drug that are necessitated by dialysis are likely to be determined by the exchange rate. In contrast, replacement doses of drugs with high molecular weights are not likely to be influenced by the exchange rate. This is because an increase in the exchange rate is offset by the decrease in dwell time and the fraction of equilibrium achieved. Consequently, the total calculated clearance would change very little.

Because the surface area of the peritoneal membrane is large and peritoneal infections are frequent, it has become a common practice to administer antibiotics directly into the peritoneal space.[87] The most common antibiotics administered intraperitoneally are the cephalosporins, aminoglycosides, and vancomycin. Techniques used to administer these drugs vary from intermittently adding large doses of drug to a single dialysate exchange to the addition of small amounts of drug in each individual exchange. When drugs are placed in each exchange, the ability to achieve peak and trough concentrations is limited. (See Part II: Aminoglycoside Antibiotics and Vancomycin for usual dosing recommendations.)

ALGORITHM FOR EVALUATING AND INTERPRETING PLASMA LEVELS

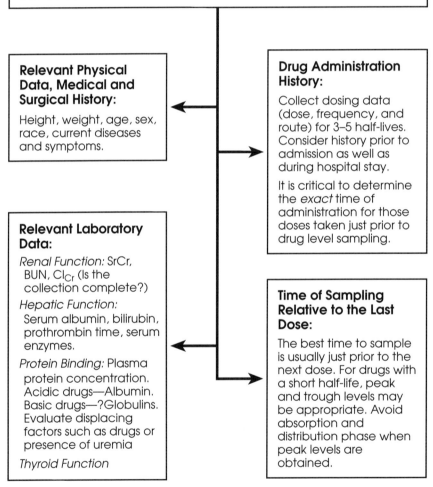

Step 1. Initial Data Collection

Before one can interpret the patient's pharmacokinetic parameters or plasma drug levels, appropriate information must be collected so that factors which may influence drug absorption and disposition can be considered.

Relevant Physical Data, Medical and Surgical History:

Height, weight, age, sex, race, current diseases and symptoms.

Relevant Laboratory Data:

Renal Function: SrCr, BUN, Cl$_{Cr}$ (Is the collection complete?)

Hepatic Function: Serum albumin, bilirubin, prothrombin time, serum enzymes.

Protein Binding: Plasma protein concentration. Acidic drugs—Albumin. Basic drugs—?Globulins. Evaluate displacing factors such as drugs or presence of uremia

Thyroid Function

Drug Administration History:

Collect dosing data (dose, frequency, and route) for 3–5 half-lives. Consider history prior to admission as well as during hospital stay.

It is critical to determine the *exact* time of administration for those doses taken just prior to drug level sampling.

Time of Sampling Relative to the Last Dose:

The best time to sample is usually just prior to the next dose. For drugs with a short half-life, peak and trough levels may be appropriate. Avoid absorption and distribution phase when peak levels are obtained.

(Continued on next page)

Step 2. Evaluation of Reported Plasma Levels

Has the patient been receiving constant dosing for more than 3 to 4 half-lives prior to obtaining the plasma sample?

Yes

No ↓

NonSteady State Plasma Concentration

The plasma level must be evaluated by considering the contribution of each dose at the time the plasma sample was obtained. Use Equation 50 for each bolus dose or Equation 53 for each "short infusion." If several different sustained infusion rates have been used during the accumulation period, Equations 37 or 41 should be used for each infusion rate.

Cp is greater than expected:

See List A.

Vd may be less than expected.

Sample was obtained during distribution phase.

Cp is less than expected:

See List B.

Vd may be greater than expected.

Sample was obtained too soon after the dose was administered and absorption was not yet complete.

List A

When drug concentrations are greater than expected, consider:

1. Increased bioavailability. This is only important if the drug's bioavailability is usually low.
2. Noncompliance. Intake is greater than prescribed.
3. Decreased clearance.
4. Increased plasma protein binding. Changes in plasma protein binding will be most important if α is ≤ 0.1 and are unlikely to be significant if α is >0.5. Increased plasma protein binding will also decrease the volume of distribution and clearance of most drugs.

List B

When drug concentrations are less than expected, consider:

1. Decreased bioavailability.
2. Noncompliance. Intake is less than prescribed.
3. Increased clearance.
4. Decreased plasma protein binding. Changes in plasma protein binding will be most important if α is ≤ 0.1. It is unlikely to be significant if α is >0.5. Decreased plasma binding will also increase the volume of distribution and the clearance of most drugs.

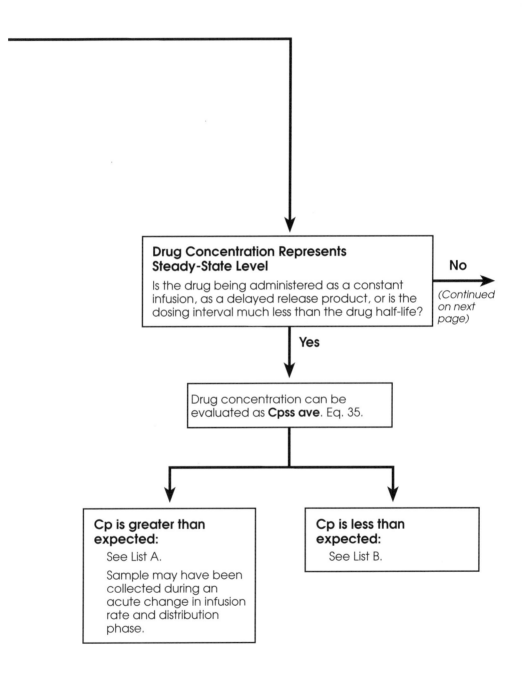

Drug Concentration Represents Steady-State Level

Is the drug being administered as a constant infusion, as a delayed release product, or is the dosing interval much less than the drug half-life?

No

(Continued on next page)

Yes

Drug concentration can be evaluated as **Cpss ave**. Eq. 35.

Cp is greater than expected:

See List A.

Sample may have been collected during an acute change in infusion rate and distribution phase.

Cp is less than expected:

See List B.

Step 2. Evaluation of Reported Plasma Levels
(Continued)

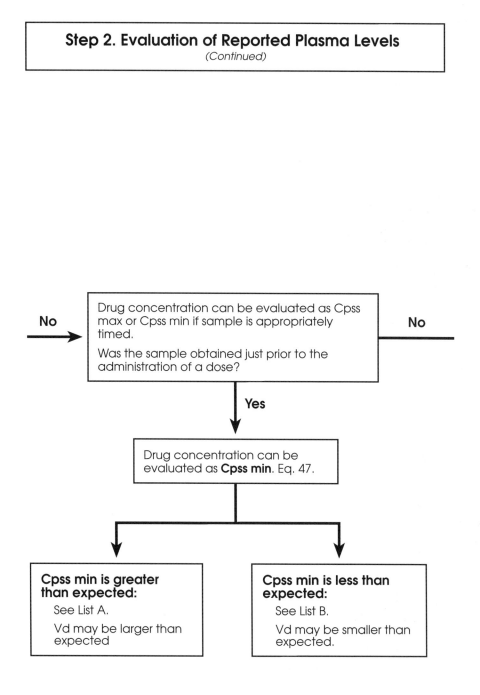

No →

Drug concentration can be evaluated as Cpss max or Cpss min if sample is appropriately timed.

Was the sample obtained just prior to the administration of a dose?

No

Yes

Drug concentration can be evaluated as **Cpss min**. Eq. 47.

Cpss min is greater than expected:

See List A.

Vd may be larger than expected

Cpss min is less than expected:

See List B.

Vd may be smaller than expected.

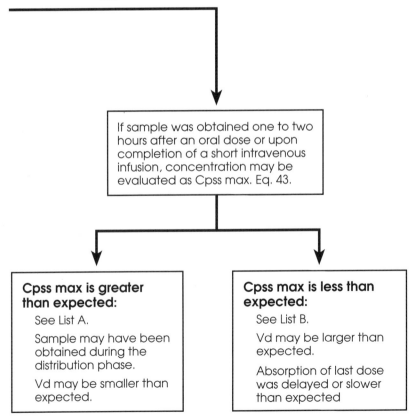

List A

When drug concentrations are greater than expected, consider:

1. Increased bioavailability. This is only important if the drug's bioavailability is usually low.
2. Noncompliance. Intake is greater than prescribed.
3. Decreased clearance.
4. Increased plasma protein binding. Changes in plasma protein binding will be most important if α is ≤ 0.1 and are unlikely to be significant if α is >0.5. Increased plasma protein binding will also decrease the volume of distribution and clearance of most drugs.

List B

When drug concentrations are less than expected, consider:

1. Decreased bioavailability.
2. Noncompliance. Intake is less than prescribed.
3. Increased clearance.
4. Decreased plasma protein binding. Changes in plasma protein binding will be most important if α is ≤ 0.1. It is unlikely to be significant if α is >0.5. Decreased plasma binding will also increase the volume of distribution and the clearance of most drugs.

No

If sample was obtained one to two hours after an oral dose or upon completion of a short intravenous infusion, concentration may be evaluated as Cpss max. Eq. 43.

Cpss max is greater than expected:

See List A.

Sample may have been obtained during the distribution phase.

Vd may be smaller than expected.

Cpss max is less than expected:

See List B.

Vd may be larger than expected.

Absorption of last dose was delayed or slower than expected

References

1. Huffman DH et al. Absorption of digoxin from different oral preparations in normal subjects during steady state. Clin Pharmacol Ther. 1974;16:310.

2. Lisalo E. Clinical pharmacokinetics of digoxin. Clin Pharmacokinet. 1977;2:1.

3. Weinberger M et al. The relation of product formulation to absorption of oral theophylline. N Engl J Med. 1978;299:852.

4. Hendeles L et al. Food-induced dose dumping from a once-a-day theophylline product as a cause of theophylline toxicity. Chest. 1985; 87:758.

5. Mallis GI et al. Superior bioavailability of digoxin solution in capsules. Clin Pharmacol Ther. 1975;18:761.

6. Marcus FI et al. Digoxin bioavailability: formulations and rates of infusions. Clin Pharmacol Ther. 1976;20:253.

7. Nahata MC, Powell DA. Bioavailability and clearance of chloramphenicol after intravenous chloramphenicol succinate. Clin Pharmacol Ther. 1981;30:368.

8. Boyer RW et al. Pharmacokinetics of lidocaine in man. Clin Pharmacol Ther. 1971;12:105.

9. Niles AS, Shand DG. Clinical pharmacology of propranolol. Circulation. 1975; 52:6.

10. Koch-Weser J, Sellers EM. Binding of drugs to serum albumin. N Engl J Med. 1976;294:311.

11. Levy RH, Shand D, ed. Clinical implications of drug-protein binding. Clin Pharmacokinet. 1984;9:(Suppl)1.

12. Fremstad D et al. Increased plasma binding of quinidine after surgery. A preliminary report. Eur J Clin Pharmacol. 1976;10:441.

13. Tucker GT et al. Binding of anilide-type local anesthetics in human plasma. Anesthesiology. 1970;33:287.

14. Borga O et al. Plasma protein binding of basic drugs. Clin Pharmacol Ther. 1977;22:539.

15. Adler DS et al. Hemodialysis of phenytoin in a uremic patient. Clin Pharmacol Ther. 1975;18:65.

16. Edwards DJ et al. Alpha-1-acid glycoprotein concentration and protein binding in trauma. Clin Pharmacol Ther. 1982;31:62.

17. Piafsky KM. Disease-induced changes in the plasma binding of basic drugs. Clin Pharmacokinet. 1980;5:246.

18. Pike E et al. Binding and displacement of basic drugs, acidic and neutral drugs in normal and orosomucoid deficient plasma. Clin Pharmacokinet. 1981;6:367.

19. Routledge PA et al. Relationship between alpha-1-acid glycoprotein and lidocaine disposition in myocardial infarction. Clin Pharmacol Ther. 1981;30:154.

20. Odar-Cederlof I, et al. Kinetics of diphenylhydantoin in uremic patients: consequence of decreased protein binding. Eur J Clin Pharmacol. 1974;7:31.

21. Koch-Weser J, Sellers EM. Binding of drugs to serum albumin. N Engl J Med. 1976;294:311.

22. Barre J et al. Problems in therapeutic drug monitoring: Free drug level monitoring. 1988;10:133–43.

23. Booker HE, Darcy B. Serum concentrations of free diphenylhydantoin and their relationship to clinical intoxication. Epilepsia. 1973;14:177–84.

24. Rowland M. Drug administration and regimens. In: Melmon K, Morelli H, eds. Clinical Pharmacology and Therapeutics, 2nd ed. New York:MacMillan; 1978: 25–70.

25. Reuning RH et al. Role of pharmacokinetics in drug dosage adjustment: I. Pharmacologic effect kinetics and apparent volume of distribution of digoxin. J Clin Pharmacol. 1973;13:127.

26. Gibaldi M, Perrier D. Drug distribution and renal failure. J Clin Pharmacol. 1972;12:201.

27. Benowitz N. Clinical application of the pharmacokinetics of lidocaine. In: Melmon K, ed. Cardiovascular Drug Therapy. Philadelphia:FM Davis; 1974:77–101.

28. Mitenko PA, Ogilvie RI. Rapidly achieved plasma concentration plateaus, with observation on theophylline kinetics. Clin Pharmacol Ther. 1972;13:329.

29. Walsh FM et al. Significance of non-steady state serum digoxin concentrations. Am J Clin Pathol. 1975;63:446.

30. Shapiro W et al. Relationship of plasma digitoxin and digoxin to cardiac response following intravenous digitalization in man. Circulation. 1970;42:1065.

31. Sheiner LB et al. Estimation of population characteristics of pharmacokinetic parameters from routine clinical data. J Pharmacokinet Biopharm. 1977;5:445.

32. Barot MH et al. Individual variation in daily dosage requirements for phenytoin sodium in patients with epilepsy. Br J Clin Pharmacol. 1978;6:267.

33. Vogelstein B et al. The pharmacokinetics of amikacin in children. J Pediatrics. 1977;91:333.

34. FDA Drug Bulletin. IV guidelines for theophylline products. 1980 (Feb); Vol 10.

35. Diem K, Lentner C, eds. Documentia Geigy: Scientific Tables, 7th ed. Switzerland:Ciba-Geigy, Ltd.; 1972.

36. Green MG. The Harriet Lane Handbook: A Manual for Pediatric House Officers. Twelfth ed. Chicago, IL:Mosby Year Book Medical Publ; 1991.

37. Ohnhaus EE et al. Protein binding of digoxin in human serum. Eur J Clin Pharmacol. 1972;5:34.

38. Pang SK, Rowland M. Hepatic clearance of drugs: I. Theoretical considerations of a "well-stirred" model and a "parallel tube" model. Influence of hepatic blood flow, plasma and blood cell binding and hepatocellular enzymatic activity on hepatic drug clearance. J Pharmacokinet Biopharm. 1977;5:625.

39. Rowland M, Tozer TN. Clinical Pharmacokinetics: Concepts and Applications. Philadelphia, PA:Lea & Febiger; 1980.

40. Powell JR et al. Theophylline disposition in acutely ill hospitalized patients. Am Rev Respir Dis. 1978;118:229.

41. Dettli L. Individualization of drug dosage in patients with renal disease. J Clin Pharmacol. 1972;12:201.

42. Welling PG et al. Prediction of drug dosage in patients with renal failure using data derived from normal subjects. Clin Pharmacol Ther. 1975;18:45.

43. Jusko WH et al. Pharmacokinetic design of digoxin dosage regimens in relation to renal function. J Clin Pharmacol. 1974;14:525.

44. Terbraak EW et al. Once-daily dosing regimen for aminoglycoside plus beta-lactam combination therapy for serious bacterial infection: comparative trial with netilmicin plus ceftriaxone. Amer J Med. 1990; 89:58–66.

45. Zeisler JA et al. Lidocaine therapy: time for re-evaluation. Clinical Pharmacy. 1993;12:527–8.

46. Chiou WL et al. Method for rapid estimation of the total body drug clearance and adjustment of dosing regimen in patients during a constant-rate intravenous infusion. J Pharmacokin Biopharm. 1978;6:135–51.

47. Vozeh S et al. Rapid prediction of steady-state serum theophylline concentration in patients treated with intravenous aminophylline. Euro J Clin Pharmacol. 1980;18:473–77.

48. Slattery JT et al. Prediction of maintenance dose required to attain a desired drug concentration at steady state from a single determination of concentration after an initial dose. Clin Pharmacokinet. 1980;5:377.

49. Koup JR. Single-point prediction methods: a critical review. Drug Intell Clin Pharm. 1982;16:855.

50. Unadkat JD et al. Further considerations of the "single-point, single-dose" method to estimate individual maintenance dosage requirements. Ther Drug Monit. 1982;4:201.

51. Patel JA et al. Abnormal theophylline levels in plasma by fluorescence polarization immunoassay in patients with renal disease. Ther Drug Monit. 1984;6:458–60.

52. Hicks JM, Brett EM. Falsely increased digoxin concentrations in samples from neonates and infants. Ther Drug Monit. 1984;6:461–64.

53. Flachsh H, Rasmussen JM. Renal disease may increase apparent phenytoin in serum as measured by enzyme-multiplied immunoassay. Clin Chem. 1980;26:361.Letter.

54. Cramer G, Isakson B. Quantitative determination of quinidine in plasma. Scand J Clin Lab Invest. 1963;15:553.

55. Kessler KM et al. Quinidine elimination in patients with congestive heart failure or poor renal function. N Engl J Med. 1974;290:706.

56. Powers J, Sadee W. Determination of quinidine by high-performance liquid chromatography. Clin Chem. 1978;24:299.

57. Conrad KA et al. Pharmacokinetic studies of quinidine in patients with arrhythmias. Circulation. 1977;55:1.

58. Gibson TP. Acetylation of procainamide in man and its relationship to isonicotinic acid-hydrazide acetylation phenotype. Clin Pharmacol Ther. 1975;17:395.

59. Drayer E. Pharmacologically active metabolites, therapeutic and toxic activities, plasma and urine data in man, accumulation in renal failure. Clin Pharmacokinet. 1976;1:426.

60. Kassirer JP. Clinical evaluation of kidney function-glomerular function. N Engl J Med. 1971;285:385.

61. Lott RS, Hayton WL. Estimation of creatinine clearance from serum creatinine concentration: a review. Drug Intell Clin Pharm. 1978; 12:140.

62. Bjornsson TD. Use of serum creatinine concentrations to determine renal function. Clin Pharmacokinet. 1979;4:200.

63. Goldman R. Creatinine excretion in renal failure. Proc Soc Biol Med. 1954;85:446.

64. Jelliffe RW. Creatinine clearance: bedside estimate. Ann Intern Med. 1973;79:604.

65. Siersbaek-Nielson K et al. Rapid evaluation of creatinine clearance (Letter). Lancet. 1971;1:1133.

66. Cockcroft DW, Gault MH. Prediction of creatinine clearance from serum creatinine. Nephron. 1976;16:31.

67. Hernandez de Acevedo L, Johnson CE. Estimation of creatinine clearance in children: comparison of six methods. Clin Pharm. 1982;1:158.

68. Dionne RE et al. Estimating creatinine clearance in morbidly obese patients. Am J Hosp Pharm. 1981;38:841–4.

69. Bauer LA et al. Influence of weight on aminoglycoside pharmacokinetics in normal weight and morbidly obese patients. Eur J Clin Pharmacol. 1983;24:643–7.

70. Smythe M et al. Estimating creatinine clearance in elderly patients with low serum creatinine concentrations. Am J Hosp Pharm. 1994; 51:198–204.

71. Bertino JS. Measured versus estimated creatinine clearance in patients with low serum creatinine values. Ann Pharmacother. 1993;27:1439–41.

72. Traub SL, Johnson CE. Comparison of methods of estimating creatinine clearance in children. Am J Hosp Pharm. 1980;37:195–200.

73. Mitch WE et al. Creatinine metabolism in chronic renal failure. Clin Sci. 1980;58:327.

74. Chow MS, Schweitzer R. Estimation of renal creatinine clearance in patients with unstable serum creatinine concentrations: comparisons of multiple methods. Drug Intell Clin Pharm. 1985;19:385–90.

75. Bleiler RE, Schedl HP. Creatinine excretion: variability and relationships to diet and body size. J Lab Clin Med. 1962;59:945.

76. Aweeka FT. Appendix: Drug reference table. In: Schrier RW, Gambertoglio JG, eds. Handbook of Drug Therapy in Liver and Kidney Disease. Little, Brown and Co. 1991.

77. Takki S et al. Pharmacokinetic evaluation of hemodialysis in acute drug overdose. Pharmacokinet Biopharm. 1978;6:427.

78. Lee CC, Marbury TC. Drug therapy in patients undergoing haemodialysis. Clinical pharmacokinetic considerations. Clin Pharmacokinet. 1984;9:42.

79. Nanese DM et al. Markedly increased clearance of vancomycin during hemodialysis using polysulfone dialyzers. Kidney Internat. 1989;35:1409–12.

80. Pollard TA et al. Vancomycin redistribution: dosing recommendations following high-flux hemodialysis. Kidney Internat. 1994;45:232–7.

81. Bickley SK. Drug dosing during continuous arteriovenous hemofiltration. Clin Pharm. 1988;7:198–206.

82. Gloper TA. Continuous arteriovenous hemofiltration in acute renal failure. Am J Kid Dis. 1985;6:373–86.

83. Pattison ME et al. Continuous arteriovenous hemodiafiltration: an aggressive approach to the management of acute renal failure. Am J Kidney Dis. 1988;11:43–7.

84. Lamier N et al. Peritoneal pharmacokinetics and pharmacological manipulation of peritoneal transport in continuous ambulatory peritoneal dialysis. In: Gokal R, ed. New York: Churchill Livingstone. 1986:56–93.

85. Matzke GR, Millikin SP. Influence of renal function and dialysis on drug disposition. In: Evans WE, Schentag JJ, Jusko WJ, eds. Applied Pharmacokinetics: Principles of Therapeutic Drug Monitoring. Third Edition. Vancouver WA: Applied Therapeutics, Inc. 1992; Chapter Eight.

86. Matzke GR. Vancomycin. In: Evans WE, Schentag JJ, Jusko WJ, eds. Applied Pharmacokinetics: Principles of Therapeutic Drug Monitoring. Third Edition. Vancouver WA: Applied Therapeutics, Inc. 1992; Chapter Fifteen.

87. O'Brien MA, Mason NA. Systemic absorption of intra-peritoneal antimicrobials in continuous ambulatory peritoneal dialysis. Clin Pharm. 1992;11:256.

88. Conford EM et al. Increased blood-brain barrier transportation of protein-bound anticonvulsant drugs in the newborn. J Cereb Blood Flow Metabol. 1983;3:280–6.

89. Craig WA, Vogelman B, Editorial: The post antibiotic effect. Ann Intern Med. 1987;106:900–2.

90. Benet LZ, Williams RL. Appendix II: Design and optimization of dosage regimens: pharmacokinetic data. In Gilman AG et al, eds. Goodman and Gilman's The Pharmacologic Basis of Therapeutics, 8th ed. New York: Pergamon Press, 1990:1650–1735.

91. LeMarie M, Tillement JP. Role of lipoproteins and erythrocytes in the *in vitro* binding and distribution of cyclosporin A in the blood. J of Pharmacy and Pharmacol. 1982;34:715–18.

92. Niederberger W et al. Distribution and binding of cyclosporine in blood and tissue. Transplant Proc. 1983;15:2419–21.

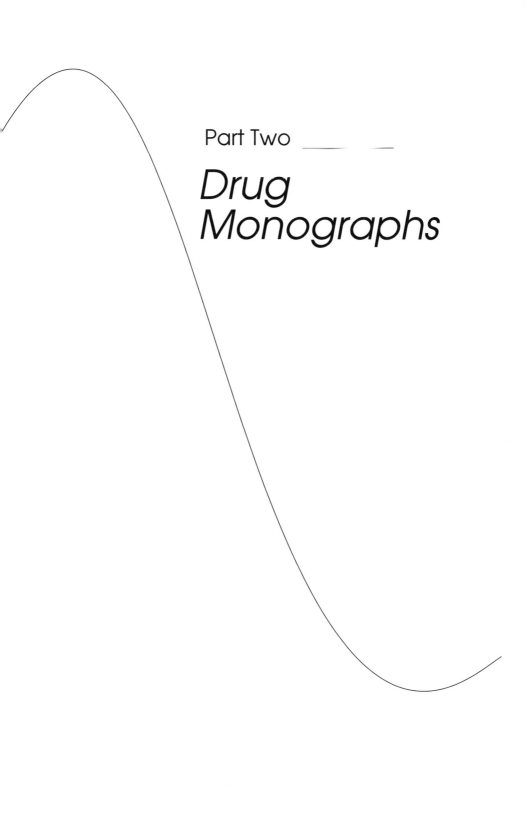

Part Two

Drug Monographs

Aminoglycoside Antibiotics   1

The aminoglycosides are bactericidal antibiotics used in the treatment of serious gram-negative infections. Since absorption from the gastrointestinal tract is poor, the aminoglycosides must be administered parenterally in order to achieve therapeutic concentrations in the systemic circulation. In most instances, the aminoglycosides are administered by intermittent intravenous (IV) infusions. The choice of an aminoglycoside dose is influenced by the specific agent (e.g., gentamicin versus amikacin), infection (e.g., site and organism), renal function, and weight or body composition of the patient. The three most commonly monitored aminoglycoside antibiotics are gentamicin, tobramycin, and amikacin. The usual dose for gentamicin and tobramycin is in the range of 50 to 120 mg (1 to 2 mg/kg), administered over 30 to 60 minutes every eight hours; the dose of amikacin is 200 to 500 mg (5 to 7.5 mg/kg), every 8 to 12 hours. The clearance, volume of distribution, and half-life of all the aminoglycosides are similar.[1] Therefore, the same pharmacokinetic model can be used for all of the aminoglycosides and the principles which are described in this chapter for any given aminoglycoside generally apply to the others as well. The aminoglycosides have different ranges of "therapeutic" serum concentrations and have different propensities for interaction with penicillin compounds.

Therapeutic and Toxic Plasma Concentrations

Peak plasma concentrations for gentamicin and tobramycin are in the range of 4 to 8 mg/L.[2–4] Peak plasma concentrations of <2 to 4 mg/L are likely to be ineffective,[3] and successful treatment of pneumonia may require peak concentrations of 8 mg/L.[2] Desirable peak concentrations for amikacin are usually 20 to 30 mg/L; trough concentrations are usually <10 mg/L.[1]

Most available data correlating aminoglycoside concentrations with oto- and nephrotoxicity refer to trough plasma concentrations, although some data suggest a correlation between peak concentrations and toxicity.[5,6] Although gentamicin trough concentrations of >2 mg/L have been associated with renal toxicity, the high trough concentrations may be the result, and not the cause, of renal dysfunction. In fact, the use of elevated trough concentrations as an indication of early renal damage has been suggested by some investigators.[7,8] Fortunately, most patients who develop renal dysfunction during aminoglycoside therapy appear to regain normal renal function after the drug has been discontinued.[9]

Key Parameters

Therapeutic Plasma Concentrations

Gentamicin, Tobramycin	Peak	4–8 mg/L
	Trough	<2 mg/L
Amikacin	Peak	20–30 mg/L
	Trough	<10 mg/L

Vd[a]	0.25 L/kg

Cl

Normal Renal Function	Equal to Cl_{Cr}
Functionally Anephric Patients[b]	0.0043 L/kg/hr
Surgically Anephric Patients[b]	0.0021 L/kg/hr
Hemodialysis[b]	1.8 L/hr

$t^{1/2}$

Normal Renal Function	2–3 hr
Functionally Anephric Patients	30–60 hr

[a] Volume of distribution should be adjusted for obesity and/or alterations in extracellular fluid status.

[b] Functionally anephric patient is a dialysis patient with kidneys intact. Surgically anephric patient is a dialysis patient with kidneys removed. Hemodialysis clearance of 1.8 L/hr refers to standard hemodialysis, not high-flux or peritoneal dialysis.

Ototoxicity has been associated with trough plasma concentrations of gentamicin exceeding 4 mg/L for more than ten days. When the trough concentration is multiplied by the number of days of therapy the risk of ototoxicity is increased when the product exceeds 40 mg-days/L. Amino-glycoside-ototoxicity also seems to be most prevalent in patients who have existing impaired renal function or have received large doses during the course of their treatment.[5–7,10,11]

Although it is the standard practice to use aminoglycoside plasma concentrations as predictors for both efficacy and toxicity, it is controversial whether this is valid.[12] One problem in using human data only to validate the therapeutic range is that doses for most patients are adjusted to achieve similar peak and trough concentrations. This makes it difficult to determine whether or not dosing regimens that produce high peak and low trough concentrations are indeed optimal. Experimental review boards are not likely to authorize a clinical study utilizing continuous infusions of aminoglycosides making it even more challenging to assess alternative dosing schemes. Some authors have recommended once daily doses of aminoglycosides[13–15] based upon the theory that aminoglycosides exhibit concentration-dependent bactericidal activity [i.e., plasma concentrations that exceed the minimum inhibitory concentration (MIC) for a given bacteria are even more effective than the MIC].[14,15] In addition to the concentration-dependent killing, there is also a postantibiotic response which results in depressed bacterial growth after plasma concentrations have fallen below minimum inhibitory concentrations.[16,17] While there is increasing evidence that once daily doses of aminoglycosides are equally efficacious and no more toxic than divided daily doses,[13,17] we do not know which patients are likely to fail on this regimen. For example, single daily dosing may not be as efficacious as divided daily doses in immunosuppressed animals.[15] Limited human data, however, counter this observation. When combined with a long-acting cephalosporin, single daily doses of amikacin appear to be at least equal in efficacy to the usual practice of divided daily doses.[13] Once-daily dosing of aminoglycosides is not yet a standard practice. It is the author's opinion that once daily dosing of aminoglycosides should only be used in those patient populations who are most likely to respond favorably to this aminoglycoside regimen.

Bioavailability (F)

The aminoglycoside antibiotics are very water soluble and poorly lipid soluble compounds. As a result, they are poorly absorbed when administered orally and must be administered parenterally for the treatment of systemic infections.

Volume of Distribution (Vd)

The volume of distribution of the aminoglycosides is ≈ 0.25 L/kg, although a relatively wide range of 0.1 to 0.5 L/kg has been reported.[18–24] Since aminoglycosides distribute very poorly into adipose tissue, lean rather than total body weight (TBW) should result in a more accurate approximation of Vd in obese patients.[25] The aminoglycoside volume of distribution in obese subjects also could be adjusted based on the patient's ideal body weight (IBW) plus 10% of his excess weight.[26,27] These adjustments in the estimation of aminoglycoside volumes of distribution in obese patients seem reasonable because aminoglycoside antibiotics appear to distribute into extracellular space, and the extracellular fluid volume of adipose tissue is approximately 10% of total body weight versus

25% for other tissues. Equation 1.1 can be used to approximate the volume of distribution (Vd) in obese patients:

$$\text{Aminoglycoside Vd (Obese Patients)} = (0.25 \text{ L/kg})(\text{IBW}) + 0.1(\text{TBW} - \text{IBW})$$

Eq. 1.1

The non-obese or ideal body weight can be approximated using Equations 65 and 66 (See Part I: Creatinine Clearance (Cl_{Cr}) on page 93.) The volume of distribution of aminoglycosides is increased in patients with ascites, edema, or other enlarged "third space" volume.[28,29] One approach to approximating the increased volume of distribution for patients with ascites or edema is to increase the Vd by 1 L for each kg of weight gain. This approach is based on the assumption that the volume of distribution of aminoglycoside antibiotics is approximately equal to the extracellular fluid volume. This is consistent with the low plasma protein binding[1] and the fact that aminoglycosides cross membranes very poorly.

$$\text{Aminoglycoside Vd (L)} = \left(\begin{array}{c} 0.25 \text{ L/kg} \times \text{Non-Obese,} \\ \text{Non-Excess Fluid Weight (kg)} \end{array}\right)$$
$$+ 0.1 \left(\begin{array}{c} \text{Excess} \\ \text{Adipose} \\ \text{Weight (kg)} \end{array}\right) + \left(\begin{array}{c} \text{Excess Third-} \\ \text{Space Fluid} \\ \text{Weight (kg)} \end{array}\right)$$

Eq. 1.2

The volume of distribution for aminoglycosides can be estimated using Equation 1.2, in which the non-obese, non-excess fluid weight usually can be estimated as the ideal body weight, and the excess adipose weight as the difference between the non-obese weight and the patient's total weight without excess third-space fluid. The excess third-space fluid weight is estimated clinically. In cases where a rapid increase in weight has occurred over several days, this weight gain is likely to represent fluid in a third space; it is therefore easily estimated by taking a difference between the initial and current weights. Some patients may exhibit significant third-spacing of fluids (apparent as either edema or ascites) upon initial evaluation. It is most difficult to estimate an aminoglycoside Vd in the obese patient with significant third-spacing of fluid. As Equation 1.2 illustrates, assigning excess third-space fluid to adipose weight could result in a significant underestimation of the volume of distribution. For this reason, it should be recognized that Equation 1.2 only approximates the Vd, and plasma concentration measurements are needed to make patient-specific adjustments.

Pediatric patients less than five years of age tend to have a volume of distribution of 0.5 L/kg. Between birth and five years of age, the volume of distribution for pediatric patients probably continues to decline from an initial value of 0.5 L/kg to the adult value of 0.25 L/kg.[30]

$$\text{Aminoglycoside Vd (L)} \atop \text{(Children)} = \left(0.5 \text{ L/kg} - \left(\frac{\text{Age in Years}}{5} \times 0.25\right)\right)\left(\text{Weight} \atop \text{in kg}\right)$$

Eq. 1.3

Because the change in volume of distribution is gradual, some clinicians have chosen to use the above algorithm to estimate the volume of distribution for patients between one and five years of age. After five years of age a Vd of 0.25 L/kg is generally used. Note that in Equation 1.3, it is assumed that the child's weight in kg represents a weight which is not obese and does contain significant excess third-space fluid. While there are no data on the subject, obese children should have a smaller-than-average volume of distribution for their age and size and children with significant third-spacing of fluid should have a larger-than-average Vd.

A one-compartment model is generally assumed for aminoglycoside pharmacokinetic calculations. The initial distribution phase following a gentamicin intravenous infusion is not a factor when the one-compartment model is utilized for gentamicin pharmacokinetic calculations.[31–33] For this reason, reported values for plasma samples obtained near the conclusion of an intravenous infusion may be higher than expected. These reported values probably have no correlation with the therapeutic or toxic effects of the drug. A third distribution phase, or gamma phase, for gentamicin has also been identified.[34] This final volume of distribution phase for gentamicin is large and because gentamicin clearance is decreased when plasma concentrations are low, the average half-life associated with this third compartment is in excess of 100 hours.[31,34] This large final volume of distribution and long terminal half-life may be significant when evaluating a patient's potential for aminoglycoside toxicity.[35]

Despite the existence of the three-compartment model for the aminoglycosides, pharmacokinetic calculations can be based upon a one-compartment model that utilizes the second volume of distribution. The errors encountered when using a single-compartment model for the aminoglycosides can be minimized if plasma drug concentrations are obtained at times that avoid the first and third distribution phases and at 24 hours after therapy has been initiated.[36] Aminoglycoside concentrations of <1 mg/L should be evaluated cautiously because the influence of the large third compartment will become greater at these low concentrations.[31]

Clearance (Cl)

The aminoglycoside antibiotics are eliminated almost entirely by the renal route.[1,23] Since the aminoglycoside and creatinine clearances are similar over a wide range of renal function, aminoglycoside clearance can be estimated from the formulas used to estimate creatinine clearance (Equations 63 and 64) when concentrations are within the therapeutic range:[1,18,23,31]

$$\frac{Cl_{Cr} \text{ for Males}}{\text{(mL/min)}} = \frac{(140 - \text{Age})(\text{Weight})}{(72)(SrCr_{ss})}$$

$$\frac{Cl_{Cr} \text{ for Females}}{\text{(mL/min)}} = (0.85)\frac{(140 - \text{Age})(\text{Weight})}{(72)(SrCr_{ss})}$$

As presented in Part I, the age is in years, weight is in kg, and serum creatinine is in mg/dL. Correct estimates of creatinine clearance can only be obtained if the patient's weight represents a normal ratio of muscle mass to total body weight, and the serum creatinine is at steady state. For this reason, pharmacokinetic calculations for obese patients and patients who have significant third-spacing of fluid should take into consideration adjustments for obesity and third-spacing. Generally, the ideal body weight for obese subjects calculated from Equations 65 and 66 can be used; adjustments for ideal body weight in patients who are <20% overweight are probably unnecessary.

$$\frac{\text{Ideal Body Weight}}{\text{for Males in kg}} = 50 + (2.3)(\text{Height in Inches} > 60)$$

$$\frac{\text{Ideal Body Weight}}{\text{for Females in kg}} = 45 + (2.3)(\text{Height in Inches} > 60)$$

In patients who are morbidly obese (i.e., actual body weight approximately double their ideal body weight), creatinine and aminoglycoside clearances are best estimated by using a weight that falls between the ideal and total body weight.[37,38] For this reason, some clinicians prefer to estimate the non-obese weight by using the following equation:

$$\text{Non-Obese Weight} \approx \text{IBW} + 0.4(\text{TBW} - \text{IBW})$$

where IBW is the ideal body weight as estimated by Equations 65 and 66, and TBW represents the patient's total body weight without the presence of excess third-space fluid.

Non-Renal Clearance. Another factor which should be considered when estimating the clearance of aminoglycosides is the non-renal clearance, which is $\approx$0.0021 L/kg/hr (or $\approx$2.5 mL/min/70 kg). The non-renal clearance of aminoglycosides is generally ignored in most patients, but it is significant in patients whose renal function is markedly diminished. In patients who are functionally anephric and on intermittent hemodialysis, a clearance value of $\approx$0.0043 L/kg/hr (5 mL/min/70 kg) represents the residual renal clearance as well as the non-renal clearance. These values, however, are only approximations and serum concentrations of aminoglycosides should be monitored in patients with poor renal function.

Penicillin Interaction. Carbenicillin, ticarcillin, and related extended-spectrum penicillins chemically inactivate gentamicin and tobramycin *in vitro*. This inactivation can become clinically significant *in vivo* in patients with renal failure. Although this interaction usually is not considered a route of aminoglycoside clearance, it does act as a mechanism for drug "elimination." This interaction is a function of the specific aminoglycoside, the penicillin compound, the concentration of the penicillin compound, and the temperature. In general, tobramycin and gentamicin interact with penicillins in a similar manner; amikacin is much less likely to interact with these penicillins.[39-44] The newer semisynthetic acylureido penicillins appear to be less reactive than carbenicillin, and the cephalosporins appear to be relatively nonreactive.[45-47] For patients with very poor renal function who are receiving carbenicillin or piperacillin, the additional gentamicin clearance can be approximated by multiplying the patient's apparent volume of distribution for the aminoglycoside by 0.017 hr^{-1}.

$$\begin{array}{l}\text{Tobramycin, Gentamicin} \\ \text{Clearance by Carbenicillin} \\ \text{(L/hr)}\end{array} = \left(0.017 \text{ hr}^{-1} \right)\left(\begin{array}{l}\text{Volume of Distribution} \\ \text{for Aminoglycosides}\end{array} \right)$$

Eq. 1.4

The elimination rate constant (Kd) of 0.017 hr^{-1} represents the approximate *in vitro* elimination rate for aminoglycosides exposed to carbenicillin concentrations of 250 to 500 mg/L at a temperature of 37° C. This clearance by carbenicillin is only an approximation and should not be used for amikacin because the interaction between amikacin and carbenicillin is relatively minor. The additional clearance secondary to inactivation by carbenicillin or other penicillins is not clinically relevant in patients with reasonably normal renal function. Enhancement of gentamicin clearance by this interaction is small even in anephric patients (0.3 L/hr or 5 mL/min). Because the third-generation cephalosporin antibiotics have, to a large degree, replaced the use of penicillin derivatives, the interaction between aminoglycoside antibiotics and penicillin derivatives is encountered infrequently in most clinical practices.

Elimination Half-Life

The elimination half-life of aminoglycoside antibiotics from the body is a function of the volume of distribution and clearance. Since renal function varies considerably among individuals, the half-life is also variable. For example, a 70 kg, 25-year-old male with a serum creatinine of 0.8 mg/dL might have an aminoglycoside clearance of 100 mL/min or more. If his volume of distribution is 0.25 L/kg, the corresponding elimination half-life will be about two hours. In contrast, a 75-year-old male with a similar Vd and a serum creatinine of 1.4 mg/dL might have an aminoglycoside clearance of ≈ 35 mL/min and a half-life of approximately six hours. For this reason, the initial aminoglycoside dose and dosing interval should be selected with care. Although initial estimates of the patient's aminoglycoside pharmacokinetic parameters may be highly variable, pharmacokinetic adjustments will hopefully optimize the achievement of therapeutic, yet nontoxic, concentrations of aminoglycoside antibiotics.

Nomograms and Computers

The wide availability of nomograms to dose aminoglycosides may lead one to question the necessity for pharmacokinetic calculations.[10]

These nomograms, however, are usually designed to achieve fixed peak and trough serum concentrations, and they do not allow the clinician to individualize the dosing regimens to account for the type of infection treated or the benefit-to-risk ratio for the individual patient. Furthermore, nomograms are based upon average pharmacokinetic parameters and do not provide a method for dose adjustment for unique patients (e.g., obese individuals or those who have significant third-spacing of fluid). Patient-specific adjustments based on measured plasma concentrations also cannot be extrapolated from these nomograms. An understanding of the basic pharmacokinetic principles used to individualize aminoglycoside doses, coupled with a rational clinical approach, will enable the clinician to provide optimal therapy for the less-than-average patient.

A number of computer programs are available to help clinicians dose aminoglycosides and other therapeutic agents. Computers tend to be more flexible than nomograms in that the user often can select dosing intervals and peak or trough concentrations based on clinical judgment. The potential problem with computers, however, is that the user must be familiar with the algorithms initially used to define the expected pharmacokinetic parameters and how patient-specific parameters are revised when plasma concentrations and dosing histories are supplied. In the revision process, the user must be able to recognize data that are obviously wrong and to interpret the computer output to ensure that the parameters and dosing recommendations are reasonable. The computer should be viewed as a labor-saving device, not as a substitute for a thorough understanding of the pharmacokinetic process.

Time to Sample

Correct timing of the sample collection is important because the aminoglycoside antibiotics have a relatively short half-life and a small but significant distribution phase. The most widely-accepted guidelines recommend that samples for peak serum concentrations be obtained one hour after the maintenance dose has been initiated. This recommendation assumes that the drug is infused over about 30 minutes; an acceptable range for the infusion period is 20 to 40 minutes. If it is longer than 40 minutes, peak concentrations should be obtained approximately 30 minutes after the end of the infusion to ensure that distribution is complete. Trough concentrations generally should be obtained within the half-hour before the administration of the next maintenance dose. In cases where the trough concentrations are expected to be lower than the assay sensitivity, an earlier sampling time may be appropriate so that measurable trough concentrations can be obtained and patient-specific pharmacokinetic parameters derived. In all cases, the exact time of sampling and dose administration should be recorded.

When aminoglycoside plasma concentrations are sampled at a time which extends beyond the expected peak, it is possible to calculate the plasma concentration at the earlier time by simply rearranging Equation 26:

$$Cp = (Cp^{\circ}) (e^{-Kdt})$$

$$Cp^{\circ} = \frac{Cp}{e^{-Kdt}}$$

In the above equation, t represents the time from the measured plasma concentration (Cp) to the earlier plasma concentration (Cp°). This equation is used to back-extrapolate a plasma concentration to the "clinical peak," which is one hour after the start of the infusion. The "clinical peak" concentration has generally been used as a guide to aminoglycoside efficacy.

The optimal time to sample within the first 24 hours of therapy is difficult to determine. For patients who are critically ill, a peak and subsequent trough serum aminoglycoside concentration obtained after the initial loading dose allows for the most rapid evaluation of patient-specific parameters and subsequent dose adjustment, if necessary. In a large number of cases, however, this early sampling is not necessary. Furthermore, these early plasma samples may not be predictive of steady-state concentrations because the patient's fluid status or renal function may change. The standard of practice in many institutions is to obtain the first aminoglycoside samples after three or four doses of aminoglycoside have been administered. The majority of patients will be approaching steady state by this time.

Although one can estimate patient-specific pharmacokinetic parameters more accurately with three or four aminoglycoside plasma concentrations, reasonable pharmacokinetic parameters can be estimated using two plasma samples in most cases.

When aminoglycoside antibiotics are administered intramuscularly (IM), the time for absorption or drug input is less predictable; however, in most patients, plasma concentrations peak about one hour after the IM injection.[48] For this reason, a peak plasma concentration should be obtained one hour after the IM dose is administered. Since the rate of absorption is uncertain, it is difficult to know whether unusual plasma concentrations following IM administration represent delayed absorption or unusual pharmacokinetic parameters (e.g., a large volume of distribution).

Question #1. R.W. is a 30-year-old, 70 kg female with a serum creatinine of 0.9 mg/dL. An initial gentamicin dose of 100 mg was infused intravenously over 30 minutes. Calculate the plasma concentration of gentamicin one hour after the infusion was started (i.e., one half-hour after the infusion was completed).

A rough estimate of the peak gentamicin concentration can be calculated using Equation 49 by treating the 30-minute infusion as a bolus dose. The 100 mg dose would be divided by the literature value for the volume of distribution ($\approx$0.25 L/kg or 17.5 L) in this 70 kg female.

$$Cp^\circ = \frac{(S)(F)(\text{Loading Dose})}{Vd}$$

$$= \frac{(1)(1)(100 \text{ mg})}{17.5 \text{ L}}$$

$$= 5.7 \text{ mg/L}$$

The salt form (S) and bioavailability (F) were both assumed to be 1.0 and the plasma concentration of 5.7 mg/L is an approximation that assumes absorption was very rapid and that no significant drug elimination took place during the time of administration. In addition, it is assumed that the drug is distributed into a single compartment. Even though there is clearly a distribution phase associated with the intravenous injection of aminoglycosides, the initially high drug concentration can be ignored as long as plasma sampling is avoided during this distribution phase.[22,23,32]

A more precise calculation of the plasma concentration one hour after the half-hour infusion has been initiated would take into account the decay of gentamicin levels from the peak concentration. In Equation 50 for Cp_1 below, t_1 is the time elapsed from the beginning of the intravenous infusion to the time of sampling at one hour, and the elimination rate constant (Kd) represents the clearance of gentamicin divided by its volume of distribution (Vd) (Equation 27).

$$Cp_1 = \frac{(S)(F)(\text{Loading Dose})}{Vd} (e^{-Kdt_1})$$

$$Kd = \frac{Cl}{Vd}$$

A creatinine clearance (and therefore gentamicin clearance) of approximately 101 mL/min or 6.06 L/hr can be calculated for R.W., using Equation 64:

$$\frac{Cl_{Cr} \text{ for Females}}{(mL/min)} = (0.85)\frac{(140 - \text{Age})(\text{Weight})}{(72)(SrCr_{ss})}$$

$$= (0.85)\left[\frac{(140 - 30)(70)}{(72)(0.9)}\right]$$

$$= 101 \text{ mL/min}$$

$$Cl_{Cr} \text{ (L/hr)} = \left[(101 \text{ mL/min})\left(\frac{60 \text{ min/hr}}{1000 \text{ mL/L}}\right)\right]$$

$$= 6.06 \text{ L/hr}$$

Using this clearance of approximately 6 L/hr and the apparent volume of distribution of 17.5 L, an elimination rate constant of 0.346 hr^{-1} can be calculated using Equation 27. This elimination rate constant when used in Equation 50 to calculate the gentamicin concentration one hour after the dose results in a predicted concentration of 4.0 mg/L.

$$Kd = \frac{Cl}{Vd}$$

$$= \frac{6.06 \text{ L/hr}}{17.5 \text{ L}}$$

$$= 0.346 \text{ hr}^{-1}$$

$$Cp_1 = \frac{(S)(F)(\text{Loading Dose})}{Vd}(e^{-Kdt_1})$$

$$= [5.7 \text{ mg/L}][e^{-(0.346 \text{ hr}^{-1})(1 \text{ hr})}]$$

$$= (5.7 \text{ mg/L})(0.71)$$

$$= 4.0 \text{ mg/L}$$

To evaluate whether or not the IV bolus dose model is appropriate, the duration of infusion (one half-hour) should be compared to the apparent drug half-life. When the duration of infusion or absorption is less than one-sixth of the half-life, then the bolus dose model can be used (see Part I: Selecting the Appropriate Equation on page 57). If, however, the duration of drug input is greater than one-half of a half-life, then an infusion model should be used. Using Equation 31 and the elimination rate constant of 0.346 hr^{-1}, R.W.'s half-life is calculated to be approximately two hours as follows:

$$t\frac{1}{2} = \frac{0.693}{Kd}$$

$$= \frac{0.693}{0.346 \text{ hr}^{-1}}$$

$$= 2.0 \text{ hr}$$

Since the duration of infusion was one half-hour, the absorption time was approximately one-fourth of the half-life. This is between one-eighth of a half-life (which would allow us to use the bolus dose model) and one-half of a half-life (which would require the use of an infusion model). This intermediate infusion time suggests that either a bolus or an infusion model can be used. In practice, an infusion time of greater than one-sixth of the half-life is often used as the criterion for requiring the infusion model. (See Part I: Selecting the Appropriate Equation on page 57.)

Question #2. Using the clearance of 6.06 L/hr, the volume of distribution of 17.5 L, the elimination rate constant of 0.346 hr^{-1}, and the short infusion model, calculate the expected gentamicin concentration for R.W. one hour after initiating the one-half hour infusion of a 100 mg dose.

Equation 53 represents the short infusion model and can be used to calculate the plasma concentration one hour after starting the half-hour infusion. The duration of infusion or t_{in} would be 0.5 hours. The plasma concentration one hour after starting the infusion, t_2, or the time of decay from the end of the infusion would then be 0.5 hours. Using these values, the plasma concentration one hour after initiation of the half-hour infusion would be 4.4 mg/L.

$$Cp_2 = \frac{(S)(F)(Dose/t_{in})}{Cl} (1 - e^{-Kdt_{in}})(e^{-Kdt_2})$$

$$= \frac{(1)(1)(100 \text{ mg}/0.5 \text{ hr})}{6.06 \text{ L/hr}} (1 - e^{-(0.346 \text{ hr}^{-1})(0.5 \text{ hr})})(e^{-(0.346 \text{ hr}^{-1})(0.5 \text{ hr})})$$

$$= (33 \text{ mg/L})(0.16)(0.84)$$

$$= (5.2 \text{ mg/L})(0.84)$$

$$= 4.4 \text{ mg/L}$$

Notice that the plasma concentration of 5.2 mg/L at the end of the half-hour infusion is lower than the calculated peak concentration of 5.7 mg/L following a bolus dose. (See Question 1.) This lower concentration at the end of the infusion reflects the clearance of drug during the infusion process. Also note that the plasma concentration of 4.4 mg/L at one hour calculated by the infusion model is greater than the comparable plasma concentration (4.0 mg/L) calculated by the bolus dose model in Question 1. Less drug remains in the body at this time when the bolus dose model is used because this model assumes that all of the drug entered the body at the beginning of the infusion. The total dose, therefore, has been exposed to the body's clearing mechanisms for a longer time.

Question #3. **In what types of patients is it more appropriate to use the infusion equation for the prediction of aminoglycoside concentrations? When can the bolus dose model be used satisfactorily?**

Since the difference between the results obtained from these two approaches is primarily related to the amount of drug cleared from the body during the infusion period, it is reasonable to assume that in patients with decreased renal function and longer aminoglycoside half-lives, the bolus dose model could be used satisfactorily. In patients with good renal function (e.g., young adults and children), use of the infusion model is more appropriate because these patients often have very short aminoglycoside half-lives.

Question #4. **R.W., the 70 kg female described in Question 1, was given 100 mg of gentamicin over one half-hour every eight hours. Predict her peak and trough plasma concentrations at steady state.**

Again, one could treat this problem as if R.W. were receiving intermittent intravenous boluses or as if she were receiving one half-hour infusions every eight hours. If the bolus dose model is applied, Equation 48 can be used to predict the peak levels, where t_1 represents the time interval between the start of the infusion and the time at which the "peak concentration" is sampled (one hour) and τ is the interval between the doses (eight hours). Using the volume of distribution of 17.5 L and the elimination rate constant of $0.346 \ hr^{-1}$, the calculated peak concentration would be 4.3 mg/L.

$$Cpss_1 = \frac{\frac{(S)(F)(Dose)}{Vd}}{(1 - e^{-Kd\tau})} (e^{-Kdt_1})$$

$$= \frac{\frac{(1)(1)(100 \ mg)}{17.5 \ L}}{[1 - e^{-(0.346 \ hr^{-1})(8 \ hr)}]} (e^{-(0.346 \ hr^{-1})(1 \ hr)})$$

$$= \left[\frac{5.7 \ mg/L}{(1 - 0.063)} \right] [0.71]$$

$$= \left[\frac{5.7 \ mg/L}{0.937} \right] [0.71]$$

$$= [6.1 \ mg/L][0.71]$$

$$= 4.3 \ mg/L$$

The trough concentration also can be calculated using Equation 48, where t_1 is the time interval between the start of the infusion and the time at which trough level is sampled (eight hours). If the trough sample is obtained just before the start of the next infusion, then Equation 47 for Cpss min also can be used. Using the appropriate values for volume of distribution, elimination rate constant, and dosing interval, the calculated trough concentration would be 0.38 mg/L:

$$\text{Cpss min} = \frac{\dfrac{(S)(F)(\text{Dose})}{Vd}}{(1 - e^{-Kd\tau})} (e^{-Kd\tau})$$

$$= \frac{\dfrac{(1)(1)(100 \text{ mg})}{17.5}}{[1 - e^{-(0.346 \text{ hr}^{-1})(8 \text{ hr})}]} (e^{-(0.346 \text{ hr}^{-1})(8 \text{ hr})})$$

$$= (6.1 \text{ mg/L})(0.063)$$

$$= 0.38 \text{ mg/L}$$

If the infusion model is used (Equation 52 for $Cp_{t_{in}}$ the term),

$$\frac{(S)(F)(\text{Dose})}{Vd}$$

in Equations 47 and 48 is replaced with a term that describes the plasma concentration that can be anticipated at the conclusion of each infusion (also see Part I: Selecting the Appropriate Equation on page 57):

$$Cp_{t_{in}} = \frac{(S)(F)(\text{Dose}/t_{in})}{Cl} (1 - e^{-Kdt_{in}})$$

where t_{in} is the duration of the infusion. This substitution results in an equation describing the intermittent infusion steady-state model (Equation 57):

$$Cpss_2 = \frac{\dfrac{(S)(F)(Dose/t_{in})}{Cl}(1 - e^{-Kdt_{in}})}{(1 - e^{-Kd\tau})} (e^{-Kdt_2})$$

where τ is the dosing interval and t_2 is the time interval between the end of the infusion and the time at which the concentration is measured. That is, when peak concentrations are measured one hour after the initiation of a half-hour infusion, t_2 is 0.5 hours. For trough concentrations that are sampled just before the start of a subsequent infusion (i.e., administered on an eight hourly schedule, t_2 is 7.5 hours.

Again, assuming S and F to be 1.0, the infusion time to be 0.5 hours, the dosing interval (τ) to be eight hours, the clearance (Cl) and the elimination rate constant (Kd) to be 6.06 L/hr and 0.346 hr^{-1} respectively, the "peak" concentration one hour after starting the half-hour infusion would be calculated using Equation 57 as follows:

$$Cpss_2 = \frac{\dfrac{(S)(F)(Dose/t_{in})}{Cl}(1 - e^{-Kdt_{in}})}{(1 - e^{-Kd\tau})} (e^{-Kdt_2})$$

$$= \frac{\dfrac{(1)(1)(100 \text{ mg}/0.5 \text{ hr})}{6.06 \text{ L/hr}}(1 - e^{-(0.346 \text{ hr}^{-1})(0.5 \text{ hr})})}{(1 - e^{-(0.346 \text{ hr}^{-1})(8 \text{ hr})})} (e^{-(0.346 \text{ hr}^{-1})(0.5 \text{ hr})})$$

$$= \frac{(33 \text{ mg/L})(0.16)}{0.937} (0.84)$$

$$= (5.6 \text{ mg/L})(0.84)$$

$$= 4.7 \text{ mg/L}$$

Note that this steady-state "peak concentration" is not the true peak value which would occur at the end of the infusion, but a concentration which is obtained one hour after starting the infusion. It is this one-hour value which is traditionally used to make the clinical correlation with aminoglycoside efficacy. Concentrations measured earlier may be considerably higher due to the two-compartment modeling associated with the intravenous administration of the aminoglycosides.

If the trough concentration is sampled just before the start of an infusion, a modification of Equation 57 can be used, where t_2 is represented by $(\tau - t_{in})$. A trough concentration of 0.42 mg/L is calculated, making the appropriate substitution of eight hours for τ and 0.5 hours for t_{in}. (See Figure 1.1.)

$$\text{Cpss min} = \frac{\dfrac{(S)(F)(Dose/t_{in})}{Cl}(1 - e^{-Kdt_{in}})}{(1 - e^{-Kd\tau})}(e^{-Kd(\tau - t_{in})})$$

Eq. 1.5

$$= \frac{\dfrac{(1)(1)(100 \text{ mg}/0.5 \text{ hr})}{6.06 \text{ L/hr}}(1 - e^{-(0.346 \text{ hr}^{-1})(0.5 \text{ hr})})}{(1 - e^{-(0.346 \text{ hr}^{-1})(8 \text{ hr})})}(e^{-(0.346 \text{ hr}^{-1})(8 \text{ hr} - 0.5 \text{ hr})})$$

$$= (5.6 \text{ mg/L})(e^{-(0.346 \text{ hr}^{-1})(7.5 \text{ hr})})$$

$$= (5.6 \text{ mg/L})(0.075)$$

$$= 0.42 \text{ mg/L}$$

Note that if the trough concentration is obtained at a time earlier than just before the next dose, Equation 1.5 should not be used. Instead, Equation 57 should be used where t_2 represents the time interval from the end of the infusion to the time of sampling. For example, if the trough concentration were obtained one half-hour before the next dose, then t_2 in Equation 57 would be seven hours rather than 7.5 hours in Equation 1.5.

Trough concentrations can also be calculated by multiplying the peak concentration one hour after the dose by the fraction of drug remaining at the time the trough level is sampled (Equation 26):

$$Cp = (Cp^\circ)(e^{-Kdt})$$

where Cp° represents the peak concentration one hour after the dose, and t is the time from the peak concentration to the time of the trough sampling (seven hours if trough samples are ob-

$$Cpss_2 = \frac{\dfrac{(S)(F)(Dose/t_{in})}{Cl}(1 - e^{-Kdt_{in}})}{(1 - e^{-Kd\tau})}(e^{-Kdt_2}) \qquad \text{(Eq. 57)}$$

Figure 1.1. Intermittent Intravenous Infusion at Steady State. The infusion is administered over t_{in} hours and τ is the dosing interval; t_2 represents the time from the end of the infusion to the time of sampling.

tained just before a dose, and 6.5 hours if trough samples are obtained one half-hour before a dose administered at a dosing interval of eight hours).

Question #5. **When aminoglycosides are administered intramuscularly, how should the steady-state peak and trough plasma concentrations be calculated?**

Although the time required to achieve peak plasma concentrations following intramuscular (IM) injection varies, aminoglycoside concentrations peak after approximately one hour in most patients.[3,23,31] Since it is difficult to estimate the rate of absorption from the site of injection, IM injections can be approached as though the patient were given an IV infusion over a period of one hour. Therefore, the intermittent infusion model (Equation 57) can be used, with a t_{in} of one hour and t_2 of 0 hours. As noted earlier, unusual measured plasma concentrations will be difficult to evaluate in this situation because one cannot determine whether they represent unusual aminoglycoside absorption characteristics or pharmacokinetic parameters.

Question #6. L.K., a 40-year-old, 50 kg female with a serum creatinine of 1 mg/dL is to be given tobramycin. Calculate a maintenance dose which will produce a "peak" concentration of 7 mg/L one hour after the infusion has been started, and a trough concentration of <2 mg/L. Assume that the tobramycin will be administered as a one-half hour infusion.

To calculate a maintenance dose that meets these objectives, one would rearrange the equation for the peak concentration (Equation 57) to solve for the dose:

$$Cpss_2 = \frac{\dfrac{(S)(F)(Dose/t_{in})}{Cl}(1 - e^{-Kdt_{in}})}{(1 - e^{-Kd\tau})}(e^{-Kdt_2})$$

$$Dose = \frac{(Cpss_2)(1 - e^{-Kd\tau})}{\dfrac{((S)(F)/t_{in})}{Cl}(1 - e^{-Kdt_{in}})(e^{-Kdt_2})}$$

Eq. 1.6

Before this equation can be solved, one must first calculate L.K.'s volume of distribution, clearance, and elimination rate constant for tobramycin. A usual dosing interval of eight hours will be assumed, and adjusted later if necessary. Note that the eight-hour dosing interval must represent the equivalent of two or more half-lives if a peak concentration of 7 mg/L and a trough concentration of <2 mg/L are to be achieved within this time frame (i.e., 7 mg/L declines to 3.5 mg/L in one half-life and to 1.75 mg/L in the second half-life).

L.K.'s volume of distribution for tobramycin should be ≈12.5 L if a Vd of 0.25 L/kg is assumed. Her tobramycin clearance will be equal to her creatinine clearance, which can be calculated by using Equation 64:

$$\frac{\text{Cl}_{Cr} \text{ for Females}}{(\text{mL/min})} = (0.85)\frac{(140 - \text{Age})(\text{Weight})}{(72)(\text{SrCr}_{ss})}$$

$$= (0.85)\left(\frac{(140 - 40)(50 \text{ kg})}{(72)(1.0 \text{ mg/dL})}\right)$$

$$= 59 \text{ mL/min}$$

or

$$\text{Cl}_{Cr} \text{ (L/hr)} = (59 \text{ mL/min})\left(\frac{60 \text{ min/hr}}{1000 \text{ mL/L}}\right)$$

$$= 3.54 \text{ L/hr}$$

An elimination rate constant of 0.283 hr^{-1} can be calculated using Equation 27; this corresponds to a half-life of ≈2.4 hours (Equation 32), indicating that it is possible to achieve a peak concentration of 7 mg/L and a trough concentration below 2 mg/L within the usual eight-hour dosing interval.

$$\text{Kd} = \frac{\text{Cl}}{\text{Vd}}$$

$$= \frac{3.54 \text{ L/hr}}{12.5 \text{ L}}$$

$$= 0.283 \text{ hr}^{-1}$$

$$t\frac{1}{2} = \frac{(0.693)(\text{Vd})}{\text{Cl}}$$

$$= \frac{(0.693)(12.5 \text{ L})}{3.54 \text{ L/hr}}$$

$$= 2.44 \text{ hr}$$

Using Equation 1.6, the dose that should meet the peak concentration criterion of 7 mg/L is $\approx$100 mg administered every eight hours.

$$Dose = \frac{(Cpss_2)(1 - e^{-Kd\tau})}{\dfrac{((S)(F)/t_{in})}{Cl}(1 - e^{-Kdt_{in}})(e^{-Kdt_2})}$$

$$= \frac{(7\ mg/L)(1 - e^{-(0.283\ hr^{-1})(8\ hr)})}{\dfrac{((1)(1)/0.5\ hr)}{(3.54\ L/hr)}(1 - e^{-(0.283\ hr^{-1})(0.5\ hr)})(e^{-(0.283\ hr^{-1})(0.5\ hr)})}$$

$$= \frac{(7\ mg)(0.9)}{(0.56)(0.13)(0.87)}$$

$$= 99.5\ mg\ or\ \approx 100\ mg$$

The trough concentration that will be produced by this dosing regimen can be calculated using Equation 26, where Cp^o is the peak concentration one hour after starting the infusion and t is the time interval between the peak and trough concentrations (seven hours).

$$Cp = (Cp^o)(e^{-Kdt})$$
$$= (7\ mg/L)(e^{-(0.283\ hr^{-1})(7\ hr)})$$
$$= (7\ mg/L)(0.14)$$
$$= 0.98\ mg/L$$

The calculated trough concentration of $\approx$1 mg/L is below the desired maximum trough of 2 mg/L. If the trough level had been above 2 mg/L, it would have been necessary to increase the dosing interval and to recalculate a dose using Equation 1.6. For convenience, the dosing intervals are usually set at 8, 12, or 24 hours.

Question #7. **If L.K. was to be given tobramycin 5 mg/kg QD, what would be the calculated steady-state peak concentration one hour after starting the half-hour infusion?**

Also predict subsequent steady-state plasma concentrations 12 hours after starting the infusion and at the trough.

Using the previously calculated tobramycin pharmacokinetic parameters of 3.54 L/hr for clearance, 12.5 L for volume, and 0.283 hr^{-1} for Kd, the expected steady-state peak concentration, one half-hour after the half-hour infusion would be $\approx$<16 mg/L as calculated from Equation 57.

$$
\begin{aligned}
Cpss_2 &= \frac{\dfrac{(S)(F)(Dose/t_{in})}{Cl}(1 - e^{-Kdt_{in}})}{(1 - e^{-Kd\tau})}(e^{-Kdt_2}) \\[2ex]
&= \frac{\dfrac{(1)(1)(250 \text{ mg}/0.5 \text{ hr})}{3.54 \text{ L/hr}}(1 - e^{-(0.283)(0.5)})}{(1 - e^{-(0.283)(24)})}(e^{-(0.283)(0.5)}) \\[2ex]
&= \frac{141.2 \text{ mg/L}(1 - 0.87)}{(1 - 0.0011)}(0.87) \\[2ex]
&= 16 \text{ mg/L}
\end{aligned}
$$

The plasma concentrations at 12 and 24 hours can be estimated using Equation 26, where Cp° would be 16 mg/L and t would be 11 hours for the mid-concentration, and 23 hours for the steady-state trough concentration.

$$
\begin{aligned}
Cp &= (Cp°)(e^{-Kdt}) \\
&= (16 \text{ mg/L})(e^{-(0.283)(11)}) \\
&= (16 \text{ mg/L})(0.044) \\
&= 0.7 \text{ mg/L}
\end{aligned}
$$

12 hours after starting the infusion and,

$$
\begin{aligned}
Cp &= (16 \text{ mg/L})(e^{-(0.283)(23)}) \\
&= (16 \text{ mg/L})(0.0015) \\
&= 0.024 \text{ mg/L } \textit{at the trough}
\end{aligned}
$$

These calculations show that the initial plasma concentrations are well above the usual accepted therapeutic range for tobramycin, and the mid-interval and trough concentrations are very low. As previously discussed, administration of aminoglycosides as a total daily dose once every 24 hours appears in many cases to be as efficacious as the usual eight-hour divided dose and does not result in increased toxicities.

One common question is whether aminoglycoside plasma concentrations should be monitored in patients receiving the drug once daily. Because once-daily aminoglycosides are still undergoing evaluation, this question is difficult to answer. It is the author's opinion that peak concentrations will have little meaning because they are likely to be well above the usual therapeutic range: $\approx$20 mg/L for gentamicin and tobramycin and about three times that value for amikacin. Trough plasma concentrations do not appear to be useful in that they are likely to be well below the usual detectable range. In patients with diminished renal function, plasma level monitoring may be warranted to guard against excessive drug accumulation. Whether plasma levels to evaluate the drug's potential for toxicity should be sampled at the mid-point of the dosing interval or at the trough is unclear. In any case, there are no established guidelines for plasma concentrations.

Question #8. Y.B., a 70 kg, 38-year-old patient with a serum creatinine of 1.8 mg/dL, has been receiving IV tobramycin, 100 mg over one half-hour Q 8 hr, for several days. A peak plasma concentration obtained one hour after the start of an infusion was 8 mg/L, and a trough concentration obtained just before the initiation of a dose was 3.0 mg/L. Estimate the apparent elimination rate constant (Kd), clearance (Cl), and volume of distribution (Vd) for tobramycin in Y.B.

The two reported plasma concentrations were measured from samples obtained during the elimination phase of the plasma concentration-versus-time curve. Since the seven-hour time interval between samples exceeds the half-life of tobramycin in Y.B. (i.e., the trough concentration is less than one-half the measured peak concentration), the two concentrations can be used to estimate the elimination rate constant, [see Part I: Elimination Rate Constant (Kd) and Half-Life (t½) on page 37 and Equation 28].

$$Kd = \frac{\ln\left(\frac{Cp_1}{Cp_2}\right)}{t}$$

$$= \frac{\ln\left(\frac{8.0}{3.0}\right)}{7 \text{ hr}}$$

$$= \frac{0.98}{7 \text{ hr}}$$

$$= 0.14 \text{ hr}^{-1}$$

Using the elimination rate constant of 0.14 hr^{-1}, the observed peak concentration of 8 mg/L, and the dosing regimen of 100 mg administered over one half-hour every eight hours, Y.B.'s clearance can be calculated by rearranging Equation 57 for Cpss$_2$ where t$_{in}$ is 0.5 hours, τ is eight hours, and t$_2$ is 0.5 hours.

$$Cpss_2 = \frac{\frac{(S)(F)(Dose/t_{in})}{Cl}(1 - e^{-Kdt_{in}})}{(1 - e^{-Kd\tau})}(e^{-Kdt_2})$$

$$Cl = \frac{\frac{(S)(F)(Dose/t_{in})}{Cpss_2}(1 - e^{-Kdt_{in}})}{(1 - e^{-Kd\tau})}(e^{-Kdt_2})$$

Eq. 1.7

$$= \frac{\frac{(1)(1)(100 \text{ mg}/0.5 \text{ hr})}{8 \text{ mg/L}}(1 - e^{-(0.14 \text{ hr}^{-1})(0.5 \text{ hr})})}{(1 - e^{-(0.14 \text{ hr}^{-1})(8 \text{ hr})})}(e^{-(0.14 \text{ hr}^{-1})(0.5 \text{ hr})})$$

$$= \left[\frac{(25 \text{ L/hr})(0.067)}{(0.67)}\right][0.93]$$

$$= 2.3 \text{ L/hr}$$

Since the clearance of 2.3 L/hr and elimination rate constant of 0.14 hr^{-1} are now known, Equation 27 can be rearranged to calculate the apparent volume of distribution:

$$Kd = \frac{Cl}{Vd}$$

$$Vd = \frac{Cl}{Kd}$$

Eq. 1.8

$$= \frac{2.3 \text{ L/hr}}{0.14 \text{ hr}^{-1}}$$

$$= 16.4 \text{ L}$$

This volume of distribution of 16.4 L corresponds to about 0.23 L/kg. The value of calculating tobramycin pharmacokinetic parameters which are specific for Y.B. is that they may now be used to calculate a dosing regimen that will produce any desired peak and trough concentrations.

Question #9. **Calculate a dosing regimen for Y.B. that will achieve a peak concentration of 7 mg/L and trough concentrations of <2 mg/L.**

As before, the dose required to achieve a specific peak concentration can be calculated from Equation 57. In order to select an appropriate dosing interval, however, one should first consider Y.B.'s apparent half-life, which can be calculated using Equation 31 and the elimination rate constant of 0.14 hr^{-1}.

$$t^{1/2} = \frac{0.693}{Kd}$$

$$= \frac{0.693}{0.14 \text{ hr}^{-1}}$$

$$= 4.9 \text{ hr}$$

As presented earlier, a dosing interval of approximately two half-lives is required if the peak concentration of 7.0 is to fall below a trough value of 2.0 within the dosing interval. Since Y.B.'s tobramycin half-life is approximately five hours, the most convenient dosing interval is 12 hours. Using this dosing interval and the appropriate clearance and elimination rate constant, Equation 1.6 indicates that a dose of 100 mg administered every 12 hours should result in a peak concentration of ≈ 7 mg/L one hour after the start of a half-hour infusion.

$$
\begin{aligned}
\text{Dose} &= \frac{(Cpss_2)(1 - e^{-Kd\tau})}{\dfrac{((S)(F)/t_{in})}{Cl}(1 - e^{-Kdt_{in}})(e^{-Kdt_2})} \\[2em]
&= \frac{(7\ \text{mg/L})(1 - e^{-(0.14\ \text{hr}^{-1})(12\ \text{hr})})}{\dfrac{[(1)(1)/0.5\ \text{hr}]}{2.3\ \text{L/hr}}(1 - e^{-(0.14\ \text{hr}^{-1})(0.5\ \text{hr})})(e^{-(0.14\ \text{hr}^{-1})(0.5\ \text{hr})})} \\[2em]
&= \frac{(7\ \text{mg})(0.81)}{(0.87)(0.067)(0.93)} \\[1em]
&= 104.6\ \text{mg}\ \ or\ \ \approx 100\ \text{mg}
\end{aligned}
$$

Equation 26 can be used to confirm that the trough concentrations will be acceptable. A "t" of 11 hours and a Cp^o of 7 mg/L should be used.

$$
\begin{aligned}
Cp &= (Cp^o)(e^{-Kdt}) \\
&= (7\ \text{mg/L})(e^{-(0.14\ \text{hr}^{-1})(11\ \text{hr})}) \\
&= (7\ \text{mg/L})(0.21) \\
&= 1.5\ \text{mg/L}
\end{aligned}
$$

Question #10. **C.I., is a 50-year-old, 60 kg male with a serum creatinine of 1.5 mg/dL, is receiving 350 mg of amikacin IV over one half-hour Q 8 hr. He had a peak concentration of 15 mg/L obtained one hour after the start of the infusion and a trough concentration of 6 mg/L obtained just before the next dose. Assuming these peak and trough concentrations represent steady-state levels, calculate C.I.'s elimination rate constant, clearance, and volume of distribution. Evaluate whether or not these parameters seem reasonable and should be used to adjust C.I.'s amikacin maintenance dose.**

The approach to calculating the revised pharmacokinetic parameters for C.I. is essentially the same as that used in the previous questions. First, the elimination rate constant of 0.13 hr^{-1} can be calculated using Equation 28 and the seven-hour time interval between the peak and trough concentrations:

$$Kd = \frac{\ln\left(\dfrac{Cp_1}{Cp_2}\right)}{t}$$

$$= \frac{\ln\left(\dfrac{15}{6}\right)}{7 \text{ hr}}$$

$$= 0.13 \text{ hr}^{-1}$$

Next, the apparent clearance can be calculated by using Equation 1.7. A dose of 350 mg, τ of eight hours, and a t_{in} of 0.5 hours can be used. The latter t_2 represents the time between the end of the infusion and the "peak concentration" sampling time.

$$Cl = \frac{\dfrac{(S)(F)(Dose/t_{in})}{Cpss_2}(1 - e^{-Kdt_{in}})}{(1 - e^{-Kd\tau})}(e^{-Kdt_2})$$

$$= \frac{\dfrac{(1)(1)(350 \text{ mg}/0.5 \text{ hr})}{15 \text{ mg/L}}(1 - e^{-(0.13 \text{ hr}^{-1})(0.5 \text{ hr})})}{(1 - e^{-(0.13 \text{ hr}^{-1})(8 \text{ hr})})}\left(e^{-(0.13 \text{ hr}^{-1})(0.5 \text{ hr})}\right)$$

$$= 4.26 \text{ L/hr}$$

Using the calculated clearance value of 4.26 L/hr, and the elimination rate constant of 0.13 hr^{-1}, a volume of distribution of 32.8 L (0.55 L/kg) can be calculated using Equation 1.8.

$$Vd = \frac{Cl}{Kd}$$

$$= \frac{4.26 \text{ L/hr}}{0.13 \text{ hr}^{-1}}$$

$$= 32.8 \text{ L}$$

Before these parameters are used to calculate an adjusted amikacin dosing regimen that will bring C.I.'s peak concentration into the range of 20 to 30 mg/L and the trough concentration below 10 mg/L, care should be taken to evaluate whether these parameters appear reasonable. The calculated clearance of 4.26 L/hr is slightly greater than the expected clearance of 3 L/hr, which would be calculated using Equation 63 and C.I.'s age, weight, and serum creatinine.

$$\frac{\text{Cl}_{Cr} \text{ for Males}}{\text{(mL/min)}} = \frac{(140 - \text{Age})(\text{Weight})}{(72)(\text{SrCr}_{ss})}$$

$$= \frac{(140 - 50)(60 \text{ kg})}{(72)(1.5 \text{ mg/dL})}$$

$$= 50 \text{ mL/min}$$

or

$$\text{Cl}_{Cr} \text{ (L/hr)} = (50 \text{ mL/min})\left(\frac{60 \text{ min/hr}}{1000 \text{ mL/L}}\right)$$

$$= 3.0 \text{ L/hr}$$

While this clearance value is greater than expected, it is not so unusual as to be considered unrealistic.

The volume of distribution value of 0.55 L/kg, however, is unusually large. In general, volumes of distribution >0.35 L/kg are only observed in patients who have significant third-spacing of fluid (e.g., ascites or edema). If there is no evidence of any third-spacing in C.I., then the volume of distribution would be unrealistically large. Therefore, the dosing history or the measured plasma concentrations are probably in error. If C.I. had received tobramycin or gentamicin, the possibility of a penicillin interaction resulting in spuriously low plasma concentrations would have to be considered; however, amikacin does not interact with penicillins to a significant extent. Therefore, this is an unlikely explanation for the unusually large volume of distribution.

In any case, when pharmacokinetic calculations lead to parameters that are very different from those expected, there may be an error in the time of sampling, assay results or dosing history. In such cases, it may be more prudent to use the expected rather than the calculated parameters to adjust doses. In some cases, however, the patient may actually have unusual parameters. When this is suspected, the dosing history should be re-evaluated and another set of plasma drug concentrations should be obtained, with special attention to precise sampling times and the dosing history.

Question #11. D.H., a 40-year-old male, was admitted to the hospital following an automobile accident. He is five feet five inches tall and on admission weighed 85 kg. He was taken for abdominal surgery and post-operatively became hypotensive and required large volumes of fluid to maintain his blood pressure. Currently, he weighs 105 kg and has a serum creatinine of 2 mg/dL. D.H. is to receive gentamicin empirically after his abdominal surgery. Estimate his pharmacokinetic parameters and dose to achieve peak gentamicin concentrations of ≈5 to 7 mg/L and steady-state trough concentrations of <2 mg/L.

To calculate D.H.'s pharmacokinetic parameters, it is first necessary to identify his non-obese, excess adipose and excess third-space fluid weight. Using Equation 65, D.H.'s ideal body weight is calculated to be ≈61.5 kg.

$$\text{Ideal Body Weight for Males in kg} = 50 + (2.3)(\text{Height in Inches} > 60)$$

$$= 50 + (2.3)(5 \text{ Inches})$$

$$= 61.5 \text{ kg}$$

Assuming D.H. did not have any excess third-space fluid on admission, his excess adipose weight is ≈23.5 kg (estimated by subtracting his ideal body weight of 61.5 kg from his admission weight of 85 kg). D.H.'s excess third-space fluid weight of 20 kg can be estimated by subtracting his initial weight of 85 kg from his current weight of 105 kg. Using these weight estimates for his body composition, Equation 1.2 can be used to estimate an aminoglycoside volume of distribution of ≈38 L:

$$\text{Aminoglycoside Vd} \atop (\text{L})} = \left(\begin{array}{c} 0.25 \text{ L/kg} \times \text{Non-Obese,} \\ \text{Non-Excess Fluid Weight (kg)} \end{array} \right)$$

$$+ \ 0.1 \left(\begin{array}{c} \text{Excess Adipose} \\ \text{Weight (kg)} \end{array} \right) + \left(\begin{array}{c} \text{Excess Third-Space} \\ \text{Fluid Weight (kg)} \end{array} \right)$$

$$= (0.25 \text{ L/kg} \times 61.5 \text{ kg}) + 0.1(23.5 \text{ kg}) + (20 \text{ kg})$$

$$= 37.7 \text{ L } \textit{or} \approx 38 \text{ L}$$

To estimate D.H.'s gentamicin clearance one would use Equation 63, his IBW of 61.5 kg, and his current serum creatinine of 2 mg/dL.

$$\begin{array}{c} \text{Cl}_{\text{Cr}} \text{ for Males} \\ (\text{mL/min}) \end{array} = \frac{(140 - \text{Age})(\text{Weight})}{(72)(\text{SrCr}_{ss})}$$

$$= \frac{(140 - 40 \text{ yr})(61.5 \text{ kg})}{(72)(2 \text{ mg/dL})}$$

$$= 42.7 \text{ mL/min}$$

$$= 42.7 \text{ mL/min} \times \frac{60 \text{ min/hr}}{1000 \text{ mL/L}}$$

$$= 2.56 \text{ L/hr}$$

Using the estimated creatinine clearance of 2.56 L/hr as the gentamicin clearance and the volume of distribution of 38 L, the elimination rate constant (Equation 27) and half-life (Equation 31) are calculated to be 0.067 hr^{-1} and 10.34 hr, respectively:

$$\text{Kd} = \frac{\text{Cl}}{\text{Vd}}$$

$$= \frac{2.56 \text{ L/hr}}{38 \text{ L}}$$

$$= 0.067 \text{ hr}^{-1}$$

$$t\frac{1}{2} = \frac{0.693}{\text{Kd}}$$

$$= \frac{0.693}{0.067 \text{ hr}^{-1}}$$

$$= 10.34 \text{ hr}$$

Given D.H.'s half-life of approximately ten hours, and an infusion time of one half-hour, Equation 48, the steady-state bolus dose model, can be used to calculate his regimen.

$$Cpss_1 = \frac{\dfrac{(S)(F)(Dose)}{Vd}}{(1 - e^{-Kd\tau})} (e^{-Kdt_1})$$

Rearranged to Solve for Dose:

$$Dose = \frac{(Cpss_1)(Vd)(1 - e^{-Kd\tau})}{(S)(F)(e^{-Kdt_1})}$$

Eq 1.9

Because aminoglycoside dosing intervals are usually two to three half-lives, a dosing interval of 24 hours is reasonable given D.H.'s half-life of approximately ten hours. Making the appropriate substitution in the rearranged equation where $Cpss_1$ is assumed to be 6 mg/L, t_1 is one hour (indicating that the peak concentration is to be obtained one hour after the start of the infusion), a dose of $\approx$200 mg is calculated.

$$= \frac{(6 \text{ mg/L})(38 \text{ L})(1 - e^{-(0.067)(24)})}{(1)(1)(e^{-(0.067)(1)})}$$

$$= \frac{(6 \text{ mg/L})(38 \text{ L})(1 - 0.2)}{(1)(1)(0.94)}$$

$$= 194 \text{ mg } \textit{or} \approx 200 \text{ mg}$$

Although a dose of 200 mg appears to be large, this is due in part to the extensive third-spacing fluid and large volume of distribution. In many cases, a somewhat lower dose might be employed; however, the peak concentration would be proportionately decreased. Also, although the dose of 200 mg seems large, D.H. is receiving this dose only once daily and based upon his non-obese or ideal body weight of $\approx$61 kg, this equates to $\approx$3 mg/kg/day, which is the lower end of the usual range (3 to 6 mg/kg/day). It is also important to ensure that trough concentrations will be <2 mg/L. Given the expected half-life of ten hours and the dosing interval of 24 hours, it should be readily apparent that after two half-lives, (i.e., 20 hours) only 25%, or a concentration of 1.5 mg/L, will remain. Alternatively, Equation 26 could be used to calculate an expected trough concentration of ≈1.3 mg/L. Note that t in Equation 26 is 23 hours rather than the dosing interval of 24 hours because one hour has been subtracted to account for the time between the start of the infusion and the time to reach the peak concentration.

$$
\begin{aligned}
Cp &= (Cp^\circ)(e^{-Kdt}) \\
&= (6\ mg/L)(e^{-(0.067)(23)}) \\
&= (6\ mg/L)(0.21) \\
&= 1.28\ or\ \approx 1.3\ mg/L
\end{aligned}
$$

Question #12. D.L., a 38-year-old, 70 kg patient with renal failure, is receiving gentamicin and carbenicillin for treatment of a fever of unknown origin. How might the concurrent administration of carbenicillin influence the pharmacokinetics of gentamicin? Are there other antibiotic combinations that may influence gentamicin dosing?

The beta lactam ring of the penicillin compounds interacts *in vivo* and *in vitro* with one of the primary amines on both gentamicin and tobramycin to form an inactive amide.[39–41] The rate of gentamicin and tobramycin inactivation by penicillins is slow, however, and this interaction probably is significant only in patients with severely impaired renal function.[40–42] In these patients, the concurrent administration of carbenicillin can decrease the half-life of gentamicin from approximately 46 to 22 hours. It has been recommended that the penicillin compounds and aminoglycosides be administered separately, and that in the case of carbenicillin, the dose be decreased to avoid excessive accumulation in patients with poor renal function. To estimate the degree to which this interaction affects gentamicin clearance, Equation 1.4 can be used to calculate an apparent carbenicillin-related clearance value for D.H. Using a standard volume of distribution of 0.25 L/kg for this 70 kg patient and the apparent rate constant for the *in vitro* interaction between carbenicillin and gentamicin of 0.017 hr^{-1}, a clearance value of 0.3 L/hr can be calculated:

$$\begin{array}{l}\text{Tobramycin, Gentamicin}\\ \text{Clearance by Carbenicillin} = (0.017 \text{ hr}^{-1})\left(\begin{array}{l}\text{Volume of Distribution}\\ \text{for Aminoglycosides}\end{array}\right)\\ \text{(L/hr)}\end{array}$$

$$= (0.017 \text{ hr}^{-1})(0.25 \text{ L/kg})(70 \text{ kg})$$

$$= 0.3 \text{ L/hr}$$

This clearance value of 0.3 L/hr would be added to the estimated gentamicin clearance associated with D.H.'s residual renal function and non-renal clearance (0.0043 L/kg/hr). This is only an estimate, however, and plasma levels must be monitored to make patient-specific adjustments.

Plasma samples for patients receiving aminoglycosides and penicillins concurrently must be obtained at a time when the *in vitro* interaction is minimal. Plasma samples for assay of aminoglycoside concentrations should be obtained when the penicillin is at its lowest concentration and assayed as soon as possible. If storage is required, samples should be frozen to minimize the continual *in vitro* effect of this interaction. Amikacin appears to be more resistant to degradation by penicillins.[39] Some of the newer penicillin compounds (e.g., azlocillin, mezlocillin) appear to interact with gentamicin and tobramycin similarly but to a lesser extent than carbenicillin and ticarcillin.[45] Furthermore, the *in vitro* interaction between the newer cephalosporins (e.g., cefazolin, cefamandole) and the aminoglycoside antibiotics appears to be minimal.[45,47] Although there is some indication that moxalactam may interact with tobramycin *in vivo*, this interaction does not appear to be chemically mediated. Further evaluation is needed to clarify the underlying mechanism and clinical significance.[49]

Although somewhat debatable, the combined use of cephalosporins and aminoglycosides may place patients at a greater risk for nephrotoxicity.[50,51]

Question #13. What is the significance of a changing serum creatinine in a patient receiving gentamicin?

A rising serum creatinine in a patient always raises the question of gentamicin-induced nephrotoxicity. In this event, the drug may be discontinued, the plasma concentration re-evaluated, and/or the dose adjusted, since gentamicin may accumulate substantially when renal function is impaired. Dose modification should be based upon plasma gentamicin levels rather than serum creatinine levels since serum creatinine concentrations which are not at steady state can be misleading. (See Part I: Creatinine Clearance (Cl_{Cr}) on page 93.) The reason for this is: Despite the similarity between gentamicin and creatinine clearances,[23,31] their volumes of distribution differ. Gentamicin's Vd of 0.25 L/kg is smaller than that of creatinine, which is 0.5 L/kg.[18,19,24,52] Since the half-life is determined by the clearance and volume of distribution (see Equation 32 below), the half-life for creatinine is approximately twice as long as that of gentamicin and the other aminoglycosides. It will, therefore, take creatinine a longer time to arrive at a new steady-state concentration after a change in renal function.

$$t\tfrac{1}{2} = \frac{(0.693)(Vd)}{Cl}$$

When the serum creatinine is rising (i.e., not at steady state), the renal function is worse than would be predicted by use of the serum creatinine, and any gentamicin dose calculated using the serum creatinine would be overestimated. Conversely, when the serum creatinine is falling, renal function may be better than that reflected by the serum creatinine, and the doses calculated on the basis of these levels would be underestimated.

Question #14. D.W., a 20-year-old, 60 kg male, is receiving 80 mg of tobramycin infused IV over a 30-minute period Q 8 hr. His serum creatinine has increased from 1 mg/dL to 2 mg/dL over the past 24 hours. Since his renal function appears to be decreasing, three plasma samples were obtained to monitor serum gentamicin concentrations as follows: just before a dose; one hour after that same dose; and eight hours after that dose (two troughs and one peak level). The serum gentamicin concentrations at these times were 4 mg/L, 8 mg/L, and 5 mg/L, respectively. Calculate the volume of distribution, elimination rate constant, and clearance of tobramycin for D.W.

Since the second trough concentration of tobramycin is higher than the first, it is apparent that the drug is accumulating. Therefore, steady-state equations should not be used to calculate D.W.'s pharmacokinetic parameters. The first step that should be taken to resolve this dilemma is to calculate the elimination rate constant from the two plasma concentrations which were obtained during the elimination phase (8 mg/L and 5 mg/L). Equation 28 can be used to estimate the elimination rate constant; however, this Kd should only be used as an estimate since the two plasma concentrations were obtained less than one half-life apart.

$$Kd = \frac{\ln\left(\frac{Cp_1}{Cp_2}\right)}{t}$$

$$= \frac{\ln\left(\frac{8 \text{ mg/L}}{5 \text{ mg/L}}\right)}{7 \text{ hr}}$$

$$= 0.067 \text{ hr}^{-1}$$

This elimination rate constant of 0.067 hr^{-1} was calculated by assuming that the peak concentration of 8 mg/L was obtained one hour after the start of the tobramycin infusion and that the trough concentration was obtained just before the next dose, resulting in a time interval of seven hours. The elimination rate constant of 0.067 hr^{-1} corresponds to a half-life of 10.3 hours (Equation 31):

$$t\frac{1}{2} = \frac{0.693}{Kd}$$

$$= \frac{0.693}{0.067 \text{ hr}^{-1}}$$

$$= 10.3 \text{ hr}$$

This half-life of 10.3 hours suggests that relatively little drug is lost during the infusion period; therefore, a bolus model is most appropriately used in this situation. The volume of distribution can be estimated by assuming that the bolus dose is administered instantaneously and calculating the theoretical peak concentration by rearranging Equation 26. Cp is the measured concentration of 8 mg/L, t is the one-hour interval between the start of the infusion and the time of sampling, and Cp° is the theoretical peak concentration for an IV bolus.

$$Cp = (Cp°)(e^{-Kdt})$$

$$Cp° = \frac{(Cp)}{(e^{-Kdt})}$$

Eq. 1.10

$$= \frac{8 \text{ mg/L}}{e^{-(0.067 \text{ hr}^{-1})(1 \text{ hr})}}$$

$$= \frac{8 \text{ mg/L}}{0.94}$$

$$= 8.5 \text{ mg/L}$$

Since the change in concentration (peak minus trough) is the result of the dose administered and the volume of distribution, the Vd can be calculated using Equation 1.11.

$$Vd = \frac{Dose}{(Cp_{peak} - Cp_{min})}$$

Eq. 1.11

$$= \frac{80 \text{ mg}}{(8.5 \text{ mg/L} - 4 \text{ mg/L})}$$

$$= 17.8 \text{ L}$$

This volume of distribution of 17.8 L can then be used with the elimination rate constant of 0.067 hr^{-1} to calculate D.W.'s clearance of 1.2 L/hr, or 20 mL/min (Equation 33):

$$Cl = (Kd)Vd$$
$$= (0.067 \text{ hr}^{-1})(17.8 \text{ L})$$
$$= 1.2 \text{ L/hr} \quad or \quad 20 \text{ mL/min}$$

Question #15. **Using the pharmacokinetic parameters calculated for D.W. in Question 14, develop a dosing regimen that will produce reasonable peak and trough concentrations of tobramycin.**

Since D.W.'s tobramycin clearance is low (1.2 L/hr), it will be necessary to reduce his maintenance dose. There are two alternatives: 1) reduce the dose and maintain the same dosing interval, or 2) adjust both the dose and the dosing interval such that the peak and trough concentrations will be approximately 8 mg/L and <2 mg/L, respectively.

Reduce the Dose and Maintain the Same Dosing Interval. This method is not acceptable for D.W. because he has such a long half-life ($\approx$12 hours). If a dose which achieves a maximum concentration of 8 mg/L is used and the dosing interval of eight hours is maintained, the trough level will be $\approx$4.7 mg/L (Equation 46). This level may place D.W. at risk for tobramycin toxicity.

$$Cpss \text{ min} = (Cpss \text{ max})(e^{-Kd\tau})$$
$$= (8 \text{ mg/L})(e^{-(0.067 \text{ hr}^{-1})(8 \text{ hr})})$$
$$= 4.68 \text{ mg/L}$$

Adjust Both the Dose and Dosing Interval to Achieve Reasonable Peak and Trough Concentrations. The only limitation to this approach is that most clinicians prefer to avoid prolonged periods of time during which the gentamicin concentration is below 1 to 2 mg/L, because of the possibility of breakthrough bacteremia. A trough concentration which is slightly higher than ideal is generally accepted as a compromise to minimize the risk of therapeutic failure. Nevertheless, some animal data suggest that doses which result in high peak and low trough concentrations are less likely to produce renal toxicity than the same dose administered as a continuous IV infusion (i.e., the same average levels).[53]

A first estimate of the dosing interval can be made by examining D.W.'s tobramycin half-life of ≈ 12 hours. If a dose which produces a peak concentration of 8 mg/L is selected, the trough concentration will be ≈ 2 mg/L after about two half-lives. Therefore, a dosing interval of 24 hours can be used. Since the half-life of tobramycin is long relative to the infusion time of one-half hour, the bolus dose model can be used. As previously stated, Equation 48 can be rearranged to calculate a dose required to achieve any steady-state peak concentration. Using Equation 1.9 with the previously derived pharmacokinetic parameters and a dosing interval of 24 hours, a dose of ≈ 120 mg is calculated. A peak concentration which occurs one hour after the infusion has been initiated is also assumed (i.e., $t_1 = 1$ hour).

$$Cpss_1 = \frac{\dfrac{(S)(F)(Dose)}{Vd}}{(1 - e^{-Kd\tau})}(e^{-Kdt_1})$$

$$
\begin{aligned}
Dose &= \frac{(Cpss_1)(Vd)(1 - e^{-Kd\tau})}{(e^{-Kdt_1})} \\
&= \frac{(8 \text{ mg/L})(17.8 \text{ L})(1 - e^{-(0.067 \text{ hr}^{-1})(24 \text{ hr})})}{e^{-(0.067 \text{ hr}^{-1})(1 \text{ hr})}} \\
&= \frac{(8 \text{ mg/L})(17.8 \text{ L})(0.8)}{(0.93)} \\
&= 122 \text{ mg } or \approx 120 \text{ mg}
\end{aligned}
$$

The trough concentration (calculated using Equation 26) would be 1.7 mg/L.

$$
\begin{aligned}
Cp &= (Cp^o)(e^{-Kdt}) \\
&= (8 \text{ mg/L})(e^{-(0.067 \text{ hr}^{-1})(23 \text{ hr})}) \\
&= 1.7 \text{ mg/L}
\end{aligned}
$$

Note that this expected trough concentration is slightly below the desired trough of <2 mg/L. A longer dosing interval could have been selected, but a relatively inconvenient dosing interval of ≈ 36 hours would have resulted. If the half-life is shorter than expected, prolonged time periods with relatively low amino-glycoside concentrations would result. Therefore, it is most appropriate to initiate the dosing regimen with the dosing interval of 24 hours and confirm these estimates with some additional tobramycin levels.

Question #16. **M.S., a 70 kg female, undergoes four hours of hemodialysis every 48 hours. She is functionally (not surgically) anephric and is to be started on gentamicin. Calculate a dosing regimen that achieves a peak concentration of 6 mg/L and then maintains average levels of 3.5 mg/L.**

Because the gentamicin half-life for a patient who is functionally anephric is probably in excess of 30 hours, very little drug will be eliminated from the body over the one-hour period following initiation of the infusion. Therefore, the loading dose may be calculated as though it were a bolus (Equation 11). Assuming S and F to be 1 and the volume of distribution to be 17.5 L (0.25 L/kg), a loading dose of ≈100 mg would be calculated as follows:

$$\text{Loading Dose} = \frac{(Vd)(Cp)}{(S)(F)}$$
$$= \frac{(17.5 \text{ L})(6 \text{ mg/L})}{(1)(1)}$$
$$= 105 \text{ mg}$$

Since gentamicin elimination in M.S. will be irregular, occurring at higher rates during the dialysis, the usual maintenance dose equation cannot be used. As presented in Part I: Dialysis of Drugs on page 104, there are two possible approaches to the resolution of this problem. One approach is to administer a daily dose such that average concentrations are maintained and then to calculate a replacement dose postdialysis. A second approach is to administer the drug after dialysis only. The dose used is the amount of drug lost during the inter- as well as intradialysis period. In both cases, the use of the patient's clearance (Cl_{pat}), dialysis clearance (Cl_{dial}) as well as the volume of distribution will be required. The reported clearance for the aminoglycosides in functionally anephric patients is ≈0.0043 L/kg/hr[19,54] and aminoglycoside clearance by hemodialysis is ≈20 to 40 mL/min, with an average value of ≈30 mL/min.[19,54–56]

If the approach of giving daily and postdialysis doses is taken, then the maintenance dose on non-dialysis days can be calculated using Equation 74, a patient clearance of 0.3 L/hr (0.0043 L/hr/kg × 70 kg), and a dosing interval of 24 hours. In most dialysis patients, a gentamicin concentration between 3 to 4 mg/L (average: 3.5 mg/L) is set as a goal. Therefore, a dose of ≈25 mg would be appropriate:

$$\text{Dose} = \frac{(\text{Cpss ave})(\text{Cl}_{pat})(\tau)}{(S)(F)}$$

$$= \frac{(3.5 \text{ mg/L})(0.3 \text{ L/hr})(24 \text{ hr})}{(1)(1)}$$

$$= 25.2 \text{ mg } or \approx 25 \text{ mg}$$

If the patient had been surgically anephric, the Cl_{pat} would have been approximately halved, and the corresponding maintenance dose would also have been one-half or ≈13 mg/day. To calculate the postdialysis replacement dose, Equation 76 can be used. Using the average Cl_{dial} and a dialysis time (T_d) of four hours, the replacement dose is calculated to be ≈25 mg.

$$\begin{array}{c}\text{PostDialysis}\\\text{Replacement}\\\text{Dose}\end{array} = (\text{Vd})(\text{Cpss ave})\left(1 - e^{-\left(\frac{\text{Cl}_{pat} + \text{Cl}_{dial}}{\text{Vd}}\right)(T_d)}\right)$$

$$= [17.5 \text{ L}][3.5 \text{ mg/L}]\left[1 - e^{-\frac{(0.3 \text{ L/hr} + 1.8 \text{ L/hr})}{17.5 \text{ L}}(4 \text{ hr})}\right]$$

$$= [17.5 \text{ L}][3.5 \text{ mg/L}][1 - 0.62]$$

$$= 23.3 \text{ mg } or \approx 25 \text{ mg}$$

Note that the dialysis clearance of 1.8 L/hr represents a clearance of ≈30 mL/min and that this is the primary route of elimination during the intradialysis period. Also, the postdialysis dose of 25 mg can be added to the maintenance dose of ≈25 mg, resulting in a gentamicin dose on dialysis days of 50 mg.

If it is decided to administer the aminoglycoside only after dialysis, Equation 78 can be used to calculate the postdialysis replacement dose. In this situation, a steady-state peak concentration of $\approx$4 to 5 mg/L is set as a goal (peak concentrations of 6 to 8 mg/L would expose M.S. to continuously elevated concentrations of gentamicin).

Using Equation 78, a Cpss peak of 5.0 mg/L, a patient clearance of 0.3 L/hr, and a t_1 of 44 hours [derived from a 48-hour interval between the dialyses and a dialysis time (T_d) of four hours] the postdialysis replacement dose is $\approx$62 mg.

$$
\begin{aligned}
\text{PostDialysis}\\
\text{Replacement}\\
\text{Dose}
\end{aligned}
= (Vd)(Cpss\ peak)\left(1 - \left[\left(e^{-\left(\frac{Clpat}{Vd}\right)(t_1)}\right)\left(e^{-\left(\frac{Clpat\ +\ Cldial}{Vd}\right)(T_d)}\right)\right]\right)
$$

$$
= [17.5\ L][5\ mg/L]\left[1 - \left(e^{-\left(\frac{0.3\ L/hr}{17.5\ L}\right)(44)}\right)\right.
$$

$$
\left.\left(e^{-\left(\frac{0.3\ L/hr\ +\ 1.8\ L/hr}{17.5\ L}\right)(4\ hr)}\right)\right]
$$

$$
= (17.5\ L)(5\ mg/L)[(1 - (0.47)(0.62)]
$$

$$
= (17.5\ L)(5\ mg/L)(1 - 0.29)
$$

$$
= 62\ mg
$$

To ensure that trough concentrations just before dialysis are not excessively low, the predialysis drug concentration should be calculated using Equation 80:

$$
\begin{aligned}
\text{Predialysis}\\
\text{Drug Concentration}
\end{aligned}
= [Cpss\ peak]\left[e^{-\left(\frac{Clpat}{Vd}\right)(t_1)}\right]
$$

$$
= [5\ mg/L]\left[e^{-\left(\frac{0.3\ L/hr}{17.5\ L}\right)(44\ hr)}\right]
$$

$$
= (5\ mg/L)(0.47)
$$

$$
= 2.35\ mg/L
$$

This predialysis concentration of $\approx$2 mg/L is higher than usually desired; however, because the gentamicin half-life is unusually long, it will be difficult to maintain peak levels in the range of 5 mg/L and predialysis trough concentrations <2 mg/L. Unfortunately, the persistence of relatively high concentrations between dialysis periods will place M.S. at greater risk for ototoxicity.[57] In addition, although postdialysis concentrations can be calculated, these lower concentrations are transient and probably do not correlate well with the incidence of ototoxicity in dialysis patients. If postdialysis concentrations are to be measured, time should be allowed for equilibration between the plasma compartment (in which concentrations have been lowered during the dialysis period) and the extracellular fluid compartment.[58]

Question #17. **How would the above situation have differed if peritoneal dialysis rather than hemodialysis had been used?**

Peritoneal dialysis is much less effective in removing gentamicin; the usual clearance value is ≈ 4 mL/min/m², with an average value of 5 to 10 mL/min for the 70 kg patient. Nonetheless, the total amount of drug removed during dialysis may be as much as 30% or more because peritoneal dialysis is usually continued for ≈ 36 hours.[54,59]

As discussed in Part I, aminoglycosides can be administered either parenterally or intraperitoneally to achieve systemic plasma concentrations. When administered intraperitoneally, an initial loading dose of ≈ 2 to 3 mg/kg is added to the first peritoneal dialysis exchange. Then, 1.2 mg/kg/day is added to one exchange daily (usually the night-time exchange), or a dose which produces a dialysate concentration of ≈ 6 to 10 mg/L is added to each dialysate exchange. Both of these regimens result in steady-state plasma concentrations of ≈ 3 mg/L with relatively little fluctuation.[60] When aminoglycoside antibiotics are placed in each peritoneal exchange, many clinicians estimate the steady-state plasma concentration to be $\approx 40\%$ of the peritoneal dialysate concentration. As an example, if 16 mg were added to each 2 L peritoneal exchange volume (8 mg/L), the steady-state plasma concentration would be ≈ 3.2 mg/L, or 40% of the 8 mg/L concentration in the dialysate exchanges.[61,62]

Question #18. **A patient with meningitis is being considered for treatment with intrathecal (IT) or intraventricular gentamicin. Which of these routes is preferred and what pharmacokinetic parameters are expected?**

Gentamicin does not cross the blood-brain barrier very effectively, and cerebrospinal fluid (CSF) levels are usually subtherapeutic unless IT or intraventricular injections are given.[63-65] The intraventricular route is preferred to ensure adequate ventricular levels and uniform concentration throughout the subarachnoid space.[63,65] The apparent CSF half-life of the aminoglycosides is approximately six hours.[63,64] The usual intraventricular dose of aminoglycosides is 5 to 10 mg, and is usually repeated on a daily basis. This dosing regimen is similar for gentamicin, tobramycin, and amikacin, even though doses administered systemically vary considerably. If the intraventricular route is to be used, neurosurgery will be required to insert a special access shunt that allows daily administration. CSF peak concentrations measured soon after intraventricular injection approach 100 mg/L or higher; trough concentrations 24 hours later are usually 5 to 15 mg/L.[65]

Question #19. **T.C. is receiving tobramycin 120 mg IV over one half-hour Q 8 hr at 1:00 a.m., 9:00 a.m., and 5:00 p.m. A steady-state trough level at 8:30 a.m. was 0.9 mg/L, and a level at 11:30 a.m. was 3.9 mg/L. Calculate the peak concentration expected at 10:00 a.m., or one hour after starting the 9:00 a.m. tobramycin infusion.**

Because the plasma concentrations were obtained at steady state, one would expect each dosing interval to be superimposable. The peak concentration obtained at 11:30 a.m. (2½ hours after the 9:00 a.m. dose) can be transposed to the corresponding time after the 1:00 a.m. dose, or to 3:30 a.m. The time interval between 3:30 a.m. and 8:30 a.m. is five hours, and Equation 28 can be used to determine the elimination rate constant for T.C.

$$
\begin{aligned}
Kd &= \frac{\ln\left(\dfrac{Cp_1}{Cp_2}\right)}{t} \\[2mm]
&= \frac{\ln\left(\dfrac{3.9 \text{ mg/L}}{0.9 \text{ mg/L}}\right)}{5 \text{ hr}} \\[2mm]
&= \frac{1.47}{5 \text{ hr}} \\[2mm]
&= 0.294 \text{ hr}^{-1}
\end{aligned}
$$

This patient-specific elimination rate constant of 0.294 hr^{-1} can be used in a rearrangement of Equation 26 to calculate the expected plasma concentration at 10:00 a.m., or (one hour after the start of the infusion) 1.5 hours before the observed peak of 3.9 mg/L.

$$Cp = Cp^{o}(e^{-Kdt})$$

or

$$Cp^{o} = \frac{Cp}{e^{-Kdt}}$$

$$= \frac{3.9 \text{ mg/L}}{e^{-(0.294)(1.5 \text{ hr})}}$$

$$= \frac{3.9 \text{ mg/L}}{0.643}$$

$$= 6.1 \text{ mg/L}$$

This peak concentration of 6.1 mg/L represents a concentration which is within the usual therapeutic range and suggests that T.C. does not require dose adjustment based upon plasma concentration measurements.

References

1. Pechere JC, Dugal R. Clinical pharmacokinetics of aminoglycoside antibiotics. Clin Pharmacokinet. 1979;4:170.

2. Noone P et al. Experience in monitoring gentamicin therapy during treatment of serious gram-negative sepsis. Br Med J. 1974;1:477.

3. Jackson GG, Riff LF. Pseudomonas bacteremia: pharmacologic and other basis for failure of treatment with gentamicin. J Infect Dis. 1971;124(Suppl):185.

4. Klastersky J et al. Antibacterial activity in serum and urine as a therapeutic guide in bacterial infections. J Infect Dis. 1974;129:187.

5. Cox CE. Gentamicin: a new aminoglycoside antibiotic: clinical and laboratory studies in urinary tract infections. J Infect Dis. 1969;119:486.

6. Jackson GG, Arcieri G. Ototoxicity of gentamicin in man: a survey and controlled analysis of clinical experience in the United States. J Infect Dis. 1971;124(Suppl):130.

7. Goodman EL et al. Prospective comparative study of variable dosage and variable frequency regimens for administrations of gentamicin. Antimicrob Agents Chemother. 1975;8:434.

8. Schentag JJ et al. Clinical and pharmacokinetic characteristics of amino-glycoside nephrotoxicity in 201 critically ill patients. Antimicrob Agents Chemother. 1982;5:721.

9. Wilfret JN et al. Renal insufficiency associated with gentamicin therapy. J Infect Dis. 1971;124(Suppl):148.

10. Mawer GE. Prescribing aids for gentamicin. Br J Clin Pharmacol. 1974;1:45.

11. Federspil P et al. Pharmacokinetics and ototoxicity of gentamicin, to-bramycin, and amikacin. J Infect Dis. 1976;134(Suppl):200.

12. McCormack JP, Jewesson PJ. A critical re-evaluation of the "therapeutic range" of aminoglycosides. Clin Infect Dis. 1992;14:320–39.

13. Calandra T et al. (The International Antimicrobial Therapy Cooperative Group of the European Organization for Research and Treatment of Cancer). Efficacy and toxicity of single daily doses of amikacin and ceftriaxone versus multiple daily doses of amikacin and ceftazidime for infection in patients with cancer and granulocytopenia. Ann Intern Med. 1993;119:584–93.

14. Moore RD et al. Clinical response to aminoglycoside therapy: importance of the ratio of peak concentration to minimal inhibitory concentration. J Infect Dis. 1987;155:93–9.

15. Kapusnik JE et al. Single, large, daily dosing versus intermittent dosing of tobramycin for treating experimental pseudomonas pneumonia. J Infect Dis. 1988;158:7–22.

16. Craig WA, Vogelman B. The post-antibiotic effect. Ann Intern Med. 1987; 106:900–2.

17. Fan ST et al. Once daily administration of netilmicin compared with thrice daily, both in combination with metronidazole, in gangrenous and perforated appendicitis. J Antimicrob Chemother. 1988;22:69–74.

18. Gyselynek AM et al. Pharmacokinetics of gentamicin: distribution and plasma and renal clearance. J Infect Dis. 1971;124(Suppl):70.

19. Christopher TG et al. Gentamicin pharmacokinetics during hemodialysis. Kidney Int. 1974;6:38.

20. Danish M et al. Pharmacokinetics of gentamicin and kanamycin during hemodialysis. Antimicrob Agents Chemother. 1974;6:841.

21. Barza M et al. Predictability of blood levels of gentamicin in man. J Infect Dis. 1975;132:165.

22. Sawchuck RJ, Zaske DE. Pharmacokinetics of dosing regimens which utilize multiple intravenous infusions: gentamicin in burn patients. J Pharmacokinet Biopharm. 1976;4:183.

23. Regamey C et al. Comparative pharmacokinetics of tobramycin and gentamicin. Clin Pharmacol Ther. 1973;14:396.

24. Siber GR et al. Pharmacokinetics of gentamicin in children and adults. J Infect Dis. 1975;132:637.

25. Hull JH, Sarubbi FA. Gentamicin serum concentrations: pharmacokinetic predictions. Ann Intern Med. 1976;85:183.

26. Blouin RA et al. Tobramycin pharmacokinetics in morbidly obese patients. Clin Pharmacol Ther. 1979;26:508.

27. Bauer LA et al. Amikacin pharmacokinetics in morbidly obese patients. Am J Hosp Pharm. 1980;37:519.

28. Sampliner R et al. Influence of ascites on tobramycin pharmacokinetics. J Clin Pharmacol.1984;24:43.

29. Hodgman T et al. Tobramycin disposition into ascitic fluid. Clin Pharm. 1984;3:203.

30. Echeverria P et al. Age-dependent dose response to gentamicin. Pediatrics. 1975;87:805.

31. Schentag JJ, Jusko WJ. Renal clearance and tissue accumulation of gentamicin. Clin Pharmacol Ther. 1977;22:364.

32. Mendelson J et al. Safety of bolus administration of gentamicin. Antimicrob Agents Chemother. 1976;9:633.

33. Lynn KL et al. Gentamicin by intravenous bolus injections. NZ Med J. 1977;80:442.

34. Schentag JJ et al. Tissue persistence of gentamicin in man. JAMA. 1977;238:327.

35. Colburn WA et al. A model for the prospective identification of the prenephrotoxic state during gentamicin therapy. J Pharmacokinet Biopharm. 1978;6:179.

36. Evans WE et al. A model for dosing gentamicin in children and adolescents that adjust for tissue accumulation with continuous dosing. Clin Pharmacokinet. 1980;5:295.

37. Dionne RE et al. Estimating creatinine clearance in morbidly obese patients. Am J Hosp Pharm.1981;38:841–4.

38. Bauer LA et al. Influence of weight on aminoglycoside pharmacokinetics in normal weight and morbidly obese patients. Eur J Clin Pharmacol. 1983:24:643–7.

39. Holt HA et al. Interactions between aminoglycoside antibiotics and carbenicillin or ticarcillin. Infection. 1976;4:107.

40. Ervin FR et al. Inactivation of gentamicin by penicillins in patients with renal failure. Antimicrob Agents Chemother. 1976;9:1004.

41. Weibert RT, Keane WF. Carbenicillin—gentamicin interaction in acute renal failure. Am J Hosp Pharm. 1977;34:1137.

42. Riff L, Jackson GG. Laboratory and clinical conditions for gentamicin inactivation by carbenicillin. Arch Intern Med. 1972;130:887.

43. Konishi H et al. Tobramycin inactivation by carbenicillin, ticarcillin, and piperacillin. Antimicrob Agents Chemother. 1983;23:653.

44. Pickering LK, Gerahart P. Effect of time and concentration upon interaction between gentamicin, tobramycin, netilmicin, or amikacin, and carbenicillin or ticarcillin. Antimicrob Agents Chemother. 1979;15:592.

45. Henderson JL et al. *In vitro* inactivation of tobramycin and netilmicin by carbenicillin, azlocillin, or mezlocillin. Am J Hosp Pharm. 1981;38:1167.

46. Earp CM, Barriere SL. The lack of inactivation of tobramycin by cefazolin, cefamandole, moxalactam *in vitro*. Drug Intell Clin Pharm. 1985;19:677.

47. Kehoe WA. Lack of effect of ceftizoxime on gentamicin serum level determinations. Hosp Pharm. 1986;21:340.

48. Fischer JH et al. Pharmacokinetics and antibacterial activity of two gentamicin products given intramuscularly. Clin Pharm. 1984;3:411.

49. Aronoff GR et al. Interactions of moxalactam and tobramycin in normal volunteers and in patients with impaired renal function. J Infect Dis. 1984;149:9.

50. Schultze RG. Possible nephrotoxicity of gentamicin. J Infect Dis. 1971;124(Suppl):145.

51. Kleinknecht D et al. Acute renal failure after high doses of gentamicin and cephalothin. Lancet. 1973;7812:1129.

52. Bleiler RE, Schedl HP. Creatinine excretion: variability and relationships to diet and body size. J Lab Clin Med. 1962;59:945.

53. Reiner NE et al. Nephrotoxicity of gentamicin and tobramycin in dogs on a continuous or once daily intravenous injection. Antimicrob Agents Chemother. 1978;4(Suppl A):85.

54. Reguer L et al. Pharmacokinetics of amikacin during hemodialysis and peritoneal dialysis. Antimicrob Agents Chemother. 1977;11:214.

55. Christopher TG et al. Hemodialyzer clearance of gentamicin, kanamycin, tobramycin, amikacin, ethambutol, procainamide, and flucytosine with a technique for planning therapy. J Pharmacokinet Biopharm. 1976;4:427.

56. Halprin BA et al. Clearance of gentamicin during hemodialysis: A comparison of four artificial kidneys. J Infect Dis. 1976;133:627.

57. Gailiunas P et al. Vestibular toxicity of gentamicin: incidence in patients receiving long-term hemodialysis therapy. Arch Intern Med. 1978;138:1621.

58. Bauer LA. Rebound gentamicin levels after hemodialysis. Ther Drug Monit. 1982;4:99.

59. Gary NE. Peritoneal clearance and removal of gentamicin. J Infect Dis. 1971;124(Suppl):96.

60. Lamiere N et al. Peritoneal pharmacokinetics and pharmacological manipulation of peritoneal transport. In: Gokal R, ed. Continuous Ambulatory Peritoneal Dialysis. New York: Churchill Livingstone: 1986;56–93.

61. O'Brien M, Mason NA. Systemic absorption of intra-peritoneal antimicrobials in continuous ambulatory peritoneal dialysis. Clin Pharm. 1992;11:246–54.

62. Horton MW et al. Treatment of peritonitis in patients undergoing continuous ambulatory peritoneal dialysis. Clin Pharm. 1990;9:102–17.

63. Kaiser AB. Aminoglycoside therapy of gram-negative bacillary meningitis. N Engl J Med. 1975;293:1215.

64. Rahal JJ et al. Combined intrathecal and intramuscular gentamicin for gram-negative meningitis. N Engl J Med. 1974;290:1394.

65. Everett ED, Stausbaugh LJ. Antimicrobial agents and the central nervous system. Neurosurg. 1980;6:691.

Carbamazepine   2

Carbamazepine is an anticonvulsant compound that is structurally similar to the tricyclic antidepressant agents. It has been the drug of choice for the treatment of trigeminal neuralgia, and is used in the treatment of generalized as well as complex partial seizures. Carbamazepine is most frequently prescribed for those patients who have failed to respond to other anticonvulsant therapy or for those who have developed significant side effects from other anticonvulsant agents. Its use has increased dramatically in recent years. Carbamazepine is available as a 200 mg oral tablet, a 100 mg chewable tablet, and a 100 mg/5 mL suspension.

It is eliminated primarily by the metabolic route, with one of the metabolites (10,11-epoxide) having some anticonvulsant activity.[1] Carbamazepine is bound to plasma albumin and α_1-acid glycoprotein to a significant extent. The free fraction is approximately 0.2 to 0.3, indicating that alterations in serum protein concentration may affect the therapeutic range or the relationship between the measured carbamazepine concentration and its pharmacologic effect.

Therapeutic and Toxic Plasma Concentrations

The range of therapeutic serum concentrations for carbamazepine is 4 to 12 mg/L. Many patients, however, will develop symptoms of toxicity when plasma concentrations exceed 9 mg/L. For this reason, many clinicians prefer to use a therapeutic range of approximately 4 to 8 mg/L.[2,3] The most common adverse effects associated with carbamazepine involve the central nervous system (CNS): nystagmus, ataxia, blurred vision, and drowsiness.[1] In most patients, the ratio of carbamazepine to its major metabolite (10,11-epoxide) is relatively constant. Under certain conditions, however, such as when felbamate is added to a patient's carbamazepine regimen, the carbamazepine concentration is reduced and the 10,11-epoxide concentration is increased. This may explain the observation of CNS side effects in some patients with relatively low carbamazepine concentrations.[4] There are a number of dermatologic and hematologic side effects that are not dose related, the most serious of which are the rare, but potentially fatal: aplastic anemia and Stevens-Johnson syndrome.[1] In the early 1970s, concern about the serious hematologic side effects limited the use of carbamazepine; however, serious adverse hematologic effects appear to be rare, although a mild leukopenia may occur.

Key Parameters

Therapeutic Plasma Concentrations	4–12 mg/L
F	80%
S	1.0
Vd[a]	1.4 L/kg
Cl[a,b]	
Monotherapy	0.064 L/kg/hr
Polytherapy	0.1 L/kg/hr
α (Free Fraction)	0.2–0.3
$t\frac{1}{2}$[b]	
Monotherapy	15 hr
Polytherapy	10 hr

[a] The values for volume of distribution and clearance are approximations based upon oral administration data and an estimate of bioavailability.
[b] The clearance and half-life values represent adult values after induction has taken place. Polytherapy represents patient receiving other enzyme inducing anticonvulsants (e.g., phenobarbital, phenytoin).

Bioavailability (F)

Carbamazepine is a lipid soluble compound which is slowly and variably absorbed from the gastrointestinal tract. Peak plasma concentrations occur approximately six hours (range: 2 to 24 hours) after oral ingestion.[1] Although the bioavailability of carbamazepine has not been directly determined, it is estimated to be greater than 70% and may approach 100%.[1] Since carbamazepine is so slowly absorbed, changes in gastrointestinal function, especially those associated with rapid transit, could decrease its bioavailability and result in variable plasma concentrations of carbamazepine. If bioavailability is assumed to be 100%, and absorption is in actuality less than complete in patients with altered gastrointestinal function, there will be proportional errors in the calculation of plasma concentrations, clearance, and volume of distribution. For clinical purposes, the author assumes the bioavailability factor (F) to be approximately 0.8 for carbamazepine when administered as the oral tablet, chewable tablet, or suspension.

Volume of Distribution (Vd)

On average, the volume of distribution for carbamazepine is approximately 1.4 L/kg. Although there is a wide range of reported values (0.8 to 1.9 L/kg), this variability is probably due to alterations in plasma binding and calculation of the volume of distribution from oral administration data.[1,5] Carbamazepine, a neutral compound that is primarily bound to albumin and α_1-acid glycoprotein, has a free fraction (alpha) of approximately 0.2 to 0.3.[6,7] Although carbamazepine has relatively significant binding to plasma proteins there are very few clinical studies exploring alterations in plasma binding characteristics. This may be because carbamazepine is bound to multiple plasma proteins and with a free fraction of 0.2 to 0.3, fairly large changes in plasma binding would be required for the change in binding to become clinically significant.

Clearance (Cl)

Carbamazepine is eliminated almost exclusively by the metabolic route, with less than 2% of an oral dose being excreted unchanged in the urine. Clearance values are difficult to estimate because bioavailability is uncertain. Nevertheless, the average clearance value appears to be approximately 0.064 L/hr/kg in patients who have received the drug chronically. In patients who are taking other enzyme inducing antiepileptic drugs concurrently, the clearance is increased to approximately 0.1 L/kg/hr.[8,9] Single-dose studies suggest a clearance value which is one-half to one-third of the value observed in patients on chronic therapy.[10,11] The increase in clearance associated with chronic therapy is apparently due to auto-induction of its metabolic enzymes. Therefore, the use of clearance values from single-dose studies is impractical in the calculation of a maintenance dose.

The auto-induction of carbamazepine metabolism has many clinical implications. It is important to initiate patients on relatively low doses to avoid side effects early in therapy. The maintenance dose can be increased at one to two week intervals. The auto-induction phenomenon also limits pharmacokinetic manipulation of carbamazepine dosing. For example, it is uncertain whether induction is an all-or-none or graded process which is dose related. While most clinicians assume that induction is complete within five to seven days, it is possible that the majority of induction occurs over the first one to three days. Finally, auto-induction of metabolism commonly cause changes in steady-state carbamazepine levels which are less than proportional to an increase in the maintenance dose.

As with many of the anticonvulsant agents, carbamazepine has been associated with cross-induction (i.e., enhanced metabolism) of other anticonvulsants. For this reason, whenever carbamazepine is added to an anti-convulsant regimen, or other agents are added to a carbamazepine regimen, additional plasma level monitoring may be appropriate to ensure that the maintenance regimen continues to result in plasma levels that are optimal for therapeutic control.[1,12]

There is one report of a disproportionately large increase in steady-state plasma concentrations of carbamazepine following dose adjustment. This study suggests that carbamazepine may undergo capacity-limited metabolism. It would be extremely difficult to predict the outcome of a dose adjustment if one had to consider capacity-limited metabolism as well as induction of metabolism.[13]

Half-Life (t½)

Although single-dose studies predict a carbamazepine half-life of approximately 30 to 35 hours, steady-state data suggest a half-life of approximately 15 hours in patients receiving carbamazepine monotherapy, and approximately 10 hours in patients receiving other enzyme-inducing antiepileptic drugs (e.g., phenytoin, phenobarbital) concurrently. Due to the auto-induction of carbamazepine, pharmacokinetic data derived from single-dose studies should not be used to calculate maintenance regimens.[10,11,14]

Time to Sample

Obtaining carbamazepine plasma samples within the first few weeks of therapy may be useful to establish a relationship between carbamazepine concentration and a patient's clinical response. However, these data should be interpreted cautiously if one is attempting to predict the long-term relationship between a carbamazepine dosing regimen and plasma levels. Once steady state has been achieved, the time of sampling within a dosing interval is somewhat arbitrary given the long half-life and relatively short dosing interval for carbamazepine. Nevertheless, it is reasonable to obtain carbamazepine plasma samples at a consistent time within the dosing interval. Since carbamazepine is slowly and variably absorbed, the actual sampling time may not be critical; however, as a general rule, samples should be obtained just before a dose (trough) unless this is markedly inconvenient for the patient. Inconvenience is most likely to be encountered in ambulatory patients who may be taking the drug on a schedule which is not consistent with their clinic appointments.

Question #1: N.S., a 36-year-old, 60 kg female, is to be given carbamazepine as an anticonvulsant agent. Calculate a daily dose that will produce an average steady-state plasma concentration of approximately 6 mg/L.

To calculate an average steady-state plasma concentration, Equation 16 would be used with an assumed bioavailability of 0.8 and an average clearance value of 3.84 L/hr (0.064 L/kg/hr × 60 kg). The fraction of the administered dose which is active drug (S) is 1.0.

$$\text{Maintenance Dose} = \frac{(Cl)(Cpss\ ave)(\tau)}{(S)(F)}$$

$$= \frac{(3.84\ L/hr)(6\ mg/L)(24\ hr/1\ day)}{(1)(0.8)}$$

$$= 691.2\ mg/day$$

This dose (approximately 700 mg/day) is that which would be required to achieve the steady-state level of 6 mg/L *after* auto-induction of carbamazepine metabolism had taken place. For this reason, N.S. should be started on a lower daily dose initially and increased at one to two week intervals based upon her clinical response. The usual initial daily dose for adult patients is 200 to 400 mg, with increases of approximately 200 mg every 7 to 14 days.

Question #2: After two months, N.S.'s carbamazepine dose had been increased to 300 mg BID. On this regimen she had some reduction in seizure frequency; however, seizure control was still considered unsatisfactory. The steady-state carbamazepine level at this time was reported to be 4 mg/L. What are possible explanations for this observed plasma level? What dose would be required to achieve a new steady-state carbamazepine level of 6 mg/L?

Using Equation 35 and a clearance of 3.84 L/hr, the anticipated carbamazepine level in N.S. for a dose of 600 mg/day would be approximately 5 mg/L.

$$\text{Cpss ave} = \frac{(S)(F)(Dose/\tau)}{Cl}$$

$$= \frac{(1)(0.8)(300 \text{ mg}/12 \text{ hr})}{3.84 \text{ L/hr}}$$

$$= 5.2 \text{ mg/L}$$

The observed level of 4.0 mg/L is within the predicted range, considering the fact that both bioavailability and clearance values derived from average literature values may not be applicable to N.S. At this point, it would be difficult to establish whether a slightly lower-than-expected bioavailability or a higher-than-average clearance was responsible for the observed level of 4.0 mg/L.

Because of carbamazepine's relatively slow absorption characteristics and long half-life, it is probable that the measured concentration of 4 mg/L represents an average value. At steady state, the average plasma concentration should be proportional to the daily dose. Therefore, to increase the plasma concentration from 4 to 6 mg/L, one would simply increase the carbamazepine dose by 50% (i.e., from 600 to 900 mg/day). An alternate approach might be to calculate the apparent carbamazepine clearance for N.S. using Equation 15 and an assumed bioavailability of 0.8.

$$Cl = \frac{(S)(F)(Dose/\tau)}{Cpss \text{ ave}}$$

$$= \frac{(1)(0.8)(600 \text{ mg}/24 \text{ hr})}{4 \text{ mg/L}}$$

$$= 5 \text{ L/hr}$$

This clearance value could then be used in Equation 16 to calculate the maintenance dose as illustrated in Question 1. However, this time the clearance value which has been derived from the patient's specific data would be used rather than an average value from the literature:

$$\text{Maintenance Dose} = \frac{(Cl)(Cpss\ ave)(\tau)}{(S)(F)}$$

$$= \frac{(5\ L/hr)(6\ mg/L)(24\ hr/1\ day)}{(1)(0.8)}$$

$$= 900\ mg/day$$

If N.S. were receiving other anticonvulsant agents, it would be appropriate to monitor their concentrations as well, since carbamazepine could induce their metabolism, thereby reducing their steady-state concentrations.

References

1. Bertilsson L. Clinical pharmacokinetics of carbamazepine. Clin Pharmacokinet. 1978;3:128.

2. Thomson T. Interdosage fluctuations in plasma carbamazepine concentration determine intermittent side effects. Arch Neurol. 1984; 41:830–4.

3. Hoppener RJ et al. Correlation between the daily fluctuations of carbamazepine serum levels and intermittent side effects. Epilepsia. 1980;21:341–50.

4. Albani F et al. Effect of felbamate on plasma levels of carbamazepine and its metabolites. Epilepsia. 1991;32:130–2.

5. Morselli PL. Carbamazepine: absorption, distribution, and excretion. In: Penry JK, Daly E, eds. Advances in Neurology, Volume II. New York: Raven Press; 1975:279–93.

6. Hooper WB et al. Plasma protein binding of carbamazepine. Clin Pharm Ther. 1975;17:433.

7. Jusko WJ, Gretch M. Plasma and tissue protein binding of drugs in pharmacokinetics. Drug Metab Rev. 1976;5:43.

8. Levy RH, Kerr BN. Clinical pharmacokinetics of carbamazepine. J Clin Psychiatry. 1988;49:(Suppl.):58–61.

9. Eichelbaum M et al. Carbamazepine metabolism in man: induction and pharmacogenetic aspects. Clin Pharmacokinet. 1985;10:80–90.

10. Gerardin AP et al. Pharmacokinetics of carbamazepine in normal humans after single and repeated oral doses. J Clin Pharmacokinet Biopharm. 1976;4:521.

11. Pitlick WH et al. Pharmacokinetic model to describe self-induced decreases in steady state concentrations of carbamazepine. J Pharm Sci. 1976;65:462.

12. Christiansen J, Dam M. Influence of phenobarbital and diphenylhydantoin on plasma carbamazepine levels in patients with epilepsy. Acta Neurol Scand. 1973;49:543.

13. Hooper WD et al. Preliminary observations on the clinical pharmacology of carbamazepine. Proc Aust Neurol. 1974; 19:189.

14. Westenberg HGM et al. Kinetics of carbamazepine and carbamazepine-epoxide determined by use of plasma and saliva. Clin Pharmacol Ther. 1978;23:320.

Cyclosporine   3

Cyclosporine is a cyclic peptide immunosuppressant used to prevent graft rejection in solid organ transplant patients and to prevent graft-versus-host disease in bone marrow transplant patients. It is not used to treat acute rejection episodes. Cyclosporine has been used in patients since 1978[1] and has been effective in improving the long-term survival of patients with renal and other solid organ transplants.

The usual initial oral dose of cyclosporine is approximately 15 mg/kg/day administered as a single daily dose or as a divided dose every 12 hours. The drug is available as liquid-filled capsules (25 mg and 100 mg) and as a solution in olive oil (100 mg/mL). The oral solution is recommended to be taken with milk or juice, but many patients prefer chocolate milk or orange juice to improve cyclosporine's palatability. Because cyclosporine is not water soluble, the solution should be mixed and delivered from a glass, and not a styrofoam container. After consumption, the container should be rinsed with an additional amount of milk or juice to ensure complete delivery of the dose. An injectable solution in alcohol and castor oil (50 mg/mL) is also available. Because the oral bioavailability is low for cyclosporine, the intravenous dose is usually one-third of the oral dose, or 5 mg/kg/day. Like the oral dosage forms, cyclosporine is injected once daily or divided into two equal doses. Both the package insert and American Hospital Formulary Service[2] suggest once daily administration. Nevertheless, many protocols direct twice daily administration of the drug. It is not known whether dividing the dose improves the therapeutic effect or diminishes the toxic effects of cyclosporine.

While it has become a standard of practice to monitor cyclosporine levels, they must be interpreted in the context of the assay methodology and the biological fluids that have been sampled. Concentrations necessary to optimize graft survival while minimizing potential toxicities vary depending upon both of these factors. Dosing techniques and time of sampling also must be carefully considered when evaluating cyclosporine levels.

Therapeutic and Toxic Plasma Concentrations

Cyclosporine is a lipid-soluble compound that is approximately 20% bound to leukocytes and 40% bound to erythrocytes; 40% remains in the plasma fraction of blood where it is highly bound to lipoproteins which comprise a relatively small fraction of the plasma proteins.[3,4] Cyclospor-

Key Parameters[a]

Therapeutic Concentration	See Table 3.1
F[b]	30%
Vd[c]	4–5 L/kg
Cl[d]	5–10 mL/min/kg
t½	6–12 hr
Fraction free (α)[e]	<10%

[a] As with the therapeutic range, pharmacokinetic parameters will vary, depending upon the biologic fluid and assay procedure used.
[b] Bioavailability is both inter- and intraindividually variable.
[c] Cyclosporine is distributed into multiple compartments; however, toxicity is not known to be associated with drug concentrations in the distribution phase.
[d] Clearance is primarily by hepatic metabolism.
[e] Cyclosporine is bound extensively to many blood elements and, in plasma, it is extensively bound to lipoproteins.

ine binding to these different blood elements is temperature dependent. Thus, assays performed on any sample (other than whole blood) must be done at 37°C. Otherwise, the therapeutic range needs to be temperature-adjusted for binding changes.

As can be seen in Table 3.1, non-specific assays measure not only cyclosporine but its metabolites as well. Polyclonal and monoclonal fluorescence polarization immunoassays are most commonly employed in clinical practice. Because the polyclonal assay cross reacts with cyclosporine metabolites, the therapeutic range is substantially higher than that for the more specific monoclonal procedure. As a general rule, high performance liquid chromatography (HPLC) assay results are approximately equal to the monoclonal procedures. While they are more difficult to perform, many institutions prefer them because they are less expensive than the monoclonal assays and it is simpler to pick up assay interference and to detect metabolites. Clearly, clinicians must make themselves aware of the assay procedure and biologic fluids used at their institutions. These problems have also made it difficult to establish therapeutic ranges. When concentrations in whole blood are measured, most clinicians accept levels of 150 to 400 µg/L (ng/mL) as that range within which the ability of the drug to suppress graft rejection is optimal and the risk of toxicity is minimized.

The goal of monitoring cyclosporine concentrations is to optimize the benefit to risk ratio so that the patient has an optimal chance of achieving a positive therapeutic outcome. Thus, low-risk patients (e.g., recipients of HLA-identical grafts or patients receiving other concurrent immunosuppressive therapy) might be acceptably controlled with lower-than-usual concentrations. On the other hand, high-risk groups (including those with poorly matched grafts) might require higher concentrations to prevent graft rejection.

Adverse Effects. The most common side effect associated with cyclosporine is renal impairment which usually reverses when the drug is discontinued or the dose decreased.[5,6] While the mechanism for nephrotoxicity is unclear, it may be related to cyclosporine-induced vasoconstriction. Because some patients develop irreversible renal failure, the cyclosporine doses and target concentrations are often lowered in patients who develop early signs of nephrotoxicity. Other common, but less frequent side effects include hypertension, central nervous system effects (tremor, headaches, paresthesia, and, rarely, seizures),[7] gastrointestinal reactions, hepatotoxicity, and hematologic disorders.[2]

Bioavailability (F)

Cyclosporine is a highly lipid-soluble compound that has limited oral bioavailability. While the reported bioavailability range is wide, most clinicians accept an average value of approximately 30% absorbed when the drug is given orally as the liquid olive oil solution or as the soft gelatin

Table 3.1	Therapeutic Range[20]	
Assay	*Serum/Plasma[a]* *(μg/mL or ng/L)*	*Whole Blood[a]* *(μg/mL or ng/L)*
Monoclonal radio immunoassay	50–125	150–400
Florescence polarization immunoassay		
Polyclonal	150–400	200–800
Monoclonal	50–125	150–400
High-performance liquid chromatography (HPLC)	50–125	150–400

[a] Therapeutic range is variable and will depend upon dosing interval (τ) time of sampling, assay technique, and temperature.

capsule.[8–10] Cyclosporine absorption varies widely within and among subjects[11] and is a potential problem any time there is a change in the clinical status of the patient.[12] The high lipid solubility of cyclosporine results in complex absorption characteristics with peak concentrations usually achieved within six hours after an oral dose. Rapid gastrointestinal transit may also reduce the bioavailability and should be considered in a patient with diarrhea who is receiving oral cyclosporine.[13] Another problem that is commonly associated with liver transplant patients during the immediate postoperative period is that they may, due to drainage catheters, have inadequate bile salts which are required for the adequate absorption of cyclosporine. This problem can be overcome by administering the drug intravenously or by refeeding the bile salts to enhance the solubility and absorption characteristics of oral cyclosporine.[14] The problems associated with cyclosporine bioavailability call for frequent and regular concentration monitoring.

Volume of Distribution (Vd)

The reported range for the volume of distribution of cyclosporine is wide, but the average value is approximately 4 to 5 L/kg. This relatively large Vd is consistent with the observation that cyclosporine is significantly bound to plasma and blood elements, that the unbound portion in the plasma is less than 10%, and that it is probably extensively bound to tissues outside the vascular space.[11,15–17] Part of the variability in reported volumes of distribution can be attributed to the fact that cyclosporine exhibits two-compartment modeling with a substantial alpha or distribution phase.[21] The assay procedure and the type of biologic fluid assayed will also influence the measured concentration and, therefore, the derived pharmacokinetic parameters. The uncertainty surrounding cyclosporine's volume of distribution does not influence its clinical use to a large degree because loading doses are seldom administered. (See Clinical Application of Cyclosporine Pharmacokinetics on page 190.)

Clearance (Cl)

Cyclosporine is eliminated almost exclusively by hepatic metabolism, and a significant number of metabolites can be found in both the urine and plasma. These metabolites are generally thought to be less active than the parent compound. The whole blood clearance of cyclosporine is approximately 5 to 10 mL/min/kg in adult patients, indicating that it is probably a drug with a low extraction ratio. In other words, its elimination is influenced primarily by the unbound cyclosporine concentration.[15,16]

These clearance values are based upon whole blood determinations and are lower than would be estimated using room temperature serum or plasma concentration data or those derived from non-specific assay techniques. There are a number of drugs which have been reported to influence the metabolism and clearance of cyclosporine. The anticonvulsants and rifampin can rapidly and significantly increase cyclosporine's metabolism.[18,19] Drugs known to reduce the metabolism and increase plasma concentrations of cyclosporine include erythromycin, ketoconazole, and the calcium channel antagonists.[18,19] There is a long list of agents that can alter cyclosporine concentrations; however, their mechanisms are not well established and the data are limited.[18,19]

Half-Life (t½)

The average half-life calculated from the values indicated in the preceding sections would suggest a value of approximately seven hours (Eq. 32).

$$t\tfrac{1}{2} = \frac{(0.693)(Vd)}{Cl}$$

$$= \frac{(0.693)(4.5 \text{ L/kg})}{\left(7.5 \text{ mL/min/kg}\right)\left(\dfrac{60 \text{ min/hr}}{1000 \text{ mL/L}}\right)}$$

$$= 6.93 \text{ hr}$$

This half-life is variable, however, due to the uncertainty associated with the volume of distribution and clearance estimates for cyclosporine. The multi-compartmental nature of cyclosporine also may result in an underestimation of the terminal half-life and associated pharmacokinetic parameters. The most commonly reported values for cyclosporine half-life are in the range of 6 to 12 hours.

Cyclosporine tends to be given on a fixed schedule once or twice daily, and the dosing interval is not usually adjusted based on the apparent half-life. This is because higher-than-expected plasma levels could be due to an increase in the bioavailability or a decrease in clearance (Eq. 35).

$$\uparrow Cpss \text{ ave} = \frac{(S)(\uparrow F)(Dose/\tau)}{\downarrow Cl}$$

If the change in plasma concentration is due to an increase in bioavailability (and therefore the dose or input rate), then the half-life would be normal. If, on the other hand, the increased plasma concentration is due to a reduced clearance, then one would anticipate the half-life to be extended. In most clinical settings it is impossible to determine which factor plays the more important role. For this reason, the dose rather than the dosing interval is adjusted in the clinical setting.

Time to Sample

While there are a number of recommended schemes for obtaining samples for cyclosporine concentrations, trough levels generally yield information that is the most reproducible and useful in clinical practice. Peak concentrations are often variable due to the uncertain rate and extent of absorption. Some authors have suggested that several drug levels be obtained within a dosing interval in order to fully characterize the plasma concentration curve. While this does have some merit, it is generally unnecessary and usually results in the same clinical outcome: an increase or decrease in the dose necessary to achieve the target concentration.

Because of the wide variability in its absorption and metabolism, most clinicians monitor cyclosporine levels every other day when therapy is initiated and begin to extend the interval between samples when it appears that steady state has been achieved. In acute care, plasma samples every three to five days for stable patients is probably the norm; in stable ambulatory care patients, monthly levels may be adequate. Most clinicians also recommend more intensive sampling any time there is a change in the route of administration, there are signs of cyclosporine toxicity, or there is a change in concurrent medications likely to alter cyclosporine pharmacokinetics.

Clinical Application of Cyclosporine Pharmacokinetics

Complex computer programs or relatively straightforward approaches can be used to evaluate a patient's pharmacokinetic parameters but, in most cases, the clinical result is essentially the same. When plasma concentrations are low the dose is increased, and when plasma concentrations are high, the dose is decreased. When cyclosporine concentrations are low, it is appropriate to evaluate patient compliance and determine if any drugs have been added to therapy which might alter cyclosporine absorption or metabolism. If there are no easily correctable problems, most clinicians would increase the dose modestly, recognizing that the change in concentration should be approximately proportional to the change in the maintenance dose. If cyclosporine concentrations are high, it is important to first determine if the sample has been appropriately obtained and that it truly represents a trough concentration. If the sample is a valid trough level, many clinicians will hold a daily dose and then restart on a proportionally lower maintenance dose to bring the plasma concentration into the desired range. It has been the author's experience that occasionally patients have isolated elevated or decreased cyclosporine concentrations for which no logical explanation can be found. For this reason, it is often appropriate to avoid overreacting to an isolated assay result.

Question #1: **R.I., a 39-year-old, 51 kg woman, received a nonrelated renal transplant 1 year ago. Following transplantation, her serum creatinine stabilized in the range of 1.4 to 1.7 mg/dL. She has been receiving cyclosporine orally, 125 mg BID over the past six months. Cyclosporine concentrations have been 85 to 110 µg/L (whole blood HPLC assay). Her last clinic appointment was three weeks ago. Other immunosuppressive medications included prednisone 25 mg/day and azathioprine 50 mg HS. She returned to clinic yesterday complaining of increasing fatigue since her last clinic appointment. Blood and urine cultures were taken and she was admitted to the hospital with a serum creatinine of 2.8 mg/dL. How would you adjust R.I.'s cyclosporine dose in order to increase the cyclosporine concentration to approximately 200 µg/L?**

First, it is important to determine whether the rise in serum creatinine is due to graft rejection or cyclosporine toxicity. If the increase in serum creatinine is presumed to be a sign of graft rejection, the patient would probably also receive additional acute immunosuppressant therapy including methylprednisolone, antithymocyte globulin (ATG), or muromonab (OKT3). Using approach number three as outlined in Part I: Interpretation of Plasma Drug Concentrations: Choosing a Model to Revise or Estimate a Patient's Clearance at Steady State on page 82, a revised set of pharmacokinetic parameters can be calculated:

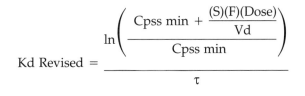

$$\text{Kd Revised} = \frac{\ln\left(\dfrac{\text{Cpss min} + \dfrac{(S)(F)(\text{Dose})}{Vd}}{\text{Cpss min}}\right)}{\tau}$$

The average cyclosporine concentration of approximately 100 µg/L would be used as the Cpss min, F would be 0.3 and the dose would be expressed as 125,000 µg. The Vd would have to be estimated (4.5 L/kg) and τ would be 12 hours. Using these values, the revised elimination rate constant is approximately 0.0807 hr^{-1} with a corresponding clearance of 18.5 L/hr and a half-life of approximately eight or nine hours.

$$\text{Kd Revised} = \frac{\ln\left(\dfrac{100 \text{ µg/L} + \dfrac{(1)(0.3)(125{,}000 \text{ µg})}{(4.5 \text{ L/kg})(51 \text{ kg})}}{100 \text{ µg/kg}}\right)}{12 \text{ hr}}$$

$$= \frac{\ln\left(\dfrac{263.4 \text{ µg/L}}{100 \text{ µg/L}}\right)}{12}$$

$$= 0.0807 \text{ hr}^{-1}$$

$$\begin{aligned}
\text{Cl} &= (\text{Kd Revised})(\text{Vd}) \\
&= (0.0807 \text{ hr}^{-1})(4.5 \text{ L/kg})(51 \text{ kg}) \\
&= (0.0807 \text{ hr}^{-1})(229.5 \text{ L}) \\
&= 18.5 \text{ L/hr}
\end{aligned}$$

$$\begin{aligned}
t\tfrac{1}{2} &= \frac{0.693}{\text{Kd}} \\
&= \frac{0.693}{0.0807 \text{ hr}^{-1}} \\
&= 8.6 \text{ hr}
\end{aligned}$$

Using the revised pharmacokinetic parameters, a new dose can be calculated by rearranging Equation 47 to solve for dose.

$$\text{Cpss min} = \frac{\dfrac{(S)(F)(\text{Dose})}{\text{Vd}}}{1 - e^{-Kd\tau}} (e^{-Kd\tau})$$

$$\text{Dose} = \frac{(\text{Cpss min})(\text{Vd})(1 - e^{Kd\tau})}{(S)(F)(e^{-Kd\tau})}$$

Making the appropriate substitutions for Cpss min, Vd, S, F, Kd, and τ, a dose of approximately 250 mg can be calculated.

$$\text{Dose} = \frac{(200 \ \mu g/L)(4.5 \ L/kg)(51 \ kg)(1 - e^{-(0.0807)(12)})}{(1)(0.3)(e^{-(0.0807)(12)})}$$

$$= \frac{(200 \ \mu g/L)(229.5)(1 - 0.38)}{(1)(0.3)(0.38)}$$

$$= 249{,}631 \ \mu g \ \ or \ \ \approx\!250 \ mg \ Q \ 12 \ hr$$

Note that this dose adjustment to 250 mg every 12 hours is double the original dose of 125 mg every 12 hours and should result in a proportional change in the steady-state trough concentration. This method of using the desired change in the plasma concentration as the same ratio change for maintenance dose is useful as long as the dosing interval is not altered. Because the dosing interval remains the same, this is the standard method of adjusting and most clinicians do not bother to calculate the elimination rate constant or clearance values associated with steady-state trough concentrations of cyclosporine. They simply make a proportional or clinically reasonable change.

Question #2: O.S., a 48-year-old, 59 kg male patient, received a living-related renal transplant 1½ years ago. He is currently receiving cyclosporine 300 mg orally as the solution BID and, in addition, prednisone 30 mg/day and azathioprine 75 mg/day. O.S.'s current serum creatinine is 2.1 mg/dL and his steady-state cyclosporine trough concentration is 590 μg/L. The physician has ruled out the possibility of rejection and feels that the recent rise in serum creatinine is due to cyclosporine toxicity. What questions would one ask O.S. and how would one adjust his cyclosporine regimen in order to achieve a new steady-state cyclosporine concentration of approximately 200 μg/L?

First, confirm that O.S. has been taking his cyclosporine 300 mg BID as prescribed and determine if any new medications have been added to his regimen. Also verify the time of sampling relative to when he took his last dose to ensure that the level is in fact a trough and not a peak concentration. If there are no easily correctable reasons for the elevated cyclosporine level at least one cyclosporine dose should be held and then O.S. should be restarted on a new regimen. The dose decrease should approximate the proportionate decrease in cyclosporine concentration that is desired:

$$\text{Desired Dose} = \frac{\text{Cpss Desired}}{\text{Cpss Current}} \times \text{Current Dose}$$

Using the current steady-state cyclosporine concentration of 590 µg/L and the new target concentration of 200 µg/L, the new cyclosporine dose is approximately 100 mg.

$$\text{Desired Dose} = \frac{200 \ \mu g/L}{590 \ \mu g/L} \times 300 \ \mu g$$

$$= 0.339 \times 300 \ mg$$

$$= 101.7 \ mg \ \ or \ \approx 100 \ mg$$

This new dose assumes that the bioavailability remains the same and that the drug will be administered at the same interval of 12 hours. It is unclear why O.S. requires a lower than average cyclosporine dose (200 mg/day or ≈3.4 mg/kg/day). He may be absorbing more than the usual 30%, his hepatic metabolism may be unusually low, or a combination of both factors may be contributing.

Question #3: M.A., a 78 kg liver transplant patient, is receiving 400 mg of cyclosporine QD as an IV infusion. Currently, his hepatic function tests appear to be stable, and for the past three days he has been improving clinically with steady-state trough cyclosporine concentrations of approximately 220 µg/L. What would be an appropriate oral cyclosporine dose for M.A.?

Because the usual bioavailability for cyclosporine is approximately 30%, most clinicians give an oral dose that is three times the parenteral dose. In this case, it would be approximately 1200 mg once daily, or 600 mg every 12 hours. Some clinicians prefer dividing the dose to reduce the volume of cyclosporine liquid or the number of capsules per dose. Dividing the dose may increase the steady-state trough concentration slightly because shortening the interval tends to lower the peak and raise the trough levels; therefore, more closely approximating the true steady-state average level. Again, pharmacokinetic calculations could have been performed; however, the outcome would have been essentially the same as adjusting the dose in proportion to the desired change in steady-state plasma concentration.

In this case we have the additional factor of a change in route and, therefore, bioavailability to consider:

$$\text{New Dose} = \frac{\text{Cpss Desired}}{\text{Cpss Current}} \times \frac{\text{F Current}}{\text{F New Dosage Form}} \times \text{Current Dose}$$

Assuming the reported cyclosporine concentration of 220 µg/L is acceptable, the new dose will be approximately 1200 mg/day.

$$\text{New Dose} = \frac{220 \ \mu g/L}{220 \ \mu g/L} \times \frac{1.0}{0.3} \times 400 \ mg$$
$$= 1 \times 3.33 \times 400 \ mg$$
$$= 1333 \ mg \ (\approx 1200 \ mg)$$

Again, if the dose is divided and given as 600 mg every 12 hours, trough levels will be somewhat higher than those produced by single daily doses. However, the bioavailability will probably be a more important influence on the trough cyclosporine concentration than dosing interval will be.

Question #4: **P.E., a 41-year-old, 60 kg woman, recently received a kidney transplant and is now receiving 150 mg cyclosporine IV BID. While her cyclosporine blood concentrations have been somewhat variable, they have been in the range of 120 to 215 µg/L over the past week. Today on rounds it was noted that her most recent cyclosporine level** was 1,200 µg/L. **What would be an appropriate course of action considering P.E.'s previous cyclosporine dosing and concentration history?**

First, there should be a careful review of P.E.'s medication history to ensure that no inhibitors of cyclosporine metabolism have been added to her therapy. Also, her hepatic function tests should be reviewed to establish that her hepatic function has remained stable. Then, determine the time at which the cyclosporine sample was obtained. An otherwise unexplained high cyclosporine concentration is often due to a plasma sample that has been obtained near the administration time. These high concentrations are common during the distribution phase and do not necessarily indicate toxic levels. P.E. should be questioned for any obvious signs of cyclosporine-induced toxicity such as gastrointestinal or neurologic side effects and a serum creatinine should be ordered. If the patient is not exhibiting any obvious side effects, and no reason for the sudden increase in cyclosporine concentration can be identified, a repeat sample is warranted before making any dose adjustments.

References

1. Borel JF. The history of Cyclosporin A and its significance. In: White DJG, ed. Cyclosporin A. New York: Elsevier;1982:5–18.

2. AHFS Drug Information 1994, Cyclosporine. American Society of Hospital Pharmacists, Inc. Bethesda, MD.

3. Le Marie M, Tillement JP. Role of lipoproteins and erythrocytes in the *in vivo* binding and distribution of Cyclosporin A in the blood. J Pharm Pharmacol. 1982;34:715–18.

4. Niederberger W et al. Distribution and binding of cyclosporine in blood and tissue. Transplant Proceedings. 1983;15:2419–21.

5. Myers VD. Cyclosporine nephrotoxicity. Kidney Int. 1986;30:964.

6. Mihatsch MJ et al. Cyclosporine nephrotoxicity. Adv Nephrol. 1988; 17:303.

7. De Groen PC et al. Central nervous system toxicity after liver transplantation: the role of cyclosporine and cholesterol. N Engl J Med. 1987;317:861–66.

8. Frey FJ et al. Trough levels and concentration time curves of cyclosporine in patients undergoing renal transplantation. Clin Pharmacol Ther. 1988;43:55.

9. Burckart GJ et al. Cyclosporine absorption following orthotopic liver transplantation. J Clin Pharmacol. 1986;26:647.

10. Nashan B et al. Effect of the application form of cyclosporine on blood levels: comparison of oral solution and capsules. Transplant Proc. 1988;20(Suppl. 2):637.

11. Lindholm A et al. Intraindividual variability in the relative systemic availability of cyclosporin after oral dosing. Eur J Clin Pharmacol. 1988;34:461.

12. Morse GD et al. Pharmacokinetics and clinical tolerance of intravenous and oral cyclosporine in the immediate postoperative period. Clin Pharmacol Ther. 1988;44:654.

13. Atkinson K et al. Oral administration of Cyclosporine A for recipients of allogeneic marrow transplants: implications of clinical gut dysfunction. Br J Haematol. 1984;56:223.

14. Merion RM et al. Bile refeeding after liver transplantation and avoidance of intravenous cyclosporine. Surgery. 1989;106:604.

15. Ptachcinski RJ et al. Cyclosporine kinetics in renal transplantation. Clin Pharmacol Ther. 1985;38:296.

16. Yee GC et al. Blood cyclosporine pharmacokinetics in patients undergoing marrow transplantation: influence of age, obesity, and hematocrit. Transplantation. 1988;46:399.

17. Lindholm A, Henricsson S. Intra- and interindividual variability in the free fraction of cyclosporine in plasma in recipients of renal transplants. Ther Drug Monit. 1989;11:623.

18. Yee GC Mcguire TR. Pharmacokinetic drug interactions with cyclosporin (part 1). Clin Pharmacokinet. 1990;19:319.

19. Yee GC, Mcguire TR. Pharmacokinetic drug interactions with cyclosporin (part 2). Clin Pharmacokinet. 1990;19:400.

20. Yee GC, Salomon DR. Cyclosporine. In: Evans WE et al., eds. Applied Pharmacokinetics. Third Edition. 1992.

21. Gupta SK et al. Pharmacokinetics of cyclosporin: influence of rate-duration profile of an intravenous infusion in renal transplant patients. Br J Clin Pharmacol. 1989;27:353.

Digoxin

4

Digoxin is an inotropic agent primarily used to treat congestive heart failure (CHF) and atrial fibrillation. It is incompletely absorbed and a substantial fraction of an absorbed dose is cleared by the kidneys. An oral digoxin loading dose of $\approx$1.0 to 1.5 mg/70 kg can be administered before the initiation of a usual maintenance dose of 0.25 mg/day. Because it has a relatively long elimination half-life, digoxin tablets are given once daily. Dosage adjustments are critical for patients who are being converted from parenteral to oral therapy or vice versa; patients with renal impairment, congestive heart failure, or thyroid abnormalities; or patients who take quinidine concurrently.

Therapeutic Plasma Concentrations

While there is considerable variation between patients, plasma digoxin concentrations of $\approx$1 to 2 μg/L (ng/mL) are considered to be within the therapeutic range.[1,2] The use of pharmacokinetics to adjust the dosing regimen can reduce the incidence of digoxin toxicity.[2–5]

Bioavailability (F)

The bioavailability of digoxin tablets ranges from 0.5 to greater than 0.9. Many clinicians use a bioavailability of 0.7 to 0.8 to minimize the possibility of overdosing patients. A bioavailability of 0.7 will be used in this text as an estimate of the average bioavailability figures reported in the literature.[6,7] Soft gelatin capsules of digoxin appear to be completely absorbed.[8,9]

Volume of Distribution (Vd)

The average volume of distribution for digoxin is $\approx$7.3 L/kg.[10] This Vd is decreased in patients with renal disease (see Question 4).

$$\text{Vd Digoxin (L/70 kg)} = 226 + \frac{(298)(\text{Cl}_{Cr} \text{ as mL/min})}{29 + \text{Cl}_{Cr} \text{ as mL/min}}$$

Eq. 4.1

$$\text{Vd Digoxin (L)} = (3.8 \text{ L/kg})(\text{Weight in kg}) + (3.1)(\text{Cl}_{Cr} \text{ as mL/min})$$

Eq. 4.2

Key Parameters

Therapeutic Range[a]	0.8–2 µg/L
F	
Tablets	0.7
Elixir	0.8
Soft Gelatin Capsule	1.0
S	1.0
Vd[b] (L)	(3.8)(Weight in kg) + (3.1)(Cl$_{Cr}$ as mL/min)
Cl[b] (mL/min)	(0.8 mL/kg/min)(Weight in kg) + (Cl$_{Cr}$ as mL/min)
Cl[b]CHF (mL/min)	(0.33 mL/kg/min)(Weight in kg) + (0.9)(Cl$_{Cr}$ as mL/min)
t½	2 days

[a] Plasma concentrations of >2 µg/L are often used in atrial fibrillation.
[b] See Table 4.1 for factors that alter Vd and Cl of digoxin.

Digoxin Vd is also decreased in hypothyroid patients (see Question 12), and in patients who are taking quinidine (see Question 14). It is increased in hyperthyroid patients (see Question 12). In addition, the volume of distribution for digoxin in obese subjects appears to be more closely related to the non-obese or ideal body weight than total body weight (TBW).[11] (See Table 4.1.)

The manner in which digoxin is distributed in the body must be considered in the interpretation of plasma levels. The distribution of digoxin follows a two-compartment model (see Part I: Volume of Distribution: Two-Compartment Models on page 22). This drug is distributed initially into Vi, the plasma compartment (and other rapidly equilibrating tissues), and then into a more slowly-equilibrating tissue compartment where it exerts its pharmacological effects on the myocardium. Since plasma samples are obtained from Vi, plasma digoxin levels do not accurately reflect the drug's pharmacologic effects until it is completely distributed into both compartments. Serum concentrations of digoxin obtained before complete distribution are often misleading. Because the initial volume of

Table 4.1	Factors That Alter Digoxin Volume of Distribution and Clearance
Volume of Distribution	*Factor[a]*
Creatinine clearance	See Equations 4.1 and 4.2
Obesity	IBW[b]
Quinidine	0.7
Thyroid	
Clinically hypothyroid	0.7
Clinically hyperthyroid	1.3
Clearance	
Creatinine clearance	See Equations 4.3 and 4.4
Congestive heart failure	See Equation 4.4
Obesity	IBW[b]
Quinidine	0.5
Amiodarone	0.5
Verapamil	0.75
Thyroid function	
Clinically hypothyroid	0.7
Clinically hyperthyroid	1.3

[a]Factor should be multiplied by calculated volume of distribution or clearance value. Multiple factors would increase the uncertainty of any volume or clearance prediction. While not tested, one might anticipate that the factors are multiplicative.

[b]IBW = ideal body weight or "non-obese weight."

distribution (Vi) of digoxin is relatively small ($\approx \frac{1}{10}$ Vt), high plasma concentrations are commonly reported immediately after a dose is administered. Since the heart behaves as though it were in the second or tissue compartment, the initial high serum concentrations that occur immediately after a dose are not reflective of either therapeutic or toxic effects. Plasma concentrations are meaningful when obtained at least four hours after an intravenous dose[12] or six hours after an oral dose.[13] The clinical effects of a dose, however, may be observed much sooner because the distribution half-life α $t\frac{1}{2}$ is only about 35 minutes.[14] Although the myocardium experiences the effects of 75% of an intravenous dose after about one hour, a plasma sample taken at this time would be misleadingly high because the remaining 25% of the dose which is not yet distributed out of

Vi would produce a plasma concentration that is high relative to that which would be observed once equilibrium between the two compartments is complete. (See Figure 4.1.)

Clearance (Cl)

Digoxin clearance varies considerably among individuals and should be estimated for each patient. Total digoxin clearance is the sum of its metabolic and renal clearances as illustrated by Equation 23:

$$Cl_t = Cl_m + Cl_r$$

In healthy individuals the metabolic clearance of digoxin is ≈ 0.57 to 0.86 mL/kg/min, and the renal clearance is about equal to or a little less than the creatinine clearance. Congestive heart failure reduces the metabolic clearance of digoxin to about one-half its usual value and may reduce the renal clearance slightly as well.[7,15–17] (Also see Part I: Clearance (Cl) on page 26.)

Using the data from Sheiner,[15] the total digoxin clearance in mL/min/kg can be calculated in patients with and without (CHF) as follows:

$$\frac{\text{Total Cl Digoxin (mL/min)}}{\text{(Patients without CHF)}} = (0.8 \text{ mL/kg/min}) \text{ (Weight in kg)} + Cl_{Cr} \text{ as mL/min}$$

Eq. 4.3

$$\frac{\text{Total Cl Digoxin (mL/min)}}{\text{(Patients with CHF)}} = (0.33 \text{ mL/kg/min}) \text{ (Weight in kg)} + (0.9)(Cl_{Cr} \text{ as mL/min})$$

Eq. 4.4

Creatinine clearance can be estimated from the patient's serum creatinine using Equations 63 and 64:

$$\frac{Cl_{Cr} \text{ for Males}}{\text{(mL/min)}} = \frac{(140 - \text{Age})(\text{Weight})}{(72)(SrCr_{ss})}$$

$$\frac{Cl_{Cr} \text{ for Females}}{\text{(mL/min)}} = (0.85) \frac{(140 - \text{Age})(\text{Weight})}{(72)(SrCr_{ss})}$$

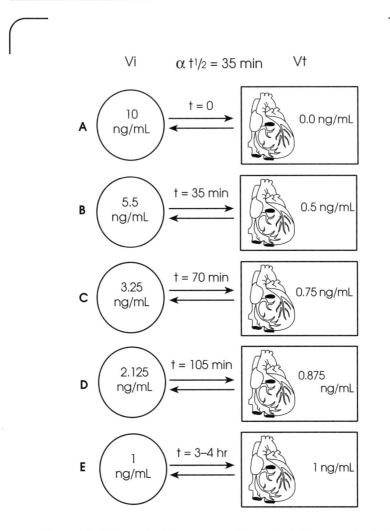

Figure 4.1. A Theoretical Two-Compartment Model for Digoxin. Note that the initial volume of distribution (Vi) is much smaller than the tissue volume of distribution (Vt). The myocardium or target organ behaves as though it were in Vt and therefore responds to the theoretical digoxin concentration in Vt. Following complete distribution, the concentrations in Vi and Vt are assumed to be equal and the pharmacologic effect maximal. Figure 4.1.A depicts digoxin distribution immediately following an intravenous bolus. All of the drug is in Vi and the plasma concentration is 10 ng/mL. Figure 4.1.E depicts complete digoxin distribution. Note that the two compartments are in equilibrium and that the digoxin concentration in both Vi and Vt is 1 ng/mL. At this point, the plasma level accurately reflects the level in the tissue compartment. Figures 4.1.B, 4.1.C, and 4.1.D depict the relative digoxin concentrations in Vi and Vt after one, two, and three distribution half-lives (αt½s). After three αt½s 87.5% of the pharmacologic effect is achieved; however, it is still much too early to obtain a digoxin level because the concentration in Vi is more than 100% higher than the final equilibrated concentration.

In obese subjects, creatinine clearance is normally calculated using ideal body weight (see Table 4.1). Similarly, IBW should also be used to estimate digoxin clearance (renal and metabolic). These and other methods for estimating digoxin clearance are illustrated in the questions which follow.

Half-Life (t½)

The half-life for digoxin is approximately two days in patients with normal renal function. In anephric patients, the half-life increases to approximately four to six days. This increase in the digoxin half-life is less than might be expected based upon the reduction in clearance because the volume of distribution is also decreased in patients with diminished renal function. (See Question 4 and Equations 4.1 and 4.2.)

Time to Sample

Plasma samples for routine digoxin level monitoring are ideally obtained 7 to 14 days after a maintenance regimen is initiated or changed. In patients with end-stage renal disease it may take 15 to 20 days to achieve steady state. Plasma samples obtained within 24 hours of an initial loading dose may help confirm the relationship between the digoxin plasma concentration and pharmacologic response or establish the apparent volume of distribution. When plasma samples are obtained this early, however, they are of little value in evaluating the maintenance regimen. Once steady state has been achieved, plasma samples for digoxin should be drawn just before the next dose (trough levels); however, any sampling time that avoids the distribution phase (at least four hours following an intravenous dose or six hours following an oral dose) is acceptable.

Patients taking digoxin who are begun on quinidine may require digoxin plasma level monitoring to determine if digoxin pharmacokinetics are altered substantially. (See Question 14.) The possibility that digoxin concentrations will fluctuate within a quinidine dosing interval also should be considered. Consequently, digoxin samples generally should be obtained at a time which corresponds to the trough of the quinidine dosing interval and which also avoids the distribution phase for digoxin.

When agents that decrease the digoxin clearance (but do not alter the volume of distribution) are added to a patient's therapy, the new digoxin half-life must be used to estimate the time required to achieve steady state. In most cases, steady state is observed within seven to ten days.

Question #1. **Estimate a digoxin loading dose that will produce a plasma concentration of 1.5 µg/L for a 70 kg patient being treated for CHF.**

Estimating a loading dose requires knowledge of the volume of distribution of the drug. In this case, the average literature value for the Vd of digoxin (7.3 L/kg) will be used. If one knew the renal function, a volume of distribution based upon renal function would be calculated instead (see Question 4 and Equations 4.1 and 4.2.)[10] Using Equation 11, the loading dose can be calculated as follows:

$$\text{Loading Dose} = \frac{(Vd)(Cp)}{(S)(F)}$$

$$= \frac{(7.3 \text{ L/kg})(70 \text{ kg})(1.5 \text{ µg/L})}{(1)(0.7)}$$

$$= \frac{(511 \text{ L})(1.5 \text{ µg/L})}{0.7}$$

$$= \frac{766.5 \text{ µg}}{0.7}$$

$$= 1095 \text{ µg } \textit{or} \approx 1000 \text{ µg}$$

In this case, it was assumed that the loading dose was to be given orally as tablets; therefore, a bioavailability (F) of 0.7 was used.[6] If the loading dose was to have been given intravenously, F would have been 1.0 and the calculated loading dose would have been 766.5 µg ($\approx$750 µg). In both cases, S is 1.0 since digoxin is not administered as a salt.

Question #2. **How should this loading dose be divided, and what would be an appropriate interval between doses?**

Loading doses of digoxin are almost always administered in divided doses so that the patient can be evaluated for toxicity and efficacy in the course of receiving the total loading dose. If the patient appears to develop toxicity or is therapeutically controlled, the remainder of the calculated loading dose is withheld. The usual procedure is to give one-half of the calculated loading dose initially, followed by one-fourth in six hours; the remaining fourth is administered six hours after the second dose.

Six hours is the usual interval between doses since it is the approximate time required for digoxin to be absorbed and distributed to the myocardium.[13] Even following an intravenous (IV) injection, two to four hours are required for a single dose of digoxin to exhibit its full effect.[12] In an emergency, clinical decisions about efficacy/toxicity can be made one to two hours following an IV dose. This is because the majority of digoxin will have been distributed into the tissue compartment and ≈75% to 90% of the pharmacologic effect can be evaluated at this time. It will still be too soon, however, to evaluate plasma concentrations due to the distribution phase. (See Figure 4.1 and Part I: Loading Dose on page 18.)

Question #3. **Assume the patient in Question 1 is R.J., a 50-year-old male with a serum creatinine of 1.0 mg/dL. Calculate a maintenance dose that will achieve an average plasma digoxin concentration of 1.5 µg/L.**

Since the objective is to achieve an average digoxin concentration of 1.5 µg/L at steady state (Cpss ave), Equation 16 can be used to calculate the maintenance dose:

$$\text{Maintenance Dose} = \frac{(\text{Cl})(\text{Cpss ave})(\tau)}{(\text{S})(\text{F})}$$

Assuming the dosing interval (τ) to be one day, the bioavailability (F) to be 0.7 for oral tablets, and the fraction of the dose which is digoxin (S) to be 1.0, the clearance (Cl) is the only remaining parameter to be calculated.

The clearance for R.J. can be determined by use of Equation 4.4:

$$\frac{\text{Total Cl Digoxin (mL/min)}}{\text{(Patients with CHF)}} = (0.33 \text{ mL/kg/min})(\text{wt in kg}) + (0.9)(\text{Cl}_{\text{Cr}} \text{ as mL/min})$$

Although the creatinine clearance (Cl_{Cr}) for R.J. is unknown, it can be estimated easily from his serum creatinine by use of Equation 63, assuming all the criteria for the use of this formula are met (i.e., serum creatinine is at steady state, and R.J.'s muscle mass is average for a 50-year-old male):

$$\frac{Cl_{Cr} \text{ for Males}}{(\text{mL/min})} = \frac{(140 - \text{Age})(\text{Weight})}{(72)(SrCr_{ss})}$$

$$= \frac{(140 - 50)\ (70)}{(72)\ (1.0)}$$

$$= 87.5 \text{ mL/min}$$

This creatinine clearance can now be used to estimate R.J.'s total digoxin clearance:

$$\frac{\text{Total Cl Digoxin (mL/min)}}{(\text{Patients with CHF})} = (0.33 \text{ mL/kg/min})(\text{wt in kg}) + (0.9)(Cl_{Cr} \text{ as mL/min})$$

$$= (0.33 \text{ mL/kg/min})(70 \text{ kg}) + (0.9)(87.5 \text{ mL/min})$$

$$= 23.1 \text{ mL/min} + 78.8 \text{ mL/min}$$

$$= 101.9 \text{ mL/min}$$

The digoxin clearance can be used to calculate the maintenance dose in ng/min, but a maintenance dose stated in µg/day is more practical. The clearance in mL/min can be converted to L/day by multiplying the value by the number of minutes per day (1440 min/day) and dividing by the number of milliliters per liter (1000 mL/L):

$$Cl \text{ (L/day)} = \frac{(Cl \text{ as mL/min})(1440 \text{ min/day})}{1000 \text{ mL/L}}$$

Eq. 4.5

$$= \frac{(101.9 \text{ mL/min})(1440 \text{ min/day})}{1000 \text{ mL/L}}$$

$$= 146.7 \text{ L/day}$$

The maintenance dose can now be calculated using Equation 16:

$$\text{Maintenance Dose} = \frac{(Cl)(Cpss\ ave)(\tau)}{(S)(F)}$$

$$= \frac{(146.7\ L/day)(1.5\ \mu g/L)(1\ day)}{(1.0)(0.7)}$$

$$= \frac{220\ \mu g}{0.7}$$

$$= 314.4\ \mu g$$

$$= 0.3144\ mg$$

One could elect to give either 0.25 or 0.375 mg/day since these are the most convenient dosage forms. Another solution is to give 0.25 and 0.375 mg on alternate days for an average dose of 0.312 mg/day.

Question #4. If the patient in Question 1 had had a serum creatinine of 5 mg/dL, would the estimated loading dose have been different?

For a number of years it was assumed that renal function influenced only the clearance of digoxin. A number of studies have indicated, however, that patients with decreased creatinine clearance also have a decreased volume of distribution for digoxin.[10,15,18]

The relationship between volume of distribution (Vd), plasma concentration (Cp), and amount of drug in the body (Ab) is described by Equation 10:

$$Vd = \frac{Ab}{Cp}$$

In uremic patients, it is assumed that digoxin is displaced from the tissue compartment. As a result, Cp is higher and Vd is smaller.

$$\downarrow Vd = \frac{Ab}{\uparrow Cp}$$

There is some controversy about the significance of this tissue displacement of digoxin. Myocardial digoxin concentrations at any given plasma digoxin level are lower relative to their non-uremic counterparts.[19] Consequently, some have suggested that no change in the loading dose is necessary.[20] Although there is no direct evidence supporting a reduction in the loading dose of digoxin in uremic individuals, elevated plasma concentrations of digoxin are associated with increased toxicity. Thus, the loading dose should be reduced in uremic patients.

Since very little digoxin is bound to plasma proteins ($\approx$30%), a change in the desired therapeutic plasma concentration is unlikely to result from plasma protein displacement.[21] (See Part I: Desired Plasma Concentration (Cp) on page 9.)

There are a number of ways to estimate the volume of distribution for digoxin in a patient with decreased renal function; Equations 4.1 and 4.2 are the most commonly used:

$$\text{Vd Digoxin (L/70 kg)} = 226 + \frac{(298)(\text{Cl}_{\text{Cr}} \text{ mL/min/70 kg})}{29 + \text{Cl}_{\text{Cr}} \text{ mL/min/70 kg}}$$

$$\text{Vd Digoxin (L)} = (3.8 \text{ L/kg})(\text{Weight in kg}) + (3.1)(\text{Cl}_{\text{Cr}} \text{ as mL/min})$$

The first of these equations is adjusted for a 70 kg person and, therefore, requires that the creatinine clearance (Cl_{Cr}) be expressed as mL/min/70 kg. If the patient is smaller or larger than 70 kg, the volume of distribution can be adjusted in proportion to the patient's body size. The second equation is for a specific patient; therefore, the estimated Cl_{Cr} should be expressed in mL/min for that patient. The volume of distribution for digoxin in uremic patients can vary considerably. For this reason, the values obtained from these equations, and the calculated loading dose, should be considered only rough estimates.

Using Equation 63 the patient's creatinine clearance is determined to be approximately 20 mL/min:

$$\begin{aligned}
\frac{\text{Cl}_{\text{Cr}} \text{ for Males}}{(\text{mL/min})} &= \frac{(140 - \text{Age})(\text{Weight})}{(72)(\text{SrCr}_{\text{ss}})} \\
&= \frac{(140 - 50)(70)}{(72)(5)} \\
&= 17.5 \text{ mL/min } or \approx 20 \text{ mL/min}
\end{aligned}$$

Using this value in Equations 4.1 and 4.2, the estimated volumes of distribution would be 347.6 L and 328 L, respectively:

$$\text{Vd Digoxin (L/70 kg)} = 226 + \frac{(298)(Cl_{Cr} \text{ as mL/min/70 kg})}{29 + Cl_{C_t} \text{ as mL/min/70 kg}}$$

$$= 226 + \frac{298(20)}{29 + 20}$$

$$= 226 + \frac{5960}{49}$$

$$= 347.6 \text{ L}$$

Since this patient weighs 70 kg, the Cl_{Cr} calculated from Equation 63 can be used directly. If the patient had not been 70 kg, the Cl_{Cr} would need to be adjusted. The Vd then generated from Equation 4.1 would represent that expected for a 70 kg person and would have to be adjusted for the patient's actual weight. Equation 4.2 takes into account the patient's actual weight:

$$\text{Vd Digoxin (L)} = (3.8 \text{ L/kg})(\text{wt in kg}) + (3.1)(Cl_{Cr} \text{ as mL/min})$$

$$= (3.8 \text{ L/kg})(70 \text{ kg}) + (3.1)(20 \text{ mL/min})$$

$$= 266 + 62$$

$$= 328 \text{ L}$$

Since both of these approaches give similar estimates, either could be used. Equation 4.2 appears to be useful over a wider range of creatinine clearance values, especially when the creatinine clearance is >100 mL/min/70 kg.[22]

If the volume of distribution is assumed to be about 330 L (as calculated from Equation 4.2), the estimated oral loading dose using Equation 11 would be approximately 750 µg:

$$\text{Loading Dose} = \frac{(\text{Vd})(\text{Cp})}{(\text{S})(\text{F})}$$

$$= \frac{(330 \text{ L})(1.5 \text{ µg/L})}{(1.0)(0.7)}$$

$$= \frac{495 \text{ µg}}{0.7}$$

$$= 707 \text{ µg } (0.707 \text{ mg}) \text{ } or \approx 750 \text{ µg}$$

Again, as in Question 1, S and F are assumed to be 1.0 and 0.7, respectively. The total loading dose should be divided and administered as described in Question 2 in case the Vd is much smaller than anticipated or the patient is more sensitive to the pharmacologic effects than expected. The Vd also may be much larger than expected, and additional doses may have to be administered in order to achieve the desired plasma concentration or pharmacologic effect.

Question #5. Estimate the daily dose that would maintain the average digoxin concentration at 1.5 µg/L in this same 70 kg, 50-year-old patient with a serum creatinine of 5.0 mg/dL.

As in Question 3, Equation 16 would be used to estimate the maintenance dose:

$$\text{Maintenance Dose} = \frac{(Cl)(Cpss\ ave)(\tau)}{(S)(F)}$$

Using the creatinine clearance estimate of 20 mL/min (see Question 4), the digoxin clearance can be estimated using Equation 4.4 (for CHF):

$$\begin{aligned}
\text{Total Cl Digoxin (mL/min)} &= (0.33\ \text{mL/kg/min})(\text{wt in kg}) + (0.9)(Cl_{Cr}\ \text{as mL/min}) \\
\text{(Patients with CHF)} \\
&= (0.33\ \text{mL/kg/min})(70) + (0.9)(20\ \text{mL/min}) \\
&= 23.1\ \text{mL/min} + 18\ \text{mL/min} \\
&= 41.1\ \text{mL/min}
\end{aligned}$$

The digoxin clearance can be converted from mL/min to L/day as described in Question 3 using Equation 4.5:

$$\begin{aligned}
\text{Cl (L/day)} &= \frac{(\text{Cl as mL/min})(1440\ \text{min/day})}{1000\ \text{mL/L}} \\
&= \frac{(41.1\ \text{mL/min})(1440\ \text{min/day})}{1000\ \text{mL/L}} \\
&= 59.2\ \text{L/day}
\end{aligned}$$

Again, assuming S to be 1.0 and F to be 0.7 for digoxin tablets, the approximate daily dose (calculated using Equation 16) would be 125 µg/day or 0.125 mg/day:

$$\text{Maintenance Dose} = \frac{(\text{Cl})(\text{Cpss ave})(\tau)}{(\text{S})(\text{F})}$$

$$= \frac{(59.2 \text{ L/day})(1.5 \text{ µg/L})(1 \text{ day})}{(1.0)(0.7)}$$

$$= \frac{88.8 \text{ µg/day}}{0.7}$$

$$= 126.8 \text{ µg/day } or \approx 0.125 \text{ mg/day}$$

Question #6. **Assume that the patient described above can take nothing by mouth and must be converted to daily intravenous doses of digoxin. Calculate an intravenous dose equivalent to the 0.125 mg tablets he ingests daily.**

If the bioavailability of digoxin is assumed to be 0.7, the equivalent intravenous dose would be 0.0875 or 0.09 mg/day as calculated from Equations 1 and 2:

$$\begin{array}{l}\text{Amount of Drug Absorbed} \\ \text{or Reaching Systemic Circulation}\end{array} = (\text{F})(\text{Dose})$$

$$= (0.7)(0.125 \text{ mg})$$

$$= 0.0875 \text{ mg}$$

$$\begin{array}{l}\text{Dose of New} \\ \text{Dosage Form}\end{array} = \frac{\begin{array}{c}\text{Amount of Drug Absorbed} \\ \text{From Current Dosage Form}\end{array}}{\text{F of New Dosage Form}}$$

$$= \frac{0.0875}{1}$$

$$= 0.0875 \text{ mg } or \approx 0.09 \text{ mg}$$

If the dose is not adjusted to account for the increased bioavailability of the intravenous dose, higher steady-state digoxin concentrations would eventually be achieved. (See Part I: Figure 16 on page 40.)

Question #7. B.G., a 62-year-old, 50 kg female, was admitted to the hospital for possible digoxin toxicity. Her serum creatinine was 3.0 mg/dL and her dosing regimen at home had been 0.25 mg of digoxin daily for many months. The digoxin plasma concentration on admission was reported to be 4.0 µg/L. How long will it take for the digoxin concentration to fall from 4.0 to 2.0 µg/L?

The answer to this question requires a knowledge of the half-life ($t^{1/2}$) or the elimination rate constant (Kd), both of which are dependent upon the clearance and volume of distribution for digoxin in B.G. The relationship between these parameters is described by Equations 27 and 32:

$$Kd = \frac{Cl}{Vd}$$

$$t^{1/2} = \frac{(0.693)(Vd)}{Cl}$$

Three basic steps are required to solve this problem: 1) estimate clearance, 2) estimate the Vd, and 3) calculate the half-life.

Step 1. If one assumes that the digoxin half-life is longer than the dosing interval, the observed digoxin plasma concentration should closely reflect the average concentration at steady state (i.e., this level is relatively independent of the volume of distribution; see Part I: Elimination Rate Constant and Half-Life on page 37). Therefore, the observed digoxin concentration could be used in Equation 15 to estimate B.G's clearance:

$$Cl = \frac{(S)(F)(Dose/\tau)}{Cpss\ ave}$$

$$= \frac{(1.0)(0.7)(250\ \mu g/day)}{4.0\ \mu g/L}$$

$$= \frac{175\ \mu g/day}{4.0\ \mu g/L}$$

$$= 43.75\ L/day$$

This digoxin clearance of 43.75 L/day which was calculated from B.G's dosing history and observed plasma level is reasonably close to what would be expected for a 50 kg, 62-year-old female with a serum creatinine of 3.0 mg/dL.

One could also estimate digoxin clearance as illustrated in previous questions by first determining B.G.'s creatinine clearance through the use of Equation 64 for women:

$$\text{Cl}_{Cr} \text{ for Females (mL/min)} = (0.85) \frac{(140 - \text{Age})(\text{Weight})}{(72)(\text{SrCr}_{ss})}$$

$$= (0.85) \frac{(140 - 62)(50 \text{ kg})}{(72)(3.0 \text{ mg/dL})}$$

$$= (0.85) \frac{(78)(50 \text{ kg})}{(72)(3.0 \text{ mg/dL})}$$

$$= 15.3 \text{ mL/min}$$

This estimation of Cl_{Cr} then can be used to determine the digoxin clearance by use of Equation 4.4 (for CHF):

$$\text{Total Cl Digoxin (mL/min) (Patients with CHF)} = (0.33 \text{ mL/kg/min})(\text{wt in kg}) + (0.9)(\text{Cl}_{Cr} \text{ as mL/min})$$

$$= (0.33 \text{ mL/kg/min})(50 \text{ kg}) + (0.9)(15.3 \text{ mL/min})$$

$$= 16.5 \text{ mL/min} + 13.8 \text{ mL/min}$$

$$= 30.3 \text{ mL/min}$$

Expressed as L/day (Equation 4.5), the clearance would be:

$$\text{Cl (L/day)} = \frac{(\text{Cl as mL/min})(1440 \text{ min/day})}{1000 \text{ mL/L}}$$

$$= \frac{(30.3 \text{ mL/min})(1440 \text{ min/day})}{1000 \text{ mL/L}}$$

$$= 43.6 \text{ L/day}$$

This expected clearance of 43.6 L/day is very close to the apparent clearance of 43.75 L/day which was obtained from B.G.'s dosing history and observed plasma level of 4.0 µg/L. Had there been a substantial difference between the expected and apparent digoxin clearance, it would have been important to decide whether there was an error in the assumptions used in Equation 15 (see Question 9) or whether B.G. was substantially different from the average individual.

Step 2. B.G.'s digoxin volume of distribution can now be estimated using Equation 4.2 and her estimated creatinine clearance (15.3 mL/min):

$$
\begin{aligned}
\text{Vd Digoxin (L)} &= (3.8 \text{ L/kg})(\text{wt in kg}) + (3.1)(\text{Cl}_{cr} \text{ as mL/min}) \\
&= (3.8 \text{ L/kg})(50 \text{ kg}) + (3.1)(15.3 \text{ mL/min}) \\
&= 237 \text{ L}
\end{aligned}
$$

Step 3. The digoxin elimination rate constant and half-life for B.G. can now be estimated from Equations 27 and 32:

$$
\begin{aligned}
\text{Kd} &= \frac{\text{Cl}}{\text{Vd}} \\
&= \frac{43.6 \text{ L/day}}{237 \text{ L}} \\
&= 0.184 \text{ day}^{-1}
\end{aligned}
$$

$$
\begin{aligned}
\text{t}^{1/2} &= \frac{(0.693)(\text{Vd})}{\text{Cl}} \\
&= \frac{(0.693)(237 \text{ L})}{43.6 \text{ L/day}} \\
&= 3.8 \text{ days}
\end{aligned}
$$

We now have the data necessary to answer the original question. The time required for B.G.'s plasma concentration of digoxin to fall from 4.0 to 2.0 µg/L (one-half the original level) is one half-life, or 3.8 days.

In most situations the arithmetic is not this easy. In such cases the Kd and a rearrangement of Equation 28 can be used to determine the time required for the plasma concentration to fall to a predetermined level. (See Part I: Elimination Rate Constant on page 41.)

$$Kd = \frac{\ln\left(\dfrac{Cp_1}{Cp_2}\right)}{t}$$

$$t = \frac{\ln\left(\dfrac{Cp_1}{Cp_2}\right)}{Kd}$$

Eq. 4.6

$$= \frac{\ln\left(\dfrac{4.0 \ \mu g/L}{2.0 \ \mu g/L}\right)}{0.184 \ days^{-1}}$$

$$= \frac{\ln(2)}{0.184 \ days^{-1}}$$

$$= 3.8 \ days$$

Question #8. **Calculate a daily dose which will maintain B.G.'s average digoxin plasma concentration at 2.0 µg/L.**

Using the clearance value of 43.6 L/day calculated from B.G.'s data, and assuming S, F, and τ to be 1.0, 0.7, and 1 day, respectively, the new maintenance dose can be estimated using Equation 16:

$$\text{Maintenance Dose} = \frac{(Cl)(Cpss \ ave)(\tau)}{(S)(F)}$$

$$= \frac{(43.6 \ L/day)(2.0 \ \mu g/L)(1 \ day)}{(1.0)(0.7)}$$

$$= \frac{87.2 \ \mu g/day}{0.7}$$

$$= 125 \ \mu g/day \ (0.125 \ mg/day)$$

Alternatively, the previous maintenance dose could be adjusted proportionately to the desired change in steady-state plasma level because clearance and other factors were assumed to be constant. Therefore, if the new steady-state level is to be one-half of the previous value, the new maintenance dose should be one-half the previous maintenance dose.

Question #9. R.N., a female who has been on the same dose of digoxin for 15 days, is seen in the clinic and is found to be doing well clinically. A digoxin plasma level drawn on the morning of her visit is reported as 3.4 μg/L (the upper limit for therapeutic levels is 2.0 μg/L). What are the possible explanations for this elevated serum digoxin concentration?

Since this serum digoxin concentration theoretically represents an average steady-state concentration (Cpss ave), one must evaluate each of the factors that could alter steady state. The relationship of each of these factors to steady state may be seen by studying Equation 35:

$$\text{Cpss ave} = \frac{(S)(F)(\text{Dose}/\tau)}{Cl}$$

a) (S)(F). R.N. may be absorbing more than 70% (average bioavailability) from the oral dosage form. Since there are no salt forms of digoxin, S should be 1.0.

b) Dose. R.N. may be taking more than the prescribed dose, although taking less than the prescribed dose is more common.[4,23]

c) τ. R.N. may be taking the proper dose more often than prescribed.

d) Cl. R.N.'s clearance or ability to eliminate the drug may be less than it was estimated to be.

e) Cpss ave. The assay could be in error. Interfering substances may be present or the plasma level may have been drawn during the distribution phase of the drug.

Plasma levels obtained during the distribution phase of digoxin are higher than anticipated because the drug is absorbed from the gastrointestinal tract faster than it is distributed into the tissues. Since the myocardium responds to digoxin as though it were in the tissue compartment (Vt), plasma levels obtained before distribution is complete do not correlate with pharmacologic effects of the drug.[4,13] Digoxin plasma levels should be obtained just before the next dose is given, or at least six hours after the oral digoxin dose.[13] (See the discussion on Digoxin Volume of Distribution and Time to Sample on pages 198 and 203, respectively.)

Question #10. Outline a reasonable plan to determine the cause of R.N.'s higher-than-predicted digoxin level.

a) Ask R.N. whether the daily digoxin dose was taken before or after the blood sample was obtained.

b) Determine R.N.'s compliance. This is difficult but must be attempted through a pill count or history.

c) Determine if any drugs interfered with the digoxin assay. Literature reports of interference by drugs having a steroid nucleus similar to that of digoxin are applicable only to the antibody assay used in the particular report and may not apply to the assay used to determine R.N.'s digoxin plasma level. Therefore, the laboratory measuring the serum level would have to be contacted about the possibility of assay interference.[17,24,25]

Patients with poor renal function and newborn infants accumulate an endogenous digoxin-like compound that can produce a falsely-elevated or false-positive digoxin assay result. The usual range of the false-positive reaction is from 0.1 to >1 µg/L,[26–28] with an average of $\approx$0.1 to 0.4 µg/L. This interference does not appear to represent a cross-reactivity with digoxin metabolites since it has been observed in patients who have never received digoxin. The assay interference in these patients with apparent renal dysfunction is assay-specific and is much more significant for some assays than for others.[27,29]

d) Radioisotopes, such as those used in nuclear medicine, can also influence radioimmunoassays.[17] R.N.'s records should be reviewed for any recent diagnostic studies such as a thyroid scan or cardiac studies that may have involved radioisotopes. Radioisotopes may cause a falsely-elevated or -depressed concentration depending on how the assay is performed. Although radioimmunoassays are seldom used in clinical practice, the laboratory would have to be consulted to determine if contamination with radioisotopes is a possibility.

e) Re-schedule a second digoxin plasma level, but be certain that it is drawn at least six hours after a dose. Preferably, obtain the sample in the morning before the daily dose is taken.

f) Evaluating R.N.'s Cl and F is difficult and costly because such evaluation would require hospitalization. Furthermore, it would only result in the obvious conclusion that the dose should be reduced if, in fact, the dosage level was too high. This approach would only be used under the most unusual circumstances. In addition, F could only increase from the assumed 0.7 to a maximum of 1.0 and could not, by itself, account for the observed elevation in Cpss ave.

Question #11. T.S., a female receiving digoxin 0.375 mg/day for several months, has a reported digoxin plasma concentration of 0.3 µg/L. Her CHF is poorly controlled. What is the most probable explanation?

The answer to this question is essentially the same as that to Question 9; the same factors should be considered. T.S. should be asked if she is receiving the same brand or dosage form of digoxin since bioavailability may vary between products. T.S. also could be one of the very rare patients who has a large metabolic and renal clearance for digoxin.[30] The most likely explanation for the subtherapeutic digoxin concentrations is noncompliance with the prescribed regimen.[23]

Question #12. In 1966, Doherty and Perkins[31] evaluated the pharmacokinetics of digoxin in hyperthyroid, hypothyroid, and euthyroid patients. Figure 4.2 is a representation of one of the graphs from this study. Using the graph, discuss the implications of thyroid disease on the loading dose, maintenance dose, and the time required to reach steady state relative to the euthyroid state. Assume that the same Cpss ave is desired in all patients.

Figure 4.2. Digoxin and Thyroid Function. Note the distribution and elimination of digoxin when administered by the intravenous route to hypothyroid, hyperthyroid, and euthyroid patients.[31]

Loading Dose. Since hypothyroid patients have higher plasma levels following a single loading dose, they must have a decreased apparent volume of distribution. Therefore, a decrease in the loading dose would be appropriate. Hyperthyroid patients have lower plasma levels and would require larger loading doses for the same reasons.

Time To Reach Steady State. The slope of all the decay curves is the same. Therefore, the half-lives and elimination rate constants are equal, and the time required to reach steady state will be the same for hyperthyroid, hypothyroid, and euthyroid patients receiving digoxin.

Maintenance Dose. Since Kd is the same in all patients, the clearance and volume of distribution must both change by the same proportion and in the same direction. (See Equation 27.)

$$\text{Kd (Same in All Patients Studied)} = \frac{\text{Cl(Variable)}}{\text{Vd(Variable)}}$$

Hypothyroid patients must have a decreased clearance, since the volume of distribution is decreased. This reduction in Cl would necessitate a reduction in maintenance doses. Hyperthyroid patients must have an increased clearance since the Vd is increased; therefore, an increase in maintenance dose would be indicated if Cpss ave is to remain the same as that used for euthyroid patients.

It is important to re-emphasize, however, that although Kd and Vd were used to estimate clearance, Vd is an independent variable which, like Clearance, is affected by thyroid disease. Since both Cl and Vd were affected in the same direction and to the same degree, the half-life (and Kd) did not change.

Two other studies[32,33] have examined the pharmacokinetics of digoxin in patients with thyroid disease. Both of these suggest that the changes in the digoxin clearance result from an increased glomerular filtration rate associated with hyperthyroidism. If this increased renal function *is* the primary factor responsible for the altered digoxin clearance observed in hyperthyroid patients, it would be possible to encounter such patients with *decreased* digoxin clearance if they also had intrinsic renal failure.

Question #13. Do patients receiving hemodialysis require additional digoxin following dialysis?

No. The dialysis clearance for digoxin is only 10 mL/min. Therefore, <3% of the total amount of drug in the body is removed during hemodialysis.[34] This dialysis clearance of 10 mL/min may seem significant when compared to the metabolic clearance of 23 mL/min/70 kg for patients with CHF,[15] but the dialysis takes place for only four to six hours every few days, while the metabolic clearance is continuous.

Dialysis, however, can induce digitalis toxicity by altering serum electrolyte concentrations and acid-base balance. For example, a high serum potassium which is protecting a patient from digitalis toxicity may be decreased during dialysis, resulting in signs of toxicity during or just following dialysis.

Question #14. V.B., a patient receiving digoxin 0.25 mg/day for atrial fibrillation, is about to be started on quinidine. What are the considerations?

Patients receiving digoxin have a rapid and sustained rise in the serum digoxin concentration following the addition of quinidine.[35,36] (See Figure 4.3, line B.) This rapid rise in digoxin within the first 24 hours apparently results from the displacement of digoxin by quinidine from tissue sites. The increased digoxin concentration reflects a decrease in digoxin's volume of distribution to 70% of the original value. The initial rise in digoxin concentrations to approximately 1.5 times the original concentration is followed by a relatively slow accumulation over the next week to a steady-state digoxin concentration that is approximately double the original value.[35,37] Many patients develop signs of digitalis toxicity (primarily gastrointestinal in nature) which subside when the dose and plasma concentrations of digoxin are adjusted.[35]

The rapid and sustained changes in digoxin concentrations (see Figure 4.3) suggest that the initial change in digoxin concentration is due to a decline in the volume of distribution which is slightly smaller than the decline in the clearance. This is illus-

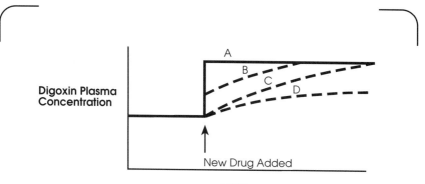

Figure 4.3. Digoxin. Figure 4.3 represents the anticipated changes in digoxin concentration following ↑ the initiation of an interacting agent. The solid line A represents the effect of a drug which changes the volume of distribution in proportion to the decrease in the digoxin clearance. Broken line B represents the effect of a drug which produces a decrease in volume of distribution that is less than proportional to the decrease in digoxin clearance (e.g., quinidine). Line C represents the effect of a drug which decreases the digoxin clearance to approximately the same extent as quinidine, but produces no apparent change in the volume of distribution (e.g., amiodarone). Line D represents the effect of a drug which decreases digoxin clearance to a lesser extent than that observed with quinidine (e.g., verapamil).

trated by the gradual rise in the serum concentration of digoxin to the final steady-state value which follows the initial rapid increase in serum digoxin concentration.

Patients receiving digoxin who are to begin quinidine therapy should be monitored very closely for the first 24 hours and subsequent 7 to 14 days following the addition of quinidine. It may even be appropriate to empirically skip a single day's dose of digoxin and then to resume a maintenance digoxin dose which is one-half of the original dose.[38–40] Although the significance of these elevated digoxin concentrations has been debated, these levels represent potentially toxic concentrations and should generally be avoided unless there is clear indication that the increased digoxin levels are warranted.[41–43]

Digoxin concentrations also may vary within a quinidine dosing interval because of varying degrees of tissue displacement. This has been demonstrated at relatively low quinidine concentrations and should be considered when obtaining digoxin plasma levels. For this reason it is generally advisable to obtain plasma digoxin concentrations just before a quinidine dose so that the digoxin plasma levels will at least be reasonably reproducible. Any change in digoxin concentration sampled in this way should represent actual changes in digoxin disposition rather than transient changes within a quinidine dosing interval.[39] (See Figure 4.4.)

Procainamide does not appear to interact with digoxin and might be considered as an alternative to quinidine. This choice might be most rational when patients require relatively high digoxin concentrations. For example, adding quinidine to a patient with a digoxin level of $\approx 1\ \mu g/L$ would be approached with less concern than adding quinidine to the therapy of a patient with a digoxin concentration of $2\ \mu g/L$ or higher. In some cases, it might even be argued that the initial low digoxin levels could be made therapeutic by the addition of a displacing agent. In contrast, the potential hazards of digitalis toxicity are increased in those patients with initially elevated digoxin levels.

Question #15. **What other drugs commonly used in patients receiving digoxin are likely to cause a marked change in its disposition?**

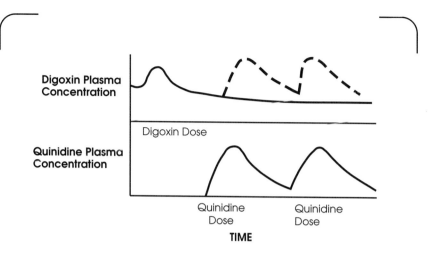

Figure 4.4. Displacement of Digoxin by Quinidine. The digoxin plasma concentration with no quinidine (—) and following the administration of two quinidine doses (- - -). Note that as the quinidine plasma concentrations rise and then fall, the digoxin levels also rise and then fall. The elevation of digoxin levels appears to be minimal at quinidine levels below 1 mg/L.[39]

Quinidine is clearly the most significant drug that interacts with digoxin.[44,45] However, other compounds, such as verapamil, also reduce digoxin clearance by about 30%.[45,46] Although this change is not remarkable, there may be individual patients in whom a modest reduction in the digoxin maintenance dose is warranted. Broken line D in Figure 4.3 depicts the anticipated rise in digoxin concentration following the institution of verapamil therapy. Note that the slow rise in digoxin concentration suggests that the volume of distribution for digoxin is not altered. The clearance, while reduced, is not reduced to the same extent as that associated with concomitant quinidine therapy; this is consistent with the smaller increase in steady-state digoxin concentrations associated with verapamil. Nifedipine and diltiazem appear to have relatively little influence on digoxin disposition; verapamil has modest effects.

Amiodarone appears to increase the digoxin concentration significantly. The average rise in digoxin appears to be similar to that observed with quinidine; however, as with verapamil, the change appears to be related primarily to a decreased clearance rather than a change in volume of distribution. This last conclusion is a little more tenuous because the accumulation of quinidine to steady state occurs within a few hours after starting therapy, but accumulation to steady state for amiodarone is likely to take several months (t½ ≈30 days). In the case of both amiodarone[47] and verapamil, if a reduction in digoxin dose is contemplated, it is not necessary to skip a daily dose. Instead, the maintenance regimen should be reduced by the appropriate amount at about the time the amiodarone or verapamil therapy is instituted.

Question #16. **A.P., a 75-year-old, 60 kg male, was admitted with complaints of increased shortness of breath (SOB) and yellow sputum production. He has a previous medical history of chronic obstructive airways disease (COAD) and CHF. During his hospital stay, he developed atrial fibrillation and was given digoxin to slow his ventricular rate. He received 250 µg IV Q 3 hr × 3 doses (starting at 9:00 p.m.) and was placed on a maintenance dose of 250 µg tablets each morning at 9:00 a.m. starting the morning after the loading dose. His serum creatinine is stable at 1.5 mg/dL. A digoxin level obtained at 9:00 a.m. on the morning of Day 4 (2.5 days after the loading dose) was reported to be 1.5 µg/L. A.P. had therefore received his initial IV loading dose and two oral maintenance doses when a plasma sample was drawn on the morning of Day 4. What would you expect his digoxin concentration to be?**

In order to calculate the expected concentration, just before the third maintenance dose, one would first need to calculate A.P.'s expected digoxin pharmacokinetic parameters. Using Equation 63 for Cl_{Cr}, Equation 4.2 for digoxin Vd, and Equation 4.4 for the digoxin clearance, the corresponding values can be obtained.

$$\frac{Cl_{Cr} \text{ for Males}}{(mL/min)} = \frac{(140 - Age)(Weight)}{(72)(SrCr_{ss})}$$

$$= \frac{(140 - 75)(60 \text{ kg})}{(72)(1.5)}$$

$$= 36.1 \text{ mL/min}$$

$$\text{Vd Digoxin (L)} = (3.8 \text{ L/kg})(\text{Weight in kg}) + (3.1)(\text{Cl}_{Cr} \text{ as mL/min})$$

$$= (3.8 \text{ L/kg})(60 \text{ kg}) + (3.1)(36.1)$$

$$= 228 \text{ L} + 111.9 \text{ L}$$

$$= 339.9 \text{ L}$$

$$\begin{array}{l} \text{Total Cl Digoxin (mL/min)} \\ \text{(Patients with CHF)} \end{array} = (0.33 \text{ mL/kg/min})(\text{Wt in kg}) + (0.9)(\text{Cl}_{Cr} \text{ as mL/min})$$

$$= (0.33 \text{ mL/kg/min})(60 \text{ kg}) + (0.9)(36.1 \text{ mL/min})$$

$$= 19.8 \text{ mL/min} + 32.5 \text{ mL/min}$$

$$= 52.3 \text{ mL/min}$$

$$\text{Cl (L/day)} = \frac{(\text{Cl as mL/min})(1440 \text{ min/day})}{1000 \text{ mL/L}}$$

$$= \frac{(52.3 \text{ mL/min})(1440 \text{ min/day})}{1000 \text{ mL/L}}$$

$$= 75.3 \text{ L/day}$$

$$\text{Kd} = \frac{\text{Cl}}{\text{Vd}}$$

$$= \frac{75.3 \text{ L/day}}{339.9 \text{ L}}$$

$$= 0.22 \text{ days}^{-1}$$

$$t\frac{1}{2} = \frac{0.693}{\text{Kd}}$$

$$= \frac{0.693}{0.22 \text{ days}^{-1}}$$

$$= 3.15 \text{ days}$$

To calculate A.P.'s digoxin plasma concentration, one needs to consider the loading dose plus the two maintenance doses. To model this series of doses, refer to Part I, Figure 27 on page 67, where the loading dose plus the two maintenance doses are depicted as D_1, D_2, and D_3. Because his loading dose was given over a total of six hours, and A.P.'s expected digoxin half-life is

3.15 days, one can group the entire loading dose together as though it were administered as a single dose [i.e., time (t_{in}) from start to end of loading is $\leq \frac{1}{6}\ t\frac{1}{2}$].

$$Cp_{(Sum)} = \frac{(S)(F)(D_1)}{Vd}(e^{-Kdt_1}) + \frac{(S)(F)(D_2)}{Vd}(e^{-Kdt_2}) + \frac{(S)(F)(D_3)}{Vd}(e^{-Kdt_3})$$

$$= \frac{(1)(1)(750\ \mu g)}{339.9\ L}(e^{-(0.22)(2.5\ days)}) + \frac{(1)(0.7)(250\ \mu g)}{339.9\ L}(e^{-(0.22)(2\ days)})$$

$$+ \frac{(1)(0.7)(250\ \mu g)}{339.9\ L}(e^{-(0.22)(1\ day)})$$

$$= (2.2\ \mu g/L)(0.58) + (0.51\ \mu g/L)(0.64) + (0.51\ \mu g/L)(0.80)$$

$$= 1.3\ \mu g/L + 0.33\ \mu g/L + 0.41\ \mu g/L$$

$$= 2.0\ \mu g/L$$

Note that the predicted digoxin concentration of 2.0 µg/L is greater than the observed value of 1.5 µg/L. Unfortunately, revision of pharmacokinetic parameters at this point would be difficult. After only 2.5 days, it is relatively easy to see that we have gone beyond one-third of the half-life since the loading dose was administered. This precludes the possibility of accurately extracting information about volume of distribution. Furthermore, A.P.'s maintenance dose has not been administered longer than two half-lives, which limits one's ability to extract information about clearance. The observed plasma concentration may reflect a larger-than-expected Vd, a higher-than-expected Cl, or some combination of both of these factors. To more accurately determine A.P.'s digoxin clearance, it will be necessary to wait several more days to obtain a plasma concentration that might reasonably be expected to yield information about clearance. Given his expected half-life of approximately three days, and the probability that his half-life is less than expected, an additional two or three days would probably be sufficient to begin to get information that will more accurately predict A.P.'s final steady-state concentration.

Question #17. C.A. is a 60-year-old, 65 kg male with a serum creatinine of 1.3 mg/dL. He had been taking 0.25 mg of digoxin orally for his CHF, and at 9:00 a.m. on the day of admission, a digoxin level of 0.8 µg/L was measured. He was continued on his outpatient maintenance dose. On the fifth day, just before his morning dose (four doses of digoxin having been administered each day at 9:00 a.m.), a second digoxin sample was obtained. Using the expected pharmacokinetic parameters, calculate C.A.'s digoxin concentration on the morning of the fifth day.

Again, in order to calculate the expected plasma concentration, one would first have to estimate C.A.'s creatinine clearance and then use the appropriate equations to calculate his volume of distribution, clearance, and elimination rate constant.

$$\frac{Cl_{Cr} \text{ for Males}}{(mL/min)} = \frac{(140 - \text{Age})(\text{Weight})}{(72)(\text{SrCr}_{ss})}$$

$$= \frac{(140 - 60)(65 \text{ kg})}{(72)(1.3)}$$

$$= 55.6 \text{ mL/min}$$

$$Vd \text{ Digoxin (L)} = (3.8 \text{ L/kg})(\text{Weight in kg}) + (3.1)(Cl_{Cr} \text{ as mL/min})$$

$$= (3.8 \text{ L/kg})(65 \text{ kg}) + (3.1)(55.6)$$

$$= 247 \text{ L} + 172.4 \text{ L}$$

$$= 419.4 \text{ L}$$

$$\frac{\text{Total Cl Digoxin (mL/min)}}{(\text{Patients with CHF})} = (0.33 \text{ mL/kg/min})(\text{Weight in kg}) + (0.9)(Cl_{Cr} \text{ as mL/min})$$

$$= (0.33 \text{ mL/kg/min})(65 \text{ kg}) + (0.9)(55.6 \text{ mL/min})$$

$$= 21.5 \text{ mL/min} + 50 \text{ mL/min}$$

$$= 71.5 \text{ mL/min}$$

$$\text{Cl (L/day)} = \frac{(\text{Cl as mL/min})(1440 \text{ min/day})}{1000 \text{ mL/L}}$$

$$= \frac{(71.5 \text{ mL/min})(1440 \text{ min/day})}{1000 \text{ mL/L}}$$

$$= 103 \text{ L/day}$$

$$Kd = \frac{Cl}{Vd}$$

$$= \frac{103 \text{ L/day}}{419.4 \text{ L}}$$

$$= 0.25 \text{ days}^{-1}$$

$$t\frac{1}{2} = \frac{0.693}{Kd}$$

$$= \frac{0.693}{0.25 \text{ days}^{-1}}$$

$$= 2.8 \text{ days}$$

In order to model the initial digoxin concentration decay and the four subsequent doses, several approaches could be used. One approach is to use Equation 26 to model the initial digoxin concentration and subsequent decay:

$$Cp = (Cp^{\circ})(e^{-Kdt})$$

The four subsequent doses decayed for the appropriate amount of time could be modeled by modifying Equation 50 to represent each individual maintenance dose rather than a loading dose.

$$Cp_1 = \frac{(S)(F)(\text{Loading Dose})}{Vd}(e^{-Kdt_1})$$

In the above equation, the loading dose would be replaced by the 250 µg dose of digoxin and t_1 would be replaced by the time interval between each of the doses and the time the second digoxin sample was obtained (i.e. one, two, three, and four days). When Equation 26 and the series from Equation 50 are combined, the equation would appear as follows and is similar to the model depicted in Part I: Figure 27 on page 67.

$$Cp_{(Sum)} = (0.8\ \mu g/L)(e^{-(0.25)(4\ days)}) + \frac{(1)(0.7)(250\ \mu g)}{419.4\ L}(e^{-(0.25)(4\ days)})$$

$$+ \frac{(1)(0.7)(250\ \mu g)}{419.4\ L}(e^{-(0.25)(3\ days)})$$

$$+ \frac{(1)(0.7)(250\ \mu g)}{419.4\ L}(e^{-(0.25)(2\ days)})$$

$$+ \frac{(1)(0.7)(250\ \mu g)}{419.4\ L}(e^{-(0.25)(1\ day)})$$

Note that because each of the four digoxin doses was the same, it is possible to factor out the dose portion and simplify the equation as follows, with the final predicted concentration of digoxin being $\approx 1.2\ \mu g/L$.

$$Cp_{(Sum)} = (0.8\ \mu g/L)(e^{-(0.25)(4\ days)})$$

$$+ \frac{(1)(0.7)(250\ \mu g)}{419.4\ L}[(e^{-(0.25)(4\ days)}) + (e^{-(0.25)(3\ days)})$$

$$+ (e^{-(0.25)(2\ days)}) + (e^{-(0.25)(1\ day)})]$$

$$= (0.8\ \mu g/L)(0.37) + (0.42\ \mu g/L)[(0.37) + (0.47) + (0.61) + (0.78)]$$

$$= (0.3\ \mu g/L) + (0.42\ \mu g/L)[2.23]$$

$$= (0.3\ \mu g/L) + (0.94\ \mu g/L)$$

$$= 1.24\ \mu g/L$$

An alternative approach is to use a model that takes advantage of digoxin's relatively long half-life and short dosing interval. In this model, one could choose to decay the initial digoxin plasma concentration using Equation 26 and then treat the four individual doses as a continuous infusion as depicted in Equation 37.

$$Cp = (Cp^{\circ})(e^{-Kdt}) + \frac{(S)(F)(Dose/\tau)}{Cl}(1 - e^{-Kdt_1})$$

It is important to choose the appropriate t_1 so that the duration of the infusion is consistent with the rate of administration and the total number of doses given. In this case, t_1 would be four days since four 250 μg doses of digoxin have been administered.

Using the appropriate doses, times, and pharmacokinetic parameters, a digoxin concentration of 1.37 μg/L is calculated.

$$Cp = (0.8\ \mu g/L)(e^{-(0.25)(4\ days)}) + \left[\frac{(1)(0.7)(250\ \mu g/day)}{103\ L/day}(1 - e^{-(0.25)(4\ days)}) \right]$$

$$= (0.8\ \mu g/L)(0.37) + [(1.7\ \mu g/L)(1 - 0.37)]$$

$$= (0.30\ \mu g/L) + (1.07\ \mu g/L)$$

$$= 1.37\ \mu g/L$$

The concentration predicted by the first method (individual bolus doses) and the second method (digoxin given as an infusion) are similar, indicating that either method is a reasonable way to predict C.A.'s digoxin concentration on the morning of the fifth day. Also note that the predicted steady-state concentration produced by a maintenance dose of 0.25 mg/day (250 μg/day) would be ≈1.7 μg/L.

Question #18. **C.A.'s digoxin level reported from the laboratory was 1.6 μg/L. Since the observed digoxin concentration is greater than the predicted level (1.2 to 1.3 μg/L), what would one expect C.A.'s digoxin clearance and subsequent steady-state digoxin concentration to be on his current regimen of 0.25 mg/day?**

Either of the two approaches in the previous question can be used to resolve this problem. Clearance could be calculated by assuming C.A.'s digoxin volume of distribution to be 419.4 L. Then, using a trial and error method or iterative search, one could substitute various clearance values and the corresponding elimination rate constant values until the equation predicted the observed digoxin concentration of 1.6 μg/L. Since this process could be laborious, an alternative approach is to use the mass balance technique (using Equation 58) and solve directly for C.A.'s clearance. The expected steady-state digoxin concentration for C.A. could then be easily calculated.

$$Cl = \frac{(S)(F)(Dose/\tau) - \dfrac{(Cp_2 - Cp_1)Vd}{t}}{Cp\ ave}$$

In this equation, t would be four days since this is the interval between Cp_1 (0.8 µg/L) and Cp_2 (1.6 µg/L). Cp ave would generally be calculated as the average of the two plasma concentrations.

$$Cp \text{ ave} = \frac{Cp_1 + Cp_2}{2}$$

$$= \frac{(0.8 \text{ µg/L}) + (1.6 \text{ µg/L})}{2}$$

$$= 1.2 \text{ µg/L}$$

Substituting the appropriate values in Equation 58, a digoxin clearance of 75.9 L/day can be calculated.

$$Cl = \frac{(1)(0.7)(250 \text{ µg/day}) - \dfrac{(1.6 \text{ µg/L} - 0.8 \text{ µg/L}) \, 419.4 \text{ L}}{4 \text{ days}}}{1.2 \text{ µg/L}}$$

$$= \frac{(175 \text{ µg/day}) - \left(\dfrac{335.52 \text{ µg}}{4 \text{ days}}\right)}{1.2 \text{ µg/L}}$$

$$= \frac{175 \text{ µg/day} - (83.9 \text{ µg/day})}{1.2 \text{ µg/L}}$$

$$= \frac{91.1 \text{ µg/day}}{1.2 \text{ µg/L}}$$

$$= 75.9 \text{ L/day}$$

Note that this calculated digoxin clearance is consistent with an expected half-life of approximately 3.8 days.

$$t\tfrac{1}{2} = \frac{(0.693)(Vd)}{Cl} \qquad \text{(Eq. 32)}$$

$$= \frac{(0.693)(419.4 \text{ L})}{75.9 \text{ L/day}}$$

$$= 3.83 \text{ days}$$

This revised half-life indicates that one has at least minimally met the time interval of one half-life between drug concentrations as one of the criteria for using the mass balance equation. The additional conditions, (i.e., $Cp_2 \leq 2 \times Cp_1$; the dosing input should be regular and consistent) have also been met. [See Part I: Nonsteady-State Revision of Clearance (Mass Balance) on page 86.]

Using the revised clearance value and Equation 35, the expected steady-state digoxin concentration of approximately 2.3 μg/L can be calculated.

$$\text{Cpss ave} = \frac{(S)(F)(\text{Dose}/\tau)}{Cl}$$

$$= \frac{(1)(0.7)(250 \ \mu g/day)}{75.9 \ L/day}$$

$$= 2.3 \ \mu g/L$$

Because this value is somewhat above the upper limit of the usually accepted therapeutic range, one might choose to reduce the digoxin maintenance dose at this time. An alternative approach is to obtain another digoxin sample after approximately one half-life (three to four days) to determine if the digoxin concentration is accumulating as anticipated. In one half-life, the digoxin concentration should accumulate to a concentration of approximately 2 μg/L, or half-way between the present concentration of 1.6 μg/L and the expected steady-state value of 2.3 μg/L. The time interval of one half-life was chosen for two reasons. First, in order to distinguish true drug accumulation from assay variability, a significant time interval is required, usually at least one half-life. Second, it is desirable to detect accumulation early enough to avoid unnecessary toxicity risks. In this case, the time interval chosen has placed C.A.'s digoxin concentration at the upper end of the therapeutic range.

References

1. Smith TW. Digitalis toxicity: epidemiology and clinical use of serum concentration measurements. Am J Med. 1975;58:470.

2. Smith TW, Haber E. Digoxin intoxication: the relationship of clinical presentation to serum digoxin concentration. J Clin Invest. 1970; 49:2377.

3. Kock-Weser J et al. Influence of serum digoxin concentration measurements on frequency of digitoxicity. Clin Pharmacol Ther. 1974; 16:284.

4. Sheiner LB et al. Instructional goals for physicians in the use of blood level data and the contribution of computers. Clin Pharmacol Ther. 1974;16:260

5. Ogilvie RI, Ruedy J. An educational program in digitalis therapy. JAMA. 1972;222:50.

6. Huffman DH et al. Absorption of digoxin from different oral preparations in normal subjects during steady state. Clin Pharmacol Ther. 1974;16:310.

7. Lisalo E. Clinical pharmacokinetics of digoxin. Clin Pharmacokinet. 1977;2:1.

8. Mallis GI et al. Superior bioavailability of digoxin solution in capsules. Clin Pharmacol Ther. 1975;18:761.

9. Marcus FI et al. Digoxin bioavailability: formulations and rates of infusions. Clin Pharmacol Ther. 1976;20:253.

10. Reuning RH et al. Role of pharmocokinetics in drug dosage adjustment: I. Pharmacologic effect kinetics and apparent volume of distribution of digoxin. J Clin Pharmacol. 1973;13:127.

11. Abernethy DR et al. Digoxin disposition in obesity: Clinical pharmacokinetic investigation. Am Heart J. 1981;102:740–4.

12. Shapiro W et al. Relationship of plasma digitoxin and digoxin to cardiac response following intravenous digitalization in man. Circulation. 1970;42:1065.

13. Walsh FM et al. Significance of non-steady state serum digoxin concentrations. Am J Clin Pathol. 1975;63:446.

14. Kramer WG et al. Pharmacokinetics of digoxin: comparison of a two and a three compartment model in man. J Pharmacokinetic Biopharm. 1974;2:299.

15. Sheiner LB et al. Estimation of population characteristics of pharmacokinetic parameters from routine clinical data. J Pharmacokinet Biopharm. 1977;5:445.

16. Sheiner LB et al. Modeling of individual pharmacokinetics for computer-aided drug dosage. Comput Biomed Res. 1972;5:441.

17. Smith TW et al. Clinical value of the radioimmunoassay of the digitalis glycosides. Pharmacol Rev. 1973;25:219.

18. Jusko WH et al. Pharmacokinetic design of digoxin dosage regimens in relation to renal function. J Clin Pharmacol. 1974;14:525.

19. Jusko WJ, Wintraub M. Myocardial distribution of digoxin and renal function. Clin Pharmacol Ther. 1974;16:449.

20. Wagner JG. Loading and maintenance doses of digoxin in patients with normal renal function and those with severely impaired renal function. J Clin Pharmacol. 1974;14:329.

21. Ohnhaus EE et al. Protein binding of digoxin in human serum. Eur J Clin Pharmacol. 1972;5:34.

22. Koup JR et al. Pharmacokinetics of digoxin in normal subjects after intravenous bolus and infusion doses. J Pharmacokinet Biopharm. 1975;3:181.

23. Wintraub M et al. Compliance as a determinant of serum digoxin concentration. JAMA. 1973;224:481.

24. Lader S et al. The measurement of plasma digoxin concentrations: a comparison of two methods. Eur J Clin Pharmacol. 1972;5:22.

25. Silber B et al. Associated digoxin radioimmunoassay interference. Clin Chem. 1979;25:48.

26. Graves SW et al. An endogenous digoxin-like substance in patients with renal impairment. Ann Intern Med. 1983;99:604.

27. Pudek MR et al. Seven different digoxin immunoassay kits compared with respect to interference by a digoxin-like immunoreactive substance in serum from premature and full-term infants. Clin Chem. 1983;29:1972.

28. Yatscoff RW et al. Digoxin-like immunoreactivity in the serum of neonates and uremic patients, as measured in the Abbott TDX (Letter). Clin Chem. 1984;30:588.

29. Avendano C et al. Interference of digoxin-like immunoreactive substances with TDx Digoxin II assay in different patients. Ther Drug Monit. 1991;13:523–7.

30. Luchi RJ, Gruber JW. Unusually large digitalis requirements. Am J Med. 1968;45:322.

31. Doherty et al. Digoxin metabolism in hypo-and hyperthyroidism. Ann Intern Med. 1966;64:489.

32. Lawrence JR. Digoxin kinetics in patients with thyroid dysfunction. Clin Pharmacol Ther. 1977;22:7.

33. Croxson MS, Ibbertson HK. Serum digoxin in patients with thyroid disease. Br Med J. 1985;3:566.

34. Ackerman GL et al. Peritoneal and hemodialysis of tritiated digoxin. Ann Intern Med. 1967;67:4:718.

35. Ejvinsson G. Effect of quinidine of plasma concentrations of digoxin. Br. Med. J. 1978;279.

36. Leahey EB Jr. et al. Interactions between quinidine and digoxin. JAMA. 1978;240:533.

37. Leahey EB et al. Quinidine-digoxin interaction: time course and pharmacokinetics. Am J Cardiol. 1981;48:1141.

38. Hager DW et al. Digoxin-quinidine interaction. N Engl J Med. 1979; 300:1238.

39. Powell JR et al. Quinidine-digoxin interaction. N Engl J Med. 1980; 302:176.

40. Doering W. Quinidine-digoxin interaction. N Engl J Med. 1979;301: 400.

41. Steiness E et al. Reduction of digoxin-induced inotropism during quinidine administration. Clin Pharmacol Ther. 1980;27:791.

42. Schenck-Gustafsson K et al. Cardiac effects of treatment with quinidine and digoxin, alone and in combination. Am J Cardiol. 1983; 51:777.

43. Belz GB et al. Quinidine-digoxin interaction; cardiac efficacy of elevated serum digoxin concentration. Clin Pharmacol Ther. 1982;31:548.

44. Fichtl B, Doering W. The quinidine-digoxin interaction in perspective. Clin Pharmacokinet. 1983;8:137.

45. Bussey HI. The influence of quinidine and other agents on digitalis glycosides. Am Heart J. 1982;104:289.

46. Pedersen KE et al. Verapamil-induced changes in digoxin kinetics and intraerythrocytic sodium concentration. Clin Pharmacol Ther. 1983; 34:8.

47. Lesko LJ. Pharmacokinetic drug interactions with amiodarone. Clin Pharmacokinet. 1989;17:130–40.

Ethosuximide 5

Ethosuximide is an anticonvulsant which has been used primarily for the treatment of absence seizures. It is available as 250 mg capsules and as a solution containing 250 mg of ethosuximide per 5 mL. Ethosuximide is eliminated by metabolism to an inactive hydroxyethyl metabolite which is excreted in the urine as the glucuronide. About 20% of the unchanged drug is excreted in the urine. The usual dosage range is 15 to 30 mg/kg/day. Children three to six years of age usually receive a single daily dose of ≈250 mg. Older children and adults generally receive their daily regimen in two divided doses, although some older patients appear to do well on once daily dosing.

Therapeutic and Toxic Plasma Concentrations

The range of therapeutic plasma concentrations for ethosuximide (measured just before the next dose) is 40 to 100 mg/L. Most patients with plasma concentrations in this range respond with a significant or complete reduction in seizure activity; patients with plasma concentrations below 40 mg/L are less likely to be well controlled.[1,2] The incidence of adverse effects associated with ethosuximide therapy is relatively low and does not correlate well with plasma concentrations. While side effects associated with ethosuximide are uncommon, those most usually encountered are related to the gastrointestinal tract and include abdominal discomfort, nausea and vomiting, and anorexia. Drowsiness, fatigue, and headaches are also observed occasionally. Many patients with plasma concentrations in excess of 100 mg/L experience no side effects.[3] Plasma levels are, therefore, primarily used to evaluate a patient's potential for clinical response and compliance. Alterations in plasma concentrations due to plasma protein binding changes are not a consideration for ethosuximide since very little is protein bound.[4]

Bioavailability (F)

Ethosuximide appears to be well absorbed following oral administration, with peak levels occurring within two to four hours after administration of a dose. Available data suggest that the bioavailability approaches 100%.[5,6] The salt factor (S) for ethosuximide is 1.

Volume of Distribution (Vd)

The volume of distribution for ethosuximide appears to be ≈0.7 L/kg.[7] There is an insignificant amount of plasma and tissue protein binding.[4,8]

Key Parameters

Therapeutic Plasma Concentrations	40–100 mg/L
F	100%
S	1.0
Vd	0.7 L/kg
Cl	
Child	0.39 L/kg/day
Adult	0.23 L/kg/day
$t\frac{1}{2}$	
Child	30 hr
Adult	50 hr

Clearance (Cl)

Ethosuximide is eliminated from the body primarily by metabolism, with a relatively small percentage of drug being excreted unchanged. Children have an average clearance value of $\approx$0.39 L/kg/day, while adults have a lower clearance value of $\approx$0.23 L/kg/day.[5,7] These clearance values vary considerably from patient to patient, making plasma level monitoring useful in designing dosing regimens. Based on ethosuximide's relatively small molecular weight (141 daltons), small volume of distribution, and negligible plasma protein binding, one would predict significant removal by hemodialysis. Data indicate that $\approx$50% of ethosuximide is removed during a standard hemodialysis run.[9]

Half-Life (t½)

The elimination half-life of ethosuximide in children is $\approx$30 hours and in adults, $\approx$50 hours. Due to the wide variation in clearance values, the half-life can be less than one-half or greater than twice these average values.[5,7] The long half-life of ethosuximide suggests that once daily dosing regimens would be appropriate; however, in some cases gastrointestinal side effects may require dividing the dose to twice daily.[10]

Time to Sample

The timing of the ethosuximide sample within a dosing interval is not critical because of its long elimination half-life.

Although trough levels are recommended for the sake of consistency, obtaining trough concentrations should not be considered crucial if it is inconvenient. Ethosuximide concentrations require approximately four to seven days to reach steady state in children. An even longer period of time will be required in adults. For this reason, early plasma level monitoring may cause confusion about the final steady-state concentration and should be avoided.

> *Question #1.* **C.A., an 8-year-old, 25 kg male, is receiving 250 mg ethosuximide BID for treatment of absence seizures. Predict C.A.'s trough plasma concentration of ethosuximide at steady state.**

In order to calculate the anticipated trough concentration of ethosuximide, the expected volume of distribution and elimination rate constant would have to be calculated and the appropriate values placed in Equation 47:

$$\text{Cpss min} = \frac{\dfrac{(S)(F)(Dose)}{Vd}}{(1 - e^{-Kd\tau})} (e^{-Kd\tau})$$

In this case, however, it is important to recognize that the difference between the trough and average concentrations will be relatively small because the dosing interval of 12 hours is short compared to the anticipated half-life of $\approx$30 hours. For this reason, an average plasma concentration of ethosuximide could be calculated by using Equation 35 and the estimated clearance value of 0.39 L/kg/day or 9.75 L/day (0.39 L/kg/day $\times$ 25 kg).

$$
\begin{aligned}
\text{Cpss ave} &= \frac{(S)(F)(Dose/\tau)}{Cl} \\
&= \frac{(1)(1)(250 \text{ mg}/0.5 \text{ days})}{9.75 \text{ L/day}} \\
&= 51.3 \text{ mg/L}
\end{aligned}
$$

This average concentration of ≈50 mg/L could then be used as an approximation of the anticipated trough concentration.

Question #2. Since C.A.'s seizure control has been poor, an ethosuximide level is ordered and reported as 35 mg/L. How would one interpret this ethosuximide concentration? What would be an appropriate course of action?

The measured ethosuximide concentration of 35 mg/L is below the usual therapeutic range; therefore, it might be assumed that increasing the plasma concentration into the therapeutic range would result in better seizure control. Before a dose is adjusted, however, C.A. or his family should be carefully questioned to ascertain whether the low ethosuximide concentration is the result of increased metabolism (clearance), or decreased compliance. If it can be determined that C.A. has been compliant, then doses should be adjusted.

Since ethosuximide concentrations should not change much during a dosing regimen, the plasma concentration of 35 mg/L probably represents an average plasma concentration. The average steady-state plasma concentration is proportional to the dosing rate, therefore, a change in the maintenance regimen should result in a proportional change in the steady-state plasma concentration. For example, if the daily dose was increased from 500 mg to 750 mg, the plasma concentration should increase by 50% (i.e., from 35 mg/L to ≈52 mg/L):

$$\text{Cpss ave (new)} = [\text{Cpss ave (old)}]\left[\frac{\text{Maintenance Dose (new)}}{\text{Maintenance Dose (old)}}\right]$$

Eq. 5.1

$$= [35 \text{ mg/L}]\left[\frac{750 \text{ mg/day}}{500 \text{ mg/day}}\right]$$

$$= [35 \text{ mg/L}][1.5]$$

$$= 52.5 \text{ mg/L}$$

An alternate approach would be to use the steady-state level of 35 mg/L to calculate C.A.'s apparent ethosuximide clearance. This could be accomplished by using the maintenance regimen of 250 mg every 12 hours (250 mg/0.5 days) and Equation 15:

$$
\begin{aligned}
Cl &= \frac{(S)(F)(Dose/\tau)}{Cpss\ ave} \\
&= \frac{(1)(1)(250\ mg/0.5\ days)}{35\ mg/L} \\
&= 14.28\ L/day
\end{aligned}
$$

This clearance value of $\approx$14.3 L/day could then be used in Equation 16 to calculate the dose that would be required to maintain any desired steady-state ethosuximide level. For example, if an average plasma concentration of 50 mg/L were inserted in this equation, the calculated maintenance dose would be 715 mg/day:

$$
\begin{aligned}
\text{Maintenance Dose} &= \frac{(Cl)(Cpss\ ave)(\tau)}{(S)(F)} \\
&= \frac{(14.3\ L/day)(50\ mg/L)(1\ day)}{(1)(1)} \\
&= 715\ mg
\end{aligned}
$$

Ethosuximide is available in 250 mg capsules; an appropriate dose would be 250 mg every eight hours or 250 mg given once daily and 500 mg given 12 hours later. Once daily therapy would not be advisable because the estimated half-life for C.A. is $\approx$20 hours, as shown below using Equation 32.

$$
\begin{aligned}
t^{1/2} &= \frac{(0.693)(Vd)}{Cl} \\
&= \frac{(0.693)(0.7\ L/kg)(25\ kg)}{14.3\ L/day}\,(24\ hr/day) \\
&= 0.848\ days\ (24\ hr/day) \\
&= 20.4\ hr
\end{aligned}
$$

References

1. Browne TR et al. Ethosuximide in the treatment of absence seizures. Neurology. 1975;25:515.

2. Sherwin AL, Robb JP. Ethosuximide: relation of plasma levels to clinical control. In: Woodbury DM, et al., eds. Anti-epileptic Drugs. New York: Raven Press; 1972:443–448.

3. Sherwin AL et al. Plasma ethosuximide levels: a new aid in the management of epilepsy. Ann R Coll Surg Can. 1971;4:48.

4. Johannessen SI. Antiepileptic drugs: pharmacokinetic and clinical aspects. Ther Drug Monit. 1981;2:17–37.

5. Buchanan RA et al. Absorption and elimination of ethosuximide in children. J Clin Pharmacol. 1969;9:393.

6. Buchanan RA, et al. The absorption and excretion of ethosuximide. Int J Clin Pharmacol. 1973;7:213–8.

7. Buchanan RA et al. The absorption and excretion of ethosuximide. Int J Clin Pharmacol Res. 1973;7:213.

8. Chang T et al. Ethosuximide: absorption, distribution and excretion. In: Woodbury DM, et al., eds. Anti-epileptic Drugs. New York: Raven Press; 1972:417–423.

9. Marbury TC, et al. Hemodialysis clearance of ethosuximide in patients with chronic renal failure. AM J Hosp Pharm. 1981;38:1757–60.

10. Dooley JM, et al. Once-daily ethosuximide in the treatment of absence epilepsy. Pediatr Neurol. 1990;6:38–9.

Lidocaine 6

Lidocaine is a local anesthetic agent with antiarrhythmic properties; it is used for the acute treatment of severe ventricular arrhythmias.[1,2] Lidocaine has poor oral bioavailability, is almost exclusively metabolized by the liver, and has a relatively short duration of action. For these reasons, lidocaine is almost always administered initially as a bolus dose of 1 to 2 mg/kg followed by a continuous infusion of approximately 1 to 4 mg/min. Because of the two-compartment modeling and rapid distribution of lidocaine, there are multiple schemes which have been used to rapidly achieve and then maintain the therapeutic effects. These usually include a combination of several small bolus doses of 0.5 to 1.0 mg/kg or an initial infusion rate of approximately 8 mg/min for 10 to 20 minutes followed by a reduction in the infusion rate to the usual maintenance rate of 1 to 4 mg/min.[3–5] Lidocaine has a narrow therapeutic index and toxic effects are generally dose or concentration related. Furthermore, conditions such as congestive heart failure, liver dysfunction, and concurrent medications may alter the pharmacokinetics of lidocaine and, therefore, the expected therapeutic responses to usual doses. The application of pharmacokinetic principles to the individualization of lidocaine dosing can be invaluable. Nevertheless, lidocaine's short half-life and use in acute treatment require a short assay turnaround time for optimal therapeutic drug monitoring.

Therapeutic and Toxic Plasma Levels

Lidocaine plasma concentrations of 1 to 5 mg/L are usually associated with therapeutic control of ventricular arrhythmias.[6–9] Minor Central Nervous System (CNS) side effects (e.g., dizziness, mental confusion, and blurred vision) can be observed in patients with plasma concentrations as low as 3 to 5 mg/L. Although seizures have occurred at plasma lidocaine concentrations as low as 6 mg/L, they are usually associated with concentrations exceeding 9 mg/L.[6–8,10,11] Lidocaine does not usually cause hemodynamic changes, but hypotension associated with myocardial depression has been observed in a patient whose plasma lidocaine concentration was 5.3 mg/L.[12] In addition, there are reports of sinus arrest following rapid intravenous injection.[13]

Volume of Distribution (Vd)

The distribution of lidocaine following an intravenous bolus can be described by a two-compartment model (see Part I: Figure 9 on page 24).

Key Parameters

Therapeutic Plasma Concentrations		1–5 mg/L	
F		1.0 (IV)	
S		0.87	

	Normal	**CHF**	**Cirrhosis**
Vi	0.5 L/kg	0.3 L/kg	0.61 L/kg
Vd	1.3 L/kg	0.88 L/kg	2.3 L/kg
$\alpha\ t\frac{1}{2}$	8 min	8 min	8 min
$\beta\ t\frac{1}{2}$	100 min	100 min	300 min
Cl	10 mL/kg/min	6 mL/kg/min	6 mL/kg/min

The initial volume of distribution (Vi) appears to be about 0.5 L/kg and the final volume following distribution (Vd) is about 1.3 L/kg.[10,11] The volume of distribution seems to increase in proportion to weight. Therefore, total body weight should be used to calculate the volume of distribution of lidocaine in obese subjects.[14] This volume of distribution, however, is not the initial or central compartment. Thus, it is not clear whether or not individual bolus doses that comprise the total loading dose ought to be adjusted. In addition, the volume of distribution reported in the previous study for both obese and non-obese subjects was approximately 2.7 L/kg. This value is larger than those normally reported and may be the result of dated analysis techniques or the specific patient populations studied. Unlike digoxin, the myocardium responds to lidocaine as though it is located in the initial volume (Vi). Therefore, the dose of each *bolus* injection of lidocaine should be based on Vi and not Vd. Plasma concentrations resulting from each bolus injection will fall as the drug distributes into the larger final volume of distribution. Therefore, the *total* loading dose should be calculated using the final volume of distribution (Vd). As stated previously, it is a common practice to initiate lidocaine therapy with a bolus dose of 1 to 2 mg/kg followed by a continuous infusion. It is often necessary to administer additional bolus doses to avoid loss of efficacy associated with the redistribution of the initial bolus into the tissue or peripheral compartment. Subsequent bolus doses are usually one-half of the initial bolus dose or in the range of 0.5 to 1.0 mg/kg. Because there is a residual lidocaine plasma concentration, smaller bolus doses minimize the potential risk of excessive distribution-phase concentrations and lidocaine toxicity.[3–5]

In *congestive heart failure (CHF)*, both volumes of distribution for lidocaine are decreased: Vi is 0.3 L/kg and Vd is 0.88 L/kg. Both the total loading dose and the individual bolus injections should be reduced in patients with CHF. In contrast, both volumes of distribution are increased with *chronic liver disease:* Vi is 0.61 L/kg and Vd is 2.3 L/kg. Thus, slightly larger loading doses may be required in these patients. Renal failure does not appear to alter the distribution of lidocaine.[11] In practice, the individual bolus dose is generally not adjusted for CHF or chronic liver disease; rather, the number of such doses required to achieve sustained antiarrhythmic effects would be expected to be fewer for patients with CHF and greater for patients with chronic liver disease. For example, the total loading dose used in post-myocardial infarction patients with congestive heart failure should be about 40% lower than that used for similar patients without congestive failure.[11]

Clearance (Cl)

Lidocaine has a high hepatic extraction ratio. Its clearance of 10 mL/kg/min (700 mL/min/70 kg) approximates plasma flow to the liver.[11,15,16] Less than 5% is cleared by the renal route. Because of the high first-pass effect, bioavailability (F) following oral administration is quite variable and F is usually in the range of 0.4.[17] This uncertainty in the systemic bioavailability by the oral route requires parenteral administration of lidocaine to ensure its efficacy.

Congestive heart failure and *hepatic cirrhosis* decrease the clearance of lidocaine to about 6 mL/kg/min; therefore, a 40% reduction in the maintenance infusion is appropriate for patients with these diseases.[11,18,19] Since the drug is not cleared renally, no dose adjustment is required for patients with diminished kidney function. In obese subjects, the clearance of lidocaine appears to correlate most closely with the ideal body weight rather than total body weight. For this reason, maintenance infusions of lidocaine should be based upon a subject's non-obese weight.[14]

Lidocaine is metabolized primarily to monoethylglycinexylidine (MEGX) and glycinexylidide (GX). MEGX appears to have activity similar to lidocaine. It is cleared by metabolism and, therefore, does not accumulate in renal failure. In contrast, approximately 50% of GX is cleared by the renal route and it, therefore, accumulates in patients with diminished renal function.[20] GX is less active than lidocaine and does not contribute to its therapeutic effect. The only known side effects of GX (i.e., headache and impaired mental performance) are dose related and occur at plasma concentrations >1.0 mg/L.[20] More serious toxicities have not been observed in patients with GX levels as high as 9 mg/L.[21]

Half-Life (t½)

The lidocaine *distribution half-life* (α t½) of eight minutes does not appear to be altered by heart failure, hepatic disease, or renal failure.

The *elimination half-life* (β t½) of lidocaine is a function of its volume of distribution and clearance as illustrated by Equation 32:

$$t\tfrac{1}{2} = \frac{(0.693)(Vd)}{Cl}$$

The usual elimination half-life for lidocaine is about 100 minutes.[11] It is unchanged in patients with congestive heart failure because both the volume of distribution and the clearance are reduced to a similar extent in these individuals.

Patients with liver disease have a lidocaine β half-life of about 300 minutes due to an increased volume of distribution and decreased clearance.[22] An elimination half-life of 200 minutes has been observed in healthy subjects following infusions lasting longer than 24 hours.[22] Because lidocaine concentrations continue to accumulate,[23,24] there is concern that patients receiving prolonged infusions of lidocaine may be at risk for lidocaine toxicity.[25] For this reason, the practice of using lidocaine prophylactically and continuing infusions longer than 24 hours is considered by some authors to carry substantial risk of lidocaine toxicity.[25,26]

Time to Sample

Unless assay turnaround time is unusually short, lidocaine plasma concentrations should not be monitored until four to eight hours have elapsed since the beginning of therapy. At this time, assay results should approximate steady-state concentrations. Plasma lidocaine concentrations obtained during the distribution phase following administration of a bolus dose may be useful to establish the relationship between lidocaine plasma concentration and efficacy. However, these plasma concentrations should not be used to adjust acute therapy unless the assay turnaround time is within minutes because plasma lidocaine concentrations change so rapidly. In most institutions, several hours and up to a day may be required for assay results; therefore, steady state for any given infusion dose will have been achieved by the time results are available (normal t½: two to three hours). For this reason, lidocaine assay results cannot be used to adjust the initial infusion or maintenance doses in most situations.

Patients with cirrhosis who have a prolonged lidocaine half-life are an exception to this generalization. In most instances, lidocaine plasma concentrations are primarily used to retrospectively confirm clinical impressions. Lidocaine levels can also be used to assist in the evaluation of patients in whom the minor central nervous system side effects of dizziness or mental confusion are difficult or impossible to assess (e.g., those who are unconscious or are receiving other CNS depressant drugs). This would be especially true when the lidocaine infusion is likely to be continued for more than 12 to 24 hours. In these individuals, lidocaine levels might be used to evaluate slow accumulation towards concentrations that could be associated with seizures. This use of lidocaine concentrations is most applicable to patients whose cardiac output and, therefore, lidocaine clearance, is declining.

> *Question #1.* P.M., a 55-year-old, 70 kg male, was admitted to the coronary care unit with a diagnosis of heart failure, probable myocardial infarction (MI), and premature ventricular contractions (PVCs). Calculate a bolus dose of lidocaine that should achieve an immediate response for P.M. At what rate should this dose be administered?

A lidocaine bolus dose can be calculated by using Equation 11 as shown below. Since lidocaine distribution follows a two-compartment model with the myocardium responding as though it were in the initial compartment, Vd in Equation 11 should be replaced with Vi (see the discussion of Lidocaine Volume of Distribution on page 242). The Vi for a patient with congestive heart failure is 0.3 L/kg (see Lidocaine Key Parameters on page 243) or 21 L for this 70 kg male.[11] S and F are assumed to be 0.87 and 1.0, respectively, for lidocaine. If it is assumed that peak levels should not exceed 3 mg/L to avoid toxicity the appropriate bolus dose would be 70 mg:

$$\text{Loading Dose} = \frac{(Vd)(Cp)}{(S)(F)}$$

$$\text{Bolus Dose} = \frac{(Vi)(Cp)}{(S)(F)}$$

Eq. 6.1

$$= \frac{(21 \text{ L})(3 \text{ mg/L})}{(0.87)(1.0)}$$

$$= 72 \text{ mg} \quad or \quad \approx 70 \text{ mg}$$

This bolus dose of 70 mg is essentially the same as the usually recommended dose of 1 to 2 mg/kg.[27] It should be given by slow IV push (25 to 50 mg/min).

Question #2. Calculate a maintenance infusion rate that will achieve a steady-state plasma lidocaine concentration of 2 mg/L for P.M.

The maintenance dose can be calculated from Equation 16. If it is assumed that a steady-state concentration of 2 mg/L is desired and if τ is assumed to be 1 min, Cl to be 420 mL/min (Lidocaine Key Parameters: 6 mL/kg/min for a patient in congestive heart failure), S (0.87), and F (1.0), the maintenance dose would be calculated as follows:

$$\text{Maintenance Dose} = \frac{(\text{Cl})(\text{Cpss ave})(\tau)}{(\text{S})(\text{F})}$$

$$= \frac{(0.42 \text{ L/min})(2 \text{ mg/L})(1 \text{ min})}{(0.87)(1.0)}$$

$$= 0.97 \text{ mg/min}$$

Although this calculated infusion is at the lower end of the frequently-recommended infusion rates of 1 to 4 mg/min,[27] it is consistent with the conservative target steady-state level of 2 mg/L and the decreased clearance expected for P.M. who has CHF.

The assumed clearance value of 6 mL/kg/min for heart failure is an average value. Zito and Reid have developed a scaling procedure in which the recommended lidocaine infusion rate is based upon the degree of heart failure.[28] (See Table 6.1). When lidocaine maintenance infusions were adjusted according to cardiac function in the clinical setting, significantly more patients were maintained within the usual therapeutic range for lidocaine. Although this study was restricted to individuals who had no evidence of heart failure or mild (clinical Class II) failure, it does point out the value of assessing cardiac status when determining a lidocaine maintenance infusion.[29]

Question #3. P.M.'s PVCs were controlled by the 70 mg bolus dose of lidocaine and an infusion of 1 mg/min was begun. Fifteen minutes later, PVCs were again noted. What might account for the reappearance of PVCs? What is an appropriate course of action at this point?

The distribution half-life of lidocaine is about eight minutes and the elimination half-life is 1.5 to 2 hours. Since three to four elimination half-lives (approximately six hours) must elapse before plasma lidocaine concentrations are at steady state, the recurrence of the PVCs 15 minutes after the bolus dose probably represents a declining plasma concentration caused by distribution rather than an inadequate maintenance dose. The plasma concentration resulting from the 70 mg bolus dose (Cp°) can be predicted by using the final volume of distribution (Vd) of 62 L (0.88 L/kg $\times$ 70 kg) in a rearranged version of Equation 11 for loading dose or Equation 49:

$$\text{Loading Dose} = \frac{(Vd)(Cp)}{(S)(F)}$$

$$Cp^\circ = \frac{(S)(F)(\text{Loading Dose})}{Vd}$$

$$= \frac{(0.87)(1)(70 \text{ mg})}{62 \text{ L}}$$

$$= 0.98 \text{ mg/L}$$

Since the predicted lidocaine concentration after distribution is approximately 1 mg/L, the total loading dose was probably too low and an additional bolus will be needed. It would be more rational to administer a second bolus dose rather than change the infusion rate. In practice, the second or third bolus doses are reduced by one-half to avoid excessive accumulation. In addition, some clinicians will increase the maintenance infusion for 20 to 30 minutes to allow for more rapid accumulation and then reduce the infusion back to the original rate.[3,5]

An alternative approach to managing these breakthrough PVCs involves calculating the total loading dose required to achieve a final lidocaine concentration of 2 mg/L in Vd. The additional amount that would be required to fill this volume (total loading dose minus bolus doses already administered) could be administered over approximately 20 minutes. This approach prevents the breakthrough arrhythmias which result from tissue distribution of the initial intravenous bolus dose, but also reduces the CNS side effects caused by transiently-elevated lidocaine concentrations associated with repeated bolus doses.[4,5,30]

If the PVCs had occurred several hours after starting the infusion, the most rational approach would have been to give a small bolus dose sufficient to increase the plasma concentration in the initial volume of distribution to 2 or 3 mg/L and to increase the infusion rate as well.

Question #4. **B.P., a 65-year-old, 70 kg male, was admitted with a diagnosis of hepatic encephalopathy and cirrhosis. On the fourth hospital day, he developed ventricular arrhythmias and lidocaine was ordered. Calculate a bolus dose and a maintenance infusion rate that will achieve a steady-state lidocaine level of 2 mg/L.**

The following lidocaine pharmacokinetic parameters would be expected for a 70 kg patient with chronic liver disease:

Vi 43 L (0.61 L/kg)

Vd 161 L (2.3 L/kg)

Cl 420 mL/min *or* 0.42 L/min *or* 25.2 L/hr (6 mL/kg/min)

Table 6.1	Lidocaine Clearance Based on Degree of Heart Failure	
Clinical Class	Symptoms	Apparent Lidocaine Clearance {mL/kg/min)
I	No heart failure	14.5
II	S_3 gallop and basilar pulmonary rales	5
III	Pulmonary edema	
IV	Cardiogenic shock	2.1

As in Question 1, the initial bolus can be calculated from Equation 6.1 which replaces the term Vd in Equation 11 with Vi. Assuming a maximum plasma concentration of 3 mg/L (μg/mL) in Vi is desired, the initial bolus should be 148 mg as calculated below:

$$\text{Bolus Dose} = \frac{(\text{Vi})(\text{Cp})}{(\text{S})(\text{F})}$$

$$= \frac{(43 \text{ L})(3 \text{ mg/L})}{(0.87)(1)}$$

$$= 148 \text{ mg}$$

This dose should be given no more rapidly than 25 to 50 mg/min. After final distribution, this 148 mg dose should result in a plasma level of 0.8 mg/L as shown below (Equation 49):

$$\text{Cp}^\circ = \frac{(\text{S})(\text{F})(\text{Loading Dose})}{\text{Vd}}$$

$$= \frac{(0.87)(1)(148 \text{ mg})}{161 \text{ L}}$$

$$= 0.8 \text{ mg/L}$$

Since this predicted plasma concentration is rather low, an additional bolus dose probably will be required. To avoid excessive accumulation, about one-half the original dose should be given.

The maintenance infusion can be calculated from Equation 16 using the expected clearance of 0.42 L/min:

$$\text{Maintenance Dose} = \frac{(\text{Cl})(\text{Cpss ave})(\tau)}{(\text{S})(\text{F})}$$

$$= \frac{(0.42 \text{ L/min})(2 \text{ mg/L})(1 \text{ min})}{(0.87)(1)}$$

$$= 0.96 \text{ mg}$$

Thus, a maintenance infusion of approximately 1 mg/min should achieve a steady-state plasma concentration of 2 mg/L.

Question #5. Eighteen hours after starting the infusion, B.P. appears to be more confused than usual. It is unclear whether his present condition is secondary to hepatic encephalopathy or lidocaine. Is it possible that the lidocaine is still accumulating and is causing the impaired mental state?

The expected half-life for lidocaine in B.P. can be calculated from his assumed lidocaine Cl and Vd using Equation 32:

$$t^{1}\!/_{2} = \frac{(0.693)(Vd)}{Cl}$$
$$= \frac{(0.693)(161\ L)}{25.2\ L/hr}$$
$$= 4.42\ hr$$

This calculated value of 4.4 hours is reasonably close to the value of 4.9 hours which is reported in the literature for patients with hepatic failure.[11] Since the expected half-life for lidocaine in this patient is four to five hours, steady-state levels may not have been achieved after 18 hours and his lidocaine levels may still be rising. (See Part I: Half-Life on page 43.) A "stat" lidocaine concentration should be ordered to evaluate the contribution of lidocaine to B.P.'s altered mental status. If B.P.'s PVCs are well controlled, the maintenance infusion can also be decreased slowly with careful cardiac monitoring.

Question #6. D.I., a 62-year-old, 60 kg male, has just had a myocardial infarction and has mild or Class II heart failure. On admission to the cardiac care unit, D.I. developed PVCs at a rate of 18/min, and was treated successfully with an IV bolus dose of lidocaine followed by an infusion of 1.5 mg/min. D.I. had lidocaine levels at 24 and 48 hours of 3.5 mg/L and 4.5 mg/L, respectively. What are possible explanations for the 1 mg/L rise in the lidocaine level?

Several studies have documented a slow rise in lidocaine concentrations in a number of patients. Even in healthy subjects, the apparent half-life of lidocaine after prolonged infusion appears to be increased.[18,19,22,23,25]

One very unlikely explanation for the slowly rising lidocaine levels is the possibility that the lidocaine level at 24 hours of 3.5 mg/L did not represent a steady-state concentration. If this were true, the volume of distribution for D.I. would have to be unrealistically large to account for the lidocaine level of 4.5 mg/L concentration at 48 hours. It would be more realistic to assume an assay error of approximately 0.5 mg/L for each of the measured concentrations. While this assay error exceeds the assumed confidence limit of 10%, it is more probable than an unusually large volume of distribution.

A change in clearance between the 24- and 48-hour time period that resulted in a change in the steady-state concentration could also explain this observation. While this is possible, it would be more probable if one could identify a factor in D.I. associated with decreased clearance, such as a declining cardiac output or the addition of a beta blocker to his medication regimen.[23]

The third and most likely explanation is that the plasma protein binding of lidocaine has changed as a result of an acute MI. Acute myocardial infarction is only one of many conditions or disease states that have been associated with altered plasma binding of basic drugs. (See Part I: Desired Plasma Concentrations on page 9.) This rise in plasma binding is due to an increase in the α_1-acid glycoprotein (AAG) and it probably accounts for the slowly increasing concentrations of lidocaine in D.I. It is interesting to note that while the total lidocaine concentration is increased, the unbound concentration of lidocaine is relatively unaltered.[29,31] The rise in plasma protein occurs over the first 7 to 14 days and then declines slowly. Plasma protein concentrations remain elevated for three weeks following the myocardial infarction.[31,32]

Question #7. **D.F. is a 68-year-old, 60 kg female with clinical class II heart failure. (See Table 6.1.) She was started on lidocaine for ventricular arrhythmias which occurred on postoperative Day 1 following her cardiac surgery. She received an initial 60 mg bolus dose of lidocaine at 10:00 a.m.**

followed by 120 mg administered over the next 15 minutes
(8 mg/min.) At 10:45 a.m. she was to be placed on a 2 mg/min
constant infusion. **Calculate her lidocaine concentration at
the start of her maintenance infusion and at steady state.**

To calculate D.F.'s lidocaine concentration, it is first necessary
to estimate her volume of distribution and clearance taking into
consideration her heart failure.

$$Vd = (0.88 \text{ L/kg})(60 \text{ kg})$$
$$= 52.8 \text{ L}$$

$$Cl = (5 \text{ mL/min/kg})(60 \text{ kg})$$
$$= 300 \text{ mL/min}$$
$$= (300 \text{ mL/min})(1 \text{ L/1000 mL})$$
$$= 0.3 \text{ L/min}$$

$$Kd = \frac{Cl}{Vd} \qquad \text{(Eq. 27)}$$
$$= \frac{0.3 \text{ L/min}}{52.8 \text{ L}}$$
$$= 0.0057 \text{ min}^{-1}$$

$$t\frac{1}{2} = \frac{0.693}{Kd} \qquad \text{(Eq. 31)}$$
$$= \frac{0.693}{0.0057 \text{ min}^{-1}}$$
$$= 122 \text{ min } or \approx 2 \text{ hr}$$

Note that the volume of distribution used was Vd rather than
Vi because the plasma concentration was obtained approximately 30 minutes after the end of the infusion when distribution should be complete. To calculate the expected concentration
at 10:45 a.m., Equations 50 and 53 can be combined. When the
appropriate doses, times, and pharmacokinetic parameters are
inserted into the equation, a lidocaine plasma concentration of
2.3 mg/L is calculated.

$$Cp = \frac{(S)(F)(Dose)}{Vd}(e^{-Kdt_1}) + \frac{(S)(F)(Dose/t_{in})}{Cl}(e^{-Kdt_{in}})(e^{-Kdt_2})$$

$$= \frac{(0.87)(1)(60 \text{ mg})}{52.8 \text{ L}}(e^{-(0.0057)(45 \text{ min})})$$

$$+ \frac{(0.87)(1)(120 \text{ mg}/15 \text{ min})}{0.3 \text{ L/min}}(1 - e^{-(0.0057)(15 \text{ min})})(e^{-(0.0057)(30 \text{ min})})$$

$$= (0.99 \text{ mg/L})(0.77) + (23.2 \text{ mg/L})(1 - 0.92)(0.84)$$

$$= (0.76 \text{ mg/L}) + (1.56 \text{ mg/L})$$

$$= 2.3 \text{ mg/L}$$

Note that the plasma concentrations immediately following the 60 mg bolus dose and during the 15 minute infusion are likely to be higher than those calculated by Equations 50 and 53. This is due to the two-compartment modeling and the fact that distribution is not yet complete.

The expected steady-state plasma concentration produced by the 2 mg/min infusion can be calculated using Equation 35.

$$Cpss \text{ ave} = \frac{(S)(F)(Dose/\tau)}{Cl}$$

$$= \frac{(0.87)(1)(2 \text{ mg/min})}{0.3 \text{ L/min}}$$

$$= 5.8 \text{ mg/L}$$

This calculated steady-state lidocaine concentration of 5.8 mg/L is somewhat high and suggests a reduction in the maintenance infusion may be warranted. Reducing the lidocaine infusion by one-half would reduce the steady-state plasma concentration by one-half to 2.9 mg/L. If the lidocaine infusion is not decreased, the patient should be carefully monitored for signs of lidocaine toxicity.

References

1. Griffith MJ et al. Relative efficacy and safety of intravenous drugs for termination of sustained ventricular tachycardia. Lancet. 1990;336: 670–3.

2. Gunnar RM et al. ACC/AHA guidelines for the early management of patients with acute myocardial infarction. Circulation. 1990;82:664–707.

3. Greenblatt DJ et al. Pharmacokinetic approach to the clinical use of lidocaine intravenously. JAMA. 1976;236:273–7.

4. Riddell JG et al. A new method for constant plasma drug concentration: application to lidocaine. Ann Intern Med. 1984;100:25–8.

5. Salzer LB et al. A comparison of methods of lidocaine administration in patients. Clin Pharmacol Ther. 1981;29:617–24.

6. Gianelly R et al. Effect of lidocaine on ventricular arrhythmias in patients with coronary heart disease. N Engl J Med. 1967;277:1215.

7. Jewett DE et al. Lidocaine in the management of arrhythmias after acute myocardial infarction. Lancet. 1968;1:266.

8. Seldon R, Sasahara AA. Central nervous system toxicity induced by lidocaine. JAMA. 1967;202:908.

9. Lie KI et al. Lidocaine in the prevention of primary ventricular fibrillation. N Engl J Med. 1974;291:1324–6.

10. Benowitz N. Clinical application of pharmacokinetics of lidocaine. In: Melmon K, ed. Cardiovascular Drug Therapy. Philadephia: FM Davis; 1974:77–101.

11. Thompson PD. Lidocaine pharmacokinetics in advanced heart failure, liver disease, and renal failure in humans. Ann Intern Med. 1973; 78:499.

12. Stannard M et al. Hemodynamic effects of lidocaine in acute myocardial infarction. Br Med J. 1968;2:468.

13. Cheng TO, Wadhwa K. Sinus standstill following intravenous lidocaine administration. JAMA. 1973;223:790.

14. Abernethy DR, Greenblatt DJ. Lidocaine disposition in obesity. Am J Cardiol. 1984;53:1183–6.

15. Wilkinson G. A physiological approach to hepatic drug clearance. Clin Pharmacol Ther. 1975;18:377.

16. Pang SK, Rowland M. Hepatic clearance of drugs: I. Theoretical considerations of a "well-stirred" model and a "parallel tube" model. Influence of hepatic blood flow, plasma and blood cell binding and hepatocellular enzymatic activity on hepatic drug clearance. J Pharmacokinet Biopharm. 1977;5:625.

17. Huet PM et al. Bioavailability of lidocaine in normal volunteers and cirrhotic patients. Clin Pharmacol Ther. 1979;25:229–30.

18. Prescott LF et al. Impaired lignocaine metabolism in patients with myocardial infarction and cardiac failure. Br Med J. 1976;1:939.

19. Prescott LF, Nimmo J. Plasma lidocaine concentrations during and after prolonged infusion in patients with myocardial infarction. In: Scott DB, Julian DG, eds. Lidocaine in the Treatment of Ventricular Arrhythmias. Edinburgh, England E & S Livingstone, Ltd.; 1971:168.

20. Collingsworth KA et al. Pharmacokinetics and metabolism of lidocaine in patients with renal failure. Clin Pharmacol Ther. 1975;18:59.

21. Strong JM et al. Pharmacological activity, metabolism, and pharmacokinetics of glycinexylidide. Clin Pharmacol Ther. 1975;17:184.

22. Le Lorier J et al. Pharmacokinetics of lidocaine after prolonged intravenous infusions in uncomplicated myocardial infarction. Ann Intern Med. 1977;87:700.

23. Ochs HR et al. Reduction in lidocaine clearance during continuous infusion and by coadministration of propranolol. N Eng J Med. 1980;303:373–7.

24. Morgan DJ et al. Prediction of acute myocardial disposition of antiarrhythmic drugs. J Pharm Sci. 1989;78:384–8.

25. Zeisler JA et al. Lidocaine therapy: time for re-evaluation. Clin Pharmacy. 1993;12:527–8.

26. Hine LK et al. Meta-analytic evidence against prophylactic use of lidocaine in acute myocardial infarction. Arch Intern Med. 1989;149: 2694–8.

27. Anderson JL et al. Anti-arrhythmic drugs: clinical pharmacology and therapeutic uses. Drugs. 1978;15:271.

28. Zito RA, Reid P. Lidocaine kinetic predicted by indocyanine green clearance. N Engl J Med. 1978; 298:1160.

29. Lopez LM et al. Optimal lidocaine dosing in patients with myocardial infarction. Ther Drug Monit. 1982;4:271.

30. Stargel WW et al. Clinical comparison of rapid infusion and multiple injection methods for lidocaine loading. Am Heart J. 1981;102:872.

31. Edwards DJ et al. Alpha-1-acid glycoprotein concentration and protein binding in trauma. Clin Pharmacol Ther. 1982;31:62.

32. Fremstad D et al. Increased plasma binding of quinidine after surgery. A preliminary report. Eur J Clin Pharmacol. 1976;10:441.

Lithium 7

Lithium salts have been used for a variety of psychiatric illnesses; however, they are most commonly used to treat patients with mania or patients with bipolar depression. Lithium is usually prescribed as the carbonate salt which contains 8.12 mEq of lithium per 300 mg tablet or capsule. It is also available as 300 mg (8.12 mEq) or 450 mg (12.18 mEq) extended-release capsules and as an oral solution which contains 8 mEq/5 mL. The usual adult dose for lithium carbonate ranges from 900 to 1200 mg/day. Lithium is not bound to plasma proteins and is distributed extensively in the intracellular compartment. Lithium elimination is influenced significantly by renal function as well as by sodium loading or depletion.

Therapeutic and Toxic Plasma Concentrations

The usual range of therapeutic plasma concentrations for lithium in patients receiving chronic therapy is 0.6 to 0.8 mEq/L. Occasionally, in patients with acute mania, slightly higher plasma levels of 0.8 to 1.2 mEq/L are desirable; however, chronic therapy at these concentrations is not usually the goal.[1–3,5,6] In general, the lowest lithium concentration which controls the manic state is the desired end-point.

The most common side effects associated with lithium therapy are nausea, vomiting, anorexia, epigastric bloating, and abdominal pain. These adverse effects seem to occur after large doses of rapidly-absorbed dosage forms are administered and may be due to high intragastrointestinal concentrations or high plasma concentrations. Many of these effects subside with continued therapy, but they occasionally persist. Gastrointestinal side effects may be minimized in some patients by use of the slow-release lithium dosage forms. Central nervous system (CNS) side effects (e.g., lethargy, fatigue, muscle weakness, and tremor) are usually associated with plasma concentrations exceeding 1.5 mEq/L.[2,3]

Bioavailability (F)

Lithium is rapidly absorbed, and plasma concentrations peak within one-half to three hours following oral administration. Gastrointestinal absorption of conventional lithium carbonate tablets or capsules appears to be virtually complete (95% to 100%). The absorption of sustained-release lithium products is more variable, and ranges from 60% to 90%.[6] Lithium

Key Parameters

Therapeutic Range[a]	0.6–0.8 mEq/L (morning trough)
F	100%
Vd	0.7 L/kg
Cl	$0.25 \times Cl_{Cr}$
t½	
α	6 hr
β	20 hr

[a] Slightly higher values (0.8–1.2 µg/L) often used for acute mania.

solution appears to be rapidly and completely absorbed and plasma concentrations peak within 60 minutes.[7,8]

Volume of Distribution (Vd)

The usual volume of distribution for lithium is approximately 0.7 L/kg.[8] Although this volume of distribution is approximately equal to that of body water, lithium concentrates in various intra-compartmental spaces and equilibrates very slowly with the extracellular fluid volume.[1] In addition, lithium distribution follows a two-compartment model with an initial volume of distribution of 0.25 to 0.3 L/kg and a final volume of distribution at equilibrium of ≈0.7 L/kg. The elevated plasma lithium concentrations during the distribution phase do not appear to correlate with either efficacy or toxicity.[3,7,8]

Clearance (Cl)

Lithium is not metabolized and is eliminated from the body almost exclusively by the renal route; negligible amounts are lost through feces and sweat. Lithium is readily filtered by the kidneys, and 80% of that which is filtered is reabsorbed.[3,8] The renal tubular reabsorption of lithium is very closely linked with sodium reabsorption and is influenced by changes in the renal clearance of sodium. In patients with a normal sodium balance, lithium clearance is ≈25% of creatinine clearance.[3,8]

While using 25% of creatinine clearance is a reasonable initial estimate for lithium clearance, there are a number of factors that alter the clearance of lithium. Therefore the use of this approach to predict lithium plasma concentration has been questioned.[4]

$$\text{Lithium Clearance} = [0.25][\text{Creatinine Clearance}]$$

Eq. 7.1

Although a number of drugs and disease states can influence lithium clearance, the most important influences on clearance are renal function and sodium balance.[3,9] Loop or thiazide diuretics, aminophylline, volume depletion, a low sodium diet, and hypothyroidism can decrease lithium clearance. The effect of the nonsteroidal anti-inflammatory drugs on lithium clearance is somewhat variable. It ranges from essentially no change in lithium clearance to a 25% to 30% reduction.[10,11] The angiotensin-covering enzyme inhibitors, enalapril and lisinopril, also appear to reduce the renal clearance of lithium by about 50%.[6,12] Lithium clearance has also been reported to be reduced in patients with acute mania, and it has been suggested that maintenance doses be reduced to about 60% of their usual value when acute episodes of mania occur.[13] An increase in lithium clearance has been associated with the later stage of pregnancy[9] as well as with sodium loading.

Half-Life (t½)

The initial distribution or alpha half-life of lithium is about six hours and the final elimination or beta half-life is 18 to 24 hours.[8]

Single-Point Predictions

A 24-hour serum lithium level following a single specified dose can be used to predict maintenance dose requirements.[14] One critical factor is the timing of the single plasma concentration measurement. For a one-compartment-model drug, the optimal time to sample is ≈1.44 half-lives.[15] For this two-compartment drug, however, the 24-hour time interval appears to be appropriate because a significant amount of lithium is eliminated during the initial distribution phase. Patients for whom the single-point determination method is least likely to be successful include those who significantly differ from the average population in body size or lithium clearance. Therefore, the single-point determination method should be used with great caution in patients who are significantly larger or smaller than average, or in patients with an unusually high or low lithium clearance (i.e., patients who are predicted to require unusually high or low maintenance doses).

Time of Sampling

Since lithium distribution follows a two-compartment model, it is imperative that samples for lithium plasma levels be obtained at consistent and reproducible times. The current standard of practice is to obtain samples just before the first morning dose of lithium and at least 12 hours after the last evening dose.[2,3,16] The terminal or β half-life of 18 hours suggests that steady-state lithium levels should be attained within three to five days. Although lithium levels appear to plateau within three and five days, full therapeutic effects are not generally observed for 14 to 21 days after therapy has been initiated. Nevertheless, dosing adjustments may be implemented based upon early steady-state plasma levels.

> *Question #1.* A.L., a 35-year-old, 65 kg, male, is being treated for acute mania. He is receiving 300 mg of lithium carbonate at 9:00 a.m., 2:00 p.m., and 9:00 p.m. His serum creatinine concentration is 0.9 mg/dL. Calculate the expected lithium concentration just before the morning dose on the day four of therapy.

Assuming A.L. has reasonably normal renal function and does not have an extended lithium half-life, steady state should be achieved in three days. The first step in calculating A.L.'s lithium concentration would be to approximate his renal function by use of Equation 63:

$$\frac{\text{Cl}_{\text{Cr}} \text{ for Males}}{(\text{mL/min})} = \frac{(140 - \text{Age})(\text{Weight})}{(72)(\text{SrCr}_{\text{ss}})}$$

$$= \frac{(140 - 35)(65)}{(72)(0.9)}$$

$$= 105 \text{ mL/min}$$

$$\text{Cl}_{\text{Cr}} \text{ (L/hr)} = (105 \text{ mL/min})\left[\frac{60 \text{ min/hr}}{1000 \text{ mL/L}}\right]$$

$$= 6.3 \text{ L/hr}$$

The corresponding lithium clearance should be calculated next, using Equation 7.1 as follows:

$$\begin{aligned} \text{Lithium Clearance} &= [0.25][\text{Creatinine Clearance}] \\ &= (0.25)(6.3 \text{ L/hr}) \\ &= 1.6 \text{ L/hr} \end{aligned}$$

A.L.'s total lithium dose of 900 mg corresponds to $\approx$24.4 mEq of lithium based upon the following calculation:

$$\begin{array}{c} \text{Lithium Dose} \\ \text{(mEq)} \end{array} = \left[\begin{array}{c} \text{Lithium Carbonate Dose} \\ \text{(mg)} \end{array} \right] \left[\dfrac{8.12 \text{ mEq}}{300 \text{ mg}} \right]$$

Eq. 7.2

$$\begin{aligned} &= [900 \text{ mg}] \left[\dfrac{8.12 \text{ mEq}}{300 \text{ mg}} \right] \\ &= 24.4 \text{ mEq} \end{aligned}$$

The average steady-state lithium concentration of 0.63 mEq/L can then be calculated by using Equation 35. Note that F is 1 and S is 1, because the salt factor for the dose of lithium carbonate has already been corrected or accounted for in Equation 7.2.

$$\begin{aligned} \text{Cpss ave} &= \dfrac{(S)(F)(\text{Dose}/\tau)}{Cl} \\ &= \dfrac{(1)(1)(24.4 \text{ mEq}/24 \text{ hr})}{1.6 \text{ L/hr}} \\ &= 0.63 \text{ mEq/L} \end{aligned}$$

Since lithium has a long β half-life, a divided daily dose schedule should not affect the average plasma concentration; however, trough concentrations obtained just before the morning dose are usually 20% to 30% lower than the average plasma level because of the significant two-compartmental distribution of lithium.[3] (See Part I: Maximum and Minimum Plasma Concentrations on page 53.) For this reason, one may choose to multiply the expected average concentration by a factor of 0.75 to calculate the actual trough concentration just before the morning dose.

Question #2. A.L.'s trough concentration on the morning of Day 4 was 0.8 mEq/L. Calculate a new dosing regimen designed to achieve a trough concentration of 1.2 mEq/L.

Assuming the lithium concentration of 0.8 mEq/L approximates the average steady-state concentration, Equation 15 can be used to estimate A.L.'s lithium clearance of 1.27 L/hr:

$$Cl = \frac{(S)(F)(Dose/\tau)}{Cpss\ ave}$$
$$= \frac{(1)(1)(24.4\ mEq/24\ hr)}{0.8\ mEq/L}$$
$$= 1.27\ L/hr$$

A.L.'s specific lithium clearance then can be used with Equation 16 to calculate the daily maintenance dose in mEq:

$$Maintenance\ Dose = \frac{(Cl)(Cpss\ ave)(\tau)}{(S)(F)}$$
$$= \frac{(1.27\ L/hr)(1.2\ mEq/L)(24\ hr)}{(1)(1)}$$
$$= 36.6\ mEq$$

Equation 7.3 can then be used to convert the lithium dose expressed as mEq/24 hours to the equivalent dose expressed in milligrams of lithium carbonate.

$$\frac{\text{Lithium Carbonate Dose}}{\text{(mg)}} = \left[\frac{\text{Lithium Dose}}{\text{(mEq)}}\right]\left[\frac{300\ \text{mg}}{8.12\ \text{mEq}}\right]$$

Eq. 7.3

$$= \left[36.6\ \text{mEq}\right]\left[\frac{300\ \text{mg}}{8.12\ \text{mEq}}\right]$$

$$= 1352\ \text{mg}\ \ or\ \ \approx\! 1350\ \text{mg}$$

This daily dose of 1350 mg of lithium carbonate could be most conveniently administered as either four (1200 mg) or five (1500 mg) 300 mg lithium carbonate tablets or capsules. Because of the large change in the maintenance dose and the high target concentration, a conservative approach would be to administer four 300 mg tablets or capsules in a divided daily regimen.

Note that the trough concentration was assumed to approximate the average lithium level. To more closely estimate the average concentration, the measured trough concentration could be divided by 0.75 to account for the significant two-compartmental distribution of lithium. However, if the new trough concentration was to be 1.2 mEq/L, a similar calculation would be made such that the associated average concentration would be 1.6 mEq/L (1.2 mEq/L ÷ 0.75). The lower clearance calculated would be associated with a higher average concentration and as a result the new dose would be essentially the same (i.e., 1352 mg/day).

Question #3. **M.C., a 55-year-old female, is receiving 300 mg of lithium carbonate at 9:00 a.m., 1:00 p.m., and 5:00 p.m. At 11:30 a.m. her lithium plasma concentration was reported to be 2.7 mEq/L. What factors should be considered in evaluating this measured lithium concentration?**

The significant two-compartmental modeling and the prolonged lithium α half-life of six hours dictate that lithium levels be obtained only before the first morning dose and at least 12 hours after the previous evening dose. In the case of M.C., it is likely that this elevated lithium concentration of 2.7 mEq/L was obtained during the distribution phase. Plasma concentrations measured in this phase do not correlate with the efficacy or toxicity of lithium. The time of the last administered lithium dose should be ascertained to assure that the elevated lithium level is in fact due to problems associated with the distribution phase. In addition, a second lithium level should be obtained the following morning just before the next administered dose. M.C.'s medical records also should be reviewed for any factors associated with diminished lithium clearance (e.g., an elevated serum creatinine, concomitant diuretic therapy, or volume depletion).

Question #4. **Are erythrocyte lithium concentration measurements useful in monitoring chronic lithium therapy?**

In theory, erythrocyte lithium concentrations are attractive because they represent an intracellular lithium concentration and may more directly correspond to the efficacy and toxicity of lithium. A number of studies have examined the relationship between efficacy and the erythrocyte lithium concentrations or the erythrocyte-plasma lithium concentration ratio. Unfortunately, the results are still inconclusive; therefore, erythrocyte lithium concentrations have relatively limited use in general clinical practice at this time and cannot be recommended for use in the routine monitoring of patients taking this drug.

References

1. Elizur A et al. Intra: extracellular lithium ratios and clinical course in affective states. Clin Pharm Ther. 1972;13:947.

2. Salem RB. A pharmacist's guide to monitoring lithium drug-drug interactions. Drug Intell Clin Pharm. 1982;16:745.

3. Amdisen A. Lithium. In: Evans WE, Schentag JJ, Jusko WJ, eds. Applied Pharmacokinetics: Principles of Therapeutic Drug Monitoring, 2nd ed. Spokane:Applied Therapeutics;1986:978–1002.

4. Browne JL, et al. Comparison of pharmacokinetic procedures for dosing lithium based on analysis of prediction error. Drug Intell Clin Pharm. 1988;22:227–31.

5. Consensus development panel. Mood disorders: pharmacologic prevention of recurrences. Am J Psychiatry. 1985;142:469–76.

6. Carson SW. Lithium in. Evans WE, et al., eds. Applied Pharmacokinetics: Principles of Therapeutic Drug Monitoring. 3rd Ed. Vancouver, WA: Applied Therapeutics Inc. 1992:34–1.

7. Sugita ET et al. Lithium carbonate absorption in humans. Clin Pharm. 1973;13:264.

8. Goth U et al. Estimation of pharmacokinetic parameters of lithium from saliva and urine. Clin Pharmacol Ther. 1974;16:490.

9. Amdisen A. Lithium and drug interactions. Drugs. 1982;24:133.

10. Frolich JC. et al. Indomethacin increases plasma lithium. Med J. 1979; 1:1115–6.

11. Ragheb M, Powell AL. Lithium interaction with sulindac and naproxen. J Clin Psychopharmacol. 1986;6:150–4.

12. Balwin CM, Safferman AZ. A case of lisinopril-induced lithium toxicity. DICP Ann Pharmacother.1990;24:946–7.

13. Almy GL, Taylor MG. Lithium retention in mania. Arch Gen Psychiatry. 1973;29:232–4.

14. Cooper TB et al. The 24-hour serum lithium level as a prognosticator of dosage requirements. Am J Psychiatry. 1973;130:601–3

15. Unadkat JD, Rowland M. Further considerations of the "single-point, single-dose"method to estimate individual maintenance dosage requirements. Ther Drug Monit. 1982;4:201.

16. Bergner PE et al. Lithium kinetics in man: effect of variation in dosage pattern. Br Pharmacol. 1973;49:328.

Methotrexate (MTX) 8

Methotrexate is a folic acid antagonist which competitively inhibits dihydrofolate reductase, the enzyme responsible for converting folic acid to the reduced or active folate cofactors. Although methotrexate has been used as an anticancer agent for a number of years, there has been a recent resurgence in its use because moderate (500 to 1500 mg) and high (>5 gm) dosing regimens have been introduced. Moderate and high-dose regimens were developed because tumors responded poorly to low-dose regimens (20 to 100 mg). Currently, methotrexate is used to treat a number of neoplasms, including leukemia, osteogenic sarcoma, Wilm's tumor, and non-Hodgkin's lymphoma. Methotrexate is always administered by the intravenous (IV) route when doses exceed 30 mg/m^2 because oral absorption is limited.[1] Current dosing regimens can range from as low as 20 to 50 mg to as high as 10 to 12 gm or more. These doses are administered over a period as short as three to six hours to as long as 40 hours.[2,3]

Approximately 50% of methotrexate is bound to plasma proteins.[1,2] Methotrexate has active metabolites, the most significant of which is the 7-hydroxy compound. Although this metabolite only has approximately 1/200th the clinical activity of methotrexate, it is one-third to one-fifth as soluble. As a result, it may precipitate in the renal tubules causing acute nephrotoxicity.[4] Due to this solubility problem, patients receiving large doses of methotrexate should be adequately hydrated and should receive sodium bicarbonate to maintain the urine pH above 7.[2,3]

Therapeutic and Toxic Plasma Concentrations

The therapeutic and toxic effects of methotrexate are closely linked to its plasma concentrations. Since the goal of therapy is to inhibit dihydrofolate reductase (DHFR) and, ultimately, to deplete the reduced folate cofactors, the relative ability to inhibit DHFR and the time course required to deplete the cofactors is critical to the relationship between the drug's efficacy and its toxicity.

Units. Methotrexate is generally administered in mg or gm doses and the plasma concentrations are reported in units of mg/L, µg/mL, and molar or micromolar units. When methotrexate concentrations are reported in molar units, they usually range from values of 10^{-8} to 10^{-2} molar. In addition, they are occasionally reported in micromolar (or 10^{-6} molar) units. To interpret methotrexate concentrations accurately, it is important to establish which units are being reported and how those units corre-

Key Parameters

Therapeutic Plasma Concentration	Variable
Toxic Concentration	
Plasma	$>1 \times 10^{-7}$ molar for >48 hr $>1 \times 10^{-6}$ molar at >48 hr requires increased rescue factor doses
CNS	Continuous CNS MTX concentrations $>10^{-8}$ molar
F	
Dose <30 mg/m^2	100%
Dose >80 mg/m^2	Variable
Vi (initial)	0.2 L/kg
Vd AUC	0.7 L/kg
Cl	$[1.6][Cl_{Cr}]$
t½	
α^a	3 hr
β^b	10 hr

[a] t½ of 3 hr generally employed with methotrexate plasma concentrations greater than 5×10^{-7} molar.
[b] t½ of 10 hr generally employed with methotrexate plasma concentrations of less than 5×10^{-7} molar.

spond to the generally-accepted therapeutic or toxic values. Methotrexate has a molecular weight of 454 gm/mole; therefore, a value of 0.454 mg/L is equal to 1×10^{-6} molar or 1 micromolar. To convert methotrexate concentrations in units of mg/L to molar concentrations, the following equation can be used:

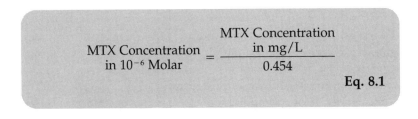

$$\text{MTX Concentration in } 10^{-6} \text{ Molar} = \frac{\text{MTX Concentration in mg/L}}{0.454}$$

Eq. 8.1

In the above equation, MTX represents the methotrexate concentration, and the factor 0.454 is the number of mg/L equal to 10^{-6} molar or 1 micromolar. Methotrexate concentrations reported in molar units should first be converted to 10^{-6} molar and then multiplied times the factor 0.454 to calculate the equivalent methotrexate concentration in units of mg/L:

$$\frac{\text{MTX Concentration}}{\text{in mg/L}} = \left(\frac{\text{MTX Concentration}}{\text{in } 10^{-6} \text{ Molar}}\right)(0.454)$$

Eq. 8.2

Methotrexate concentrations in the units of molar, micromolar, or mg/L are interchangeable, as long as the correct unit adjustment and interpretation of the reported concentration are made. For example, a methotrexate concentration of 1 micromolar would be equivalent to the following:

$$0.01 \times 10^{-4} \text{ molar}$$

$$0.1 \times 10^{-5} \text{ molar}$$

$$1.0 \times 10^{-6} \text{ molar}$$

$$1 \text{ μM (micromolar)}$$

$$10 \times 10^{-7} \text{ molar}$$

$$0.454 \text{ mg/L}$$

Note that while all of the concentrations listed above represent the same value, the units differ. For example, the concentration, 0.01×10^{-4} molar, is expressed in units that are 100 times more concentrated than 10^{-6}. Therefore, when interpreting methotrexate plasma concentrations, it is important to determine whether a value of 1.0 represents micromolar units (10^{-6} molar) or some other unit value.

Therapeutic Plasma Concentrations. Most therapeutic regimens are designed to achieve concentrations above 1×10^{-7} molar for <48 hours. Concentrations of methotrexate that have been associated with successful treatment of various neoplasms range from 10^{-6} up to 10^{-3} or 10^{-2} molar. Although the relationship of the methotrexate concentration to tumor kill is somewhat empiric, Evans et al. have documented that methotrexate concentrations in the range of 16×10^{-6} molar are successful in the treatment of leukemic patients.[5] These high methotrexate levels are not usually associated with serious methotrexate toxicity as long as adequate hydration and renal function are maintained, and the methotrexate concentration falls below 1×10^{-7} molar within 48 hours following the initiation of therapy or the discontinuation of rescue factor.

Toxic Plasma Concentration. Plasma concentrations exceeding 1×10^{-8} to 1×10^{-7} molar for 48 hours or more are associated with methotrexate toxicity.[6] The most common toxic effects of methotrexate include myelosuppression, oral and gastrointestinal mucositis, and acute hepatic dysfunction.[1,2,6]

Leucovorin Rescue. In order to ensure that methotrexate toxicities do not occur, rescue factor (citrovorin factor or leucovorin) is administered every four to six hours in doses that range from 10 to 50 mg/m^2.[2,3,6] The usual course of rescue therapy is from 12 to 72 hours, or until the plasma concentration of methotrexate falls below the critical value of 1×10^{-7} molar. In some rescue protocols, concentrations of less than 1×10^{-7} molar (e.g., 5×10^{-8}) have been considered to be the value indicating the rescue is complete.[3] Most protocols, however, utilize the value of 1×10^{-7} molar as the concentration at which rescue is completed.

Methotrexate concentrations in excess of 1×10^{-6} molar at 48 hours are associated with an increased incidence of methotrexate toxicity, even in the face of leucovorin rescue doses of 10 mg/m^2. When the methotrexate concentration exceeds 1×10^{-6} molar at 48 hours, increasing the leucovorin rescue dose to 50 to 100 mg/m^2 or more reduces methotrexate toxicity.[6] Presumably, this increased dose enables leucovorin factor to compete successfully with methotrexate for intracellular transport; it thereby rescues host tissues.

Although rescue regimens vary considerably, most employ a leucovorin dosing regimen of $\approx$10 mg/m^2 administered every six hours for 72 hours. If the methotrexate concentration falls below 1×10^{-7} molar before the completion of the 72-hour rescue period, then the rescue factor can be discontinued. If the methotrexate concentrations are still greater than 1×10^{-7} but less than 1×10^{-6} at 48 hours, then rescue with leucovorin is continued at doses of $\approx$10 mg/m^2 every six hours until the methotrexate concentration falls below the rescue value of 1×10^{-7} molar.

Goals of Monitoring. One of the primary goals of methotrexate plasma monitoring is to ensure that all patients receive adequate doses of rescue factor to prevent serious toxicity. Since most high-dose rescue regimens are designed to "save" the average patient, the vast majority of methotrexate plasma levels that are obtained for monitoring will be routine and are unlikely to require intervention. Nevertheless, plasma concentration monitoring can be used to detect unusual methotrexate disposition characteristics that could result in serious toxicity.

Methotrexate Assays. There are a number of methotrexate assays, which use differing methodologies; however, none of these appear to be clearly superior to the others. All assays used should have the ability to measure plasma concentrations below the rescue value of 1×10^{-7} molar and above 1×10^{-6} molar. When methotrexate plasma levels are still elevated at 48 hours, the dose of rescue factor must be increased.[7,8]

Bioavailability (F)

Methotrexate oral absorption is complete and rapid, with peak concentrations occurring one to two hours following doses of <30 mg/m². At doses >80 mg/m², the extent of methotrexate absorption declines, and bioavailability is incomplete.[1] For this reason, moderate and high-dose methotrexate regimens must be administered by the IV route. Low-dose methotrexate (<30 mg/m²) may be administered parenterally or orally.

Volume of Distribution (Vd)

The relationship between methotrexate plasma concentrations and volume of distribution is complex. The drug displays at least a bi-exponential elimination curve, indicating that there is an initial plasma volume of distribution of about 0.2 L/kg and a second larger volume of distribution of 0.5 to 1.0 L/kg following complete distribution.[9,10] The evaluation of the apparent volume of distribution for methotrexate is further complicated by the fact that it appears to increase at higher plasma concentrations.[9] This phenomenon may reflect an active transport system which becomes saturated at high plasma concentrations and reverts to passive intracellular diffusion of methotrexate. The multi-compartmental modeling, as well as the variable relationship between the plasma concentration and apparent volume of distribution of methotrexate, make calculation of methotrexate loading doses somewhat speculative. Nevertheless, when loading doses are required, a volume of distribution of 0.2 to 0.5 L/kg is usually employed.

The presence of third-space fluids such as ascites, edema, or pleural effusions can also influence the volume of distribution of methotrexate.[11] Although pleural effusions do not substantially increase the volume of distribution, the high concentrations of methotrexate which accumulate in these spaces can be important because equilibration with plasma is delayed. In patients with pleural effusions, the initial elimination half-life appears to be normal; however, the second elimination phase is prolonged.[12] Prolongation of this terminal elimination phase is significant because the time required for patients to achieve a methotrexate plasma concentration of less than 1×10^{-7} can be extended. In this situation, additional doses of rescue factor may have to be administered beyond the usual rescue period. [See Figure 8.1 and Methotrexate Half-Life (t½).]

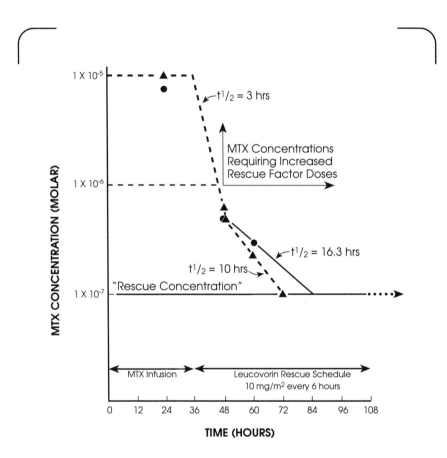

Figure 8.1. Methotrexate. Figure 8.1 represents a semilog plot of the expected (▲) and measured (●) methotrexate (MTX) plasma concentrations during and following a 36 hour infusion. Levels were obtained at 24, 48, and 60 hours after the start of the infusion. Note that leucovorin rescue should be continued as long as the methotrexate concentration is greater than the rescue value (represented here as 1×10^{-7} molar or 0.1 micromolar) and that the rescue dose should be increased for methotrexate levels greater than 1×10^{-6} molar at 48 hours and beyond.

Clearance (Cl)

The vast majority of methotrexate is eliminated by the renal route.[12,13] Methotrexate clearance ranges from one to as much as two times the creatinine clearance.[2,4,12,13] (The author uses a factor of 1.6 to estimate methotrexate clearance in the clinical setting.) Methotrexate clearance by an active transport mechanism that may be saturable results in a renal clearance value which varies (relative to creatinine clearance) with methotrexate plasma concentrations.[4]

The renal clearance of methotrexate also is influenced by a number of compounds (e.g., probenecid and salicylates influence weak acid secretion). In addition, sulfisoxazole and other weak acids have been reported to diminish the renal transport of methotrexate.[4,14] Since methotrexate renal clearance may be inhibited, all drugs should be added cautiously to the regimen of a patient receiving methotrexate therapy. Although early reports attributed salicylate-induced methotrexate toxicity to plasma protein displacement of methotrexate, the most likely mechanism is an alteration in renal clearance. An alteration in plasma binding is an unlikely explanation because methotrexate is only 50% protein-bound to plasma proteins.[4,14]

Changes in renal function are important when designing and monitoring methotrexate therapy. Therefore, all patients receiving moderate and high-dose methotrexate therapy should have their plasma level of methotrexate and their renal function monitored. While the therapeutic dose of methotrexate may range over several grams, serious toxicity and death have been attributed to doses as low as 10 mg of methotrexate when administered to a patient with inadequate renal function.[15,16]

Concomitant administration of the prostaglandin inhibitors, indomethacin and ketoprofen, with methotrexate has been associated with an acute decrease in renal function and a greatly prolonged exposure to high methotrexate concentrations.[17,18] This interaction presumably results from the combined renal effects of the nonsteroidal anti-inflammatory agent with methotrexate. Although this interaction has not been described for all nonsteroidal anti-inflammatory agents, these agents probably should be avoided in patients receiving methotrexate therapy.

A relatively small percentage of methotrexate is metabolized; nevertheless, significant amounts of methotrexate metabolites can be found in the urine when large doses are administered. This is especially true during the late phase of methotrexate elimination when the majority of the parent compound has been eliminated. The most extensively studied metabolite is the 7-hydroxy methotrexate compound, which is considered to be potentially nephrotoxic because of its low water solubility.[4]

Half-Life (t½)

The relationship between methotrexate's volume of distribution and clearance is complex. Because of the potential for capacity-limited intracellular transport as well as capacity-limited renal clearance, the apparent half-lives for methotrexate are determined by both a changing volume of distribution and clearance. Consequently, the elimination of methotrexate is not accurately described by linear pharmacokinetic modeling. Given these problems, a relatively simple, two-compartment model with an initial α half-life of two to three hours and a β or terminal half-life of approximately ten hours appears to represent the elimination phase reasonably well.[10,12,13] The terminal or β half-life of approximately ten hours often does not become apparent until plasma concentrations decline into the range of 5×10^{-7} molar (0.5×10^{-6} or 0.5 micromolar). Since the terminal phase is also independent of the dose administered, it probably reflects a change in the distribution and elimination of methotrexate.

While the apparent terminal half-life of methotrexate is somewhat variable, it does not appear to increase with increasing doses. Unlike most other two-compartmental drugs, significant methotrexate is eliminated during the α phase. In fact, a very large percentage of the total methotrexate may be eliminated during the α phase. Nevertheless, the terminal phase is also important, because retention of even a very small amount of the administered dose can be potentially toxic to the patient.[10,11]

Pleural effusions can significantly prolong the terminal half-life of methotrexate, and leucovorin rescue regimens may need to be extended over a longer period of time in this situation. Some patients may unexpectedly develop acute changes in renal function or, in a few cases, prolonged elimination characteristics which are unpredictable and independent of renal function. For this reason, continued monitoring of methotrexate is essential, even if early plasma level monitoring indicates that an adjustment of the methotrexate dose or rescue factor regimen is unnecessary.

Time to Sample

Methotrexate plasma concentrations can be used to evaluate the potential efficacy of a given dosing regimen and to determine if the quantity and/or duration of leucovorin rescue is adequate. There are two situations when monitoring methotrexate levels for efficacy is useful. The first is in patients who are to receive prolonged methotrexate infusions, since in these cases the infusion rate can be adjusted. The second is in patients who are going to receive repeated methotrexate doses, in which case future doses can be adjusted to achieve the desired target concentration.

When using methotrexate levels to evaluate the rescue dosage regimen, samples are obtained 24 to 48 hours following the initiation of therapy to determine whether additional leucovorin will be required, either in quantity or duration of administration. For example, plasma levels greater than 1×10^{-6} molar at 48 hours are usually associated with increased methotrexate toxicity unless leucovorin rescue doses are increased from 10 mg/m² every six hours to 50 to 100 mg/m² every 4 to 6 hours. For patients with plasma levels below 1×10^{-6} but above 1×10^{-7} molar, a leucovorin rescue dose of 10 mg/m² every six hours is generally adequate to prevent toxicity if continued until the plasma concentration drops below 1×10^{-7} molar.

Plasma samples obtained before the critical 48-hour time period may indicate whether the elimination of methotrexate is normal; however, because of the potential toxicity associated with even small amounts of retained methotrexate, all patients should have documented methotrexate concentrations below 1×10^{-7} molar before leucovorin rescue is discontinued. Calculating the critical rescue value may be acceptable in some cases, but extrapolating the data to more than one or two methotrexate half-lives is hazardous because the half-life of methotrexate tends to increase during the final decay periods. In most protocols, methotrexate levels are monitored sometime during the IV infusion, at 48 hours, and then every 24 hours until levels drop below the concentration at which the patient is considered to be "rescued," usually 1×10^{-7} molar.

Question #1. P.J., a 60-year-old, 70 kg male (SrCr = 1.2 mg/dL), is to receive a course of methotrexate therapy. His regimen will consist of a 30 mg methotrexate loading dose to be administered over 10 to 15 minutes, followed by an IV infusion of 30 mg/hr for the next 36 hours. He will then receive a 20 mg (≈10 mg/m²) dose of leucovorin every six hours intravenously for the first four doses followed by eight doses orally at six-hour intervals. The leucovorin regimen will begin immediately after the 36-hour methotrexate infusion has been discontinued and is scheduled to continue for the next 72 hours, ending 108 hours after initiation of the methotrexate therapy. Methotrexate levels are scheduled to be obtained 24 hours after the beginning of the 30 mg/hr infusion, at 48 hours (12 hours after the end of the

36-hour infusion), and at 60 hours (24 hours after the end of the methotrexate infusion). Calculate the anticipated methotrexate concentrations at the scheduled sampling times.

Determine MTX Clearance. Before the anticipated methotrexate concentrations can be calculated, it is first necessary to determine P.J.'s creatinine clearance, using Equation 63:

$$\begin{array}{l} \text{Cl}_{\text{Cr}} \text{ for Males} \\ \text{(mL/min)} \end{array} = \frac{(140 - \text{Age})(\text{Weight})}{(72)(\text{SrCr}_{\text{ss}})}$$

$$= \frac{(140 - 60)(70)}{(72)(1.2)}$$

$$= 64.8 \text{ mL/min}$$

Using this creatinine clearance of $\approx$65 mL/min and Equation 8.3, a methotrexate clearance of 6.24 L/hr can be calculated as shown below. P.J.'s creatinine clearance is first converted from mL/min to L/hr and then multiplied by a factor of 1.6 (see Methotrexate Clearance (Cl) on page 272).

$$\begin{array}{l} \text{Cl}_{\text{Cr}} \\ \text{(L/hr)} \end{array} = \left[\begin{array}{c} \text{Cl}_{\text{Cr}} \\ \text{(mL/min)} \end{array} \right] \left[\frac{60 \text{ min/hr}}{1000 \text{ mL/L}} \right]$$

$$= \left[64.8 \text{ mL/min} \right] \left[\frac{60 \text{ min/hr}}{1000 \text{ mL/L}} \right]$$

$$= 3.88 \text{ L/hr}$$

$$\text{Cl}_{\text{MTX}} = (1.6)(\text{Cl}_{\text{Cr}})$$

Eq. 8.3

$$= [1.6][3.9 \text{ L/hr}]$$

$$= 6.24 \text{ L/hr}$$

Calculate the 24-Hour Concentration. The 24-hour concentration represents an average steady-state level. The steady-state level of methotrexate in mg/L can then be calculated by using Equation 35:

$$\text{Cpss ave} = \frac{(S)(F)(\text{Dose}/\tau)}{Cl}$$

$$= \frac{(1)(1)(30 \text{ mg}/1 \text{ hr})}{6.24 \text{ L/hr}}$$

$$= 4.8 \text{ mg/L}$$

The values of S and F were assumed to be 1, and this methotrexate concentration in mg/L can be converted to a concentration in the units of micromoles or 10^{-6} molar by use of Equation 8.1:

$$\text{MTX Concentration in } 10^{-6} \text{ Molar} = \frac{\text{MTX Concentration in mg/L}}{0.454}$$

$$= \frac{4.8 \text{ mg/L}}{0.454}$$

$$= 10.57 \times 10^{-6} \text{ molar } or \ 1.057 \times 10^{-5} \text{ molar}$$

The resultant methotrexate concentration of approximately 10 $\times 10^{-6}$ or 1×10^{-5} molar assumes that steady state has been achieved 24 hours after the infusion rate of 30 mg/hr has been initiated. Steady state is assumed to have been achieved because the methotrexate plasma concentrations are relatively high. At concentrations greater than 10^{-7} molar, a half-life of two to three hours appears to determine the elimination and accumulation of most of the methotrexate in the body. As noted earlier, this model is not consistent with the traditional view of a two-compartment model in which the terminal half-life plays an important role in the accumulation toward steady state. Although there is the possibility of some continued accumulation, this generally appears to be minor and use of the shorter, two to three hour methotrexate half-life in evaluating initial methotrexate loss or accumulation is satisfactory in most cases.

Calculate the 48-Hour Level. Assuming, then, that the plasma concentration at the end of the 36-hour infusion is 10×10^{-6} molar, a plasma concentration of 0.625×10^{-6} molar (6.25×10^{-7} molar) at 48 hours (or 12 hours after the infusion has been discontinued) can be calculated using Equation 26:

$$Cp = (Cp°)(e^{-Kdt})$$

$Cp°$ is the methotrexate plasma concentration at the end of the infusion and t is the 12-hour time interval spanning from the end of the 36-hour infusion to the time of sampling at 48 hours. Kd is the elimination rate constant calculated from a rearrangement of Equation 31 using the shorter elimination half-life of three hours.

$$Kd = \frac{0.693}{t_{1/2}} \qquad \textbf{Eq. 8.4}$$

$$= \frac{0.693}{3 \text{ hr}}$$

$$= 0.231 \text{ hr}^{-1}$$

$$Cp = (Cp°)(e^{-Kdt})$$

$$Cp_1 = (10 \times 10^{-6} \text{ molar})(e^{-(0.231 \text{ hr}^{-1})(12 \text{ hr})})$$

$$= (10 \times 10^{-6} \text{ molar})(0.0625)$$

$$= 0.625 \times 10^{-6} \text{ molar } or \ 6.25 \times 10^{-7} \text{ molar}$$

Because this methotrexate concentration is below 1×10^{-6} molar 48 hours after starting the methotrexate therapy, the leucovorin rescue dose does not have to be increased, but should be continued until the concentration falls below 1×10^{-7} molar.

Calculate the 60-Hour Level. Calculation of the methotrexate concentration 60 hours after the infusion has been initiated (24 hours after the infusion has been concluded) is more problematic. The half-life for methotrexate tends to increase as the methotrexate concentration approaches 0.2 to 0.7×10^{-6} (2 to

7×10^{-7}) molar. Therefore, use of a traditional two-compartment model for this drug is inappropriate because the more prolonged terminal half-life correlates more closely with a specific concentration range than with a specific time interval following discontinuation of the infusion. This unusual phenomenon may be related to changes in the active transport system that is influenced by plasma concentration.

One technique that is used to predict methotrexate concentrations several hours after the infusion has been discontinued is to decay the methotrexate concentration to a range of 0.2 to 0.7×10^{-6} molar using a half-life of three hours. The longer or β half-life of ten hours is used to predict subsequent decay. If a plasma concentration of 0.5×10^{-6} is arbitrarily selected as the cut-off concentration for using a half-life of three hours, the time required for the initial decay can be calculated using Equation 4.6:

$$t = \frac{\ln\left(\dfrac{Cp_1}{Cp_2}\right)}{Kd}$$

Cp_1 represents the initial plasma concentration of 10×10^{-6} molar; Cp_2, the arbitrary cut-off plasma concentration of 0.5×10^{-6} molar; and Kd, the elimination rate constant corresponding to the initial half-life of three hours ($0.231 \ \text{hr}^{-1}$). Using Equation 4.6, the time (t) required for the methotrexate concentration to fall to 0.5×10^{-6} molar would be 13 hours after the end of the infusion or 49 hours after the methotrexate regimen is begun:

$$t = \frac{\ln\left(\dfrac{10 \times 10^{-6} \ \text{molar}}{0.5 \times 10^{-6} \ \text{molar}}\right)}{0.231 \ \text{hr}^{-1}}$$

$$= \frac{3}{0.231 \ \text{hr}^{-1}}$$

$$= 13 \ \text{hr}$$

To calculate the plasma concentration at 60 hours, the plasma level at 49 hours (36-hour infusion, 13-hour decay) would have to be decayed using Equation 26 for an additional 11 hours. In this case, however, the elimination rate constant that corresponds to the terminal elimination half-life of ten hours would be used (Equation 8.4):

$$Kd = \frac{0.693}{t\frac{1}{2}}$$

$$= \frac{0.693}{10 \ hr}$$

$$= 0.0693 \ hr^{-1}$$

Using these values and Equation 26, a methotrexate concentration of 1.6×10^{-7} molar can be calculated.

$$Cp = (Cp°)(e^{-Kdt})$$

$$= (0.5 \times 10^{-6} \ molar)(e^{-(0.0693 \ hr^{-1})(11 \ hr)})$$

$$= 0.23 \times 10^{-6} \ molar \quad or \quad 2.3 \times 10^{-7} \ molar$$

Since this concentration will decay to a concentration below 1×10^{-7} (the rescue value) in a little more than one half-life (≈ 10 hours), it would appear from our calculations that P.J. will have been rescued by leucovorin successfully.

Equation 26 suggests that an additional 12 hours will be required to decay the concentration to 1×10^{-7} molar; therefore, the rescue concentration will be achieved before leucovorin is scheduled to be discontinued. Nevertheless, these predicted concentrations are only approximations and cannot replace measured methotrexate concentrations. A graphical representation of the expected methotrexate concentrations [▲] is plotted in Figure 8.1. Unless there is a dramatic increase in the methotrexate half-life, the concentration will be well below 1×10^{-7} molar long before the leucovorin is scheduled to be discontinued.

Question #2. **P.J.'s methotrexate levels were reported as 8×10^{-6} molar at 24 hours, 0.5×10^{-6} molar (5×10^{-7} molar) at 48 hours, and 0.3×10^{-6} molar (3×10^{-7} molar)** at 60 hours. How would one interpret each of these methotrexate values? What would be an appropriate course of action regarding P.J.'s rescue therapy?

Evaluating the 24-Hour Concentration. The initial plasma concentration of 8×10^{-6} is lower than the predicted concentration calculated in Question 1 (10.57×10^{-6} molar). The lower-than-predicted concentration suggests that P.J.'s methotrexate clearance is greater than expected; however, the difference between the predicted and actual concentrations is well within the expected variation.

Evaluating the 48-Hour Concentration. The plasma level of 5×10^{-7} molar at 48 hours (12 hours after the infusion) suggests that P.J. is progressing as expected during the initial elimination phase. The difference between the expected (6.25×10^{-7} molar) and observed concentrations is minimal, considering the fact that the initial plasma level was slightly lower than predicted (see Figure 8.1). Because the observed plasma level is below 1×10^{-6} molar at 48 hours, it is unnecessary to increase the leucovorin dose.

Evaluating the 60-Hour Concentration. The measured methotrexate concentration of 3×10^{-7} molar at 60 hours is greater than the predicted concentration of 2.3×10^{-7} molar. Although the differences are not remarkable, it is of some concern that P.J.'s half-life is longer than anticipated. P.J.'s elimination rate constant and half-life are $0.046 \ hr^{-1}$ and 16.3 hr, respectively. These are calculated from the methotrexate concentrations at 48 and 60 hours using Equations 28 and 31, and a time interval of 12 hours:

$$Kd = \frac{\ln\left(\dfrac{Cp_1}{Cp_2}\right)}{t}$$

$$= \frac{\ln\left[\dfrac{5 \times 10^{-7} \ molar}{3 \times 10^{-7} \ molar}\right]}{12 \ hr}$$

$$= \frac{0.51}{12 \ hr}$$

$$= 0.0426 \ hr^{-1}$$

$$t\tfrac{1}{2} = \frac{0.693}{Kd}$$

$$= \frac{0.693}{0.0426 \ hr^{-1}}$$

$$= 16.3 \ hr$$

Although the increased methotrexate half-life appears to be substantial, the accuracy of the half-life calculation is uncertain because the plasma levels used are separated by a time interval that is less than one half-life. The increase in this terminal half-life of methotrexate could be attributed to any of the following: an assay error; accumulation of methotrexate in a pleural effusion or other third-space fluid; a drug-induced reduction in the renal clearance of methotrexate (e.g., salicylates); or a normal variance in methotrexate elimination.

Regardless of the cause, it is important to determine whether P.J. will achieve a plasma concentration of less than 1×10^{-7} molar by the time the leucovorin rescue is scheduled to be discontinued. Using the patient-specific or revised elimination rate constant of $0.0426 \ hr^{-1}$ and Equation 4.6, it appears as though P.J.'s methotrexate concentration will fall to 1.0×10^{-7} molar after an additional 25 hours (85 hours after starting the methotrexate therapy). This is well before the time scheduled for the discontinuation of leucovorin (108 hours after starting the methotrexate infusion).

$$t = \frac{\ln\left(\dfrac{Cp_1}{Cp_2}\right)}{Kd}$$

$$= \frac{\ln\left[\dfrac{3 \times 10^{-7} \ molar}{1 \times 10^{-7} \ molar}\right]}{0.0426 \ hr^{-1}}$$

$$= \frac{1.1}{0.0426 \ hr^{-1}}$$

$$= 25.8 \ hr$$

This calculation should not be used as the sole criterion for evaluating the success of rescue therapy because the elimination rate constant calculation is uncertain and the methotrexate terminal half-life may become more prolonged as the plasma concentration declines. In this particular case, additional methotrexate plasma levels should be obtained to ensure that the actual plasma concentration is below the critical value of 1×10^{-7} before the leucovorin rescue is discontinued. If this critical value has not been achieved by 108 hours, then additional doses of leucovorin will have to be administered until P.J. has achieved a plasma level below 1×10^{-7} molar. (See Figure 8.1.) Note that the observed methotrexate levels suggest P.J. has a more prolonged terminal half-life.

Question #3. **C.T., a 50-year-old, 60 kg male with a serum creatinine of 1.0 mg/dL, is to receive 12 gm IV methotrexate infused over four hours. Calculate the methotrexate concentration at the end of the four-hour infusion, 12 hours after the end of the infusion, and 48 hours after the start of the infusion (44 hours after ending the infusion).**

In order to calculate the expected concentrations, one first needs to estimate C.T.' s methotrexate clearance by calculating his creatinine clearance (Equation 63) and then his corresponding methotrexate clearance (Equation 8.3).

$$\frac{\text{Cl}_{\text{Cr}} \text{ for Males}}{\text{(mL/min)}} = \frac{(140 - \text{Age})(\text{Weight})}{(72)(\text{SrCr}_{ss})}$$

$$= \frac{(140 - 50)(60 \text{ kg})}{(72)(1.0 \text{ mg/dL})}$$

$$= 75 \text{ mL/min}$$

$$\frac{\text{Cl}_{\text{Cr}}}{\text{(L/hr)}} = \left[\frac{\text{Cl}_{\text{Cr}}}{\text{(mL/min)}}\right]\left[\frac{60 \text{ min/hr}}{1000 \text{ mL/L}}\right]$$

$$= \left[75 \text{ mL/min}\right]\left[\frac{60 \text{ min/hr}}{1000 \text{ mL/L}}\right]$$

$$= 4.5 \text{ L/hr}$$

$$Cl_{MTX} = (1.6)(Cl_{Cr})$$

$$= (1.6)(4.5 \text{ L/hr})$$

$$= 7.2 \text{ L/hr}$$

To calculate the methotrexate concentration obtained at the end of the infusion and 12 hours after the infusion, the shorter elimination half-life of three hours should be used to calculate the elimination rate constant (Equation 8.4).

$$Kd = \frac{0.693}{t\frac{1}{2}}$$

$$= \frac{0.693}{3 \text{ hr}}$$

$$= 0.231 \text{ hr}^{-1}$$

To predict the methotrexate concentration at the end of the infusion and 12 hours later, Equation 53 can be used, where $t_2 = 0$ for the level drawn at the end of the infusion, and $t_2 = 12$ hours for the level drawn 12 hours later.

$$Cp_2 = \frac{(S)(F)(Dose/t_{in})}{Cl}(1 - e^{-Kdt_{in}})(e^{-Kdt_2})$$

$$= \frac{(1)(1)(12,000 \text{ mg/4 hr})}{7.2 \text{ L/hr}}(1 - e^{-(0.231)(4 \text{ hr})})(e^{-(0.231)(t)})$$

$$= (416.7 \text{ mg/L})(1 - 0.4)(e^{-(0.231)(t)})$$

Where t = 0 hr:

$$= 250 \text{ mg/L } (e^{-(0.231)(0)})$$

$$= 250 \text{ mg/L}$$

At the End of the Infusion Where t = 12 hr:

$$= 250 \text{ mg/L } (e^{-(0.231)(12)})$$

$$= 250 \text{ mg/L } (0.063)$$

$$= 15.75 \text{ mg/L}$$

Using Equation 8.1, one can convert the methotrexate concentrations from mg/L to micromolar (10^{-6} molar) at the end of the 4 hour infusion:

$$\text{MTX Concentration in } 10^{-6} \text{ Molar} = \frac{\text{MTX Concentration in mg/L}}{0.454}$$

$$= \frac{250 \text{ mg/L}}{0.454}$$

$$= 550 \times 10^{-6} \text{ molar}$$

And 12 Hours Later:

$$= \frac{15.75 \text{ mg/L}}{0.454}$$

$$= 34.7 \times 10^{-6} \text{ molar}$$

To calculate the plasma concentration at 48 hours (44 hours after ending the infusion), it will be necessary to use Equation 4.6 to decay the plasma concentration to the point where the half-life changes from three hours to approximately ten hours.

$$t = \frac{\ln\left(\dfrac{Cp_1}{Cp_2}\right)}{Kd}$$

$$= \frac{\ln\left(\dfrac{34.7 \times 10^{-6} \text{ molar}}{0.5 \times 10^{-6} \text{ molar}}\right)}{0.231 \text{ hr}^{-1}}$$

$$= \frac{\ln(69.4)}{0.231 \text{ hr}^{-1}}$$

$$= \frac{4.2}{0.231 \text{ hr}^{-1}}$$

$$= 18 \text{ hr}$$

Therefore, 18 hours after the 12-hour sample, or at $\approx$34 hours from the start of the infusion (4 hour infusion + 12 hours + 18 hours), the methotrexate concentration would be approximately 0.5×10^{-6} molar. To calculate the concentration at 48 hours, the plasma concentration of 0.5×10^{-6} molar should be decayed for another 14 hours. At this concentration range, however, one anticipates the half-life of methotrexate to be approximately ten hours, corresponding to an elimination rate constant of 0.0693 hr^{-1} (Equation 8.4).

$$Kd = \frac{0.693}{t^{1/2}}$$

$$= \frac{0.693}{10 \text{ hr}}$$

$$= 0.0693 \text{ hr}^{-1}$$

Now, using Equation 26 and the new elimination rate constant, the methotrexate concentration 14 hours later (48 hours after starting the infusion) can be calculated.

$$Cp = (Cp^\circ)(e^{-Kdt})$$

$$= (0.5 \times 10^{-6} \text{ molar})(e^{-(0.0693)(14 \text{ hr})})$$

$$= (0.5 \times 10^{-6} \text{ molar})(0.38)$$

$$= 0.19 \times 10^{-6} \text{ molar } \textit{ or } \approx 0.2 \text{ micromolar}$$

The expected methotrexate concentration of approximately 0.2 micromolar is well below concentration range at which an increase in the leucovorin rescue dose is required, but still above the concentration range at which it could be discontinued. Assuming the rescue concentration is approximately 0.1 micromolar, it can be seen that approximately one more half-life (ten hours) will be required to reach the concentration of methotrexate at which the leucovorin can be discontinued.

Because methotrexate pharmacokinetic parameters are subject to considerable variability, these estimated plasma concentrations will have to be confirmed with actual plasma level measurements. In most clinical institutions, an early plasma concentration is obtained near the end of the methotrexate infusion to ensure that high and potentially therapeutic methotrexate levels are achieved. Additional levels are drawn approximately every 24 hours to track the methotrexate decline and to guide the leucovorin dosing requirements.

Question #4. **R.J., an 18-year-old, 50 kg female with leukemia, is to be treated every seven days with intrathecal MTX to prevent central nervous system (CNS) spread of her bone marrow disease. What would be an appropriate dose for R.J., considering her age and body size?**

There is considerable evidence that, regardless of body size, patients older than three years of age should receive a standard 12 mg dose of intrathecal methotrexate. This dose disregards body size, because the cerebrospinal fluid volume approaches 80% to 90% of its maximum value within the first three years of life. Furthermore, the size of the CNS compartment does not correlate well with either total body weight or body surface area.[19,20]

Question #5. **When patients are receiving intrathecal MTX, what factors should be considered in evaluating the risk of methotrexate toxicity?**

Intrathecally-administered doses of methotrexate are first cleared from the central nervous system (CNS) into the systemic circulation and then eliminated from the systemic circulation by the usual renal route. Since the standard intrathecal dose of methotrexate is only 12 mg, the risk of systemic methotrexate toxicity is relatively low unless the patient develops renal dysfunction. Therefore, the patient's renal function should be evaluated. It is also important to assure that the patient has not received drugs that are known to inhibit the renal clearance of methotrexate. In patients with severe renal dysfunction, serious systemic toxicity and even death can result from intrathecally-administered methotrexate due to the patient's inability to eliminate the drug from the body.[15,16]

Central nervous system toxicities can be mild to severe and include mild weakness, minor transient paralysis, and, in rare instances, severe leukoencephalopathy.[21,22] Serious CNS toxicities are associated with CNS methotrexate levels that are continuously maintained at a concentration above 10^{-8} molar.[21] For this reason, CNS methotrexate levels should be monitored to ensure that the CNS level has declined to an acceptable value before the weekly dose is administered. Patients who are most likely to retain methotrexate and have high CNS concentrations after intrathecal or intraventricular injections are those with active CNS disease (e.g., meningeal leukemia) or other defects in cerebrospinal flow.[19,21,22] An additional point to be made, although not a pharmacokinetic one, is that intraventricular or intrathecal doses of methotrexate are frequently given concomitantly with intravenous vincristine to increase tumor cell kill. Vincristine cannot be administered intraventricularly, as this route of vincristine administration is reported to be 100% fatal. It is therefore critical to recognize that, although these two drugs are frequently given at the same time during a course of therapy, vincristine is never administered directly into the CNS.[23]

References

1. Wan SH et al. Effect route of administration and effusions on methotrexate pharmacokinetics. Cancer Res. 1974;34:3487.

2. Bleyer WA. The clinical pharmacology of methotrexate. Cancer. 1978;41:36.

3. Bleyer WA. Methotrexate, clinical pharmacology, current status and therapeutic guidelines. Cancer Treat Rev. 1977;4:87.

4. Shen DD, Azarnoff DL. Clinical pharmacokinetics of methotrexate. Clin Pharmacokinet. 1978;3:1.

5. Evans WE et al. Clinical pharmacodynamics of high-dose methotrexate in acute lymphocytic leukemia. N Engl J Med. 1986;314:471.

6. Stoller RG et al. Use of plasma pharmacokinetics to predict and prevent methotrexate toxicity. N Engl J Med. 1977;297:630.

7. Buice RG. Evaluation of enzyme immunoassay, radioassay and radioimmunoassay of serum methotrexate, as compared with liquid chromatography. Clin Chem. 1980;26:1902.

8. Crom WR, Evans WE. Methotrexate. In: Evans WE et al., eds. Applied Pharmacokinetics: Principles of Therapeutic Drug Monitoring, 3rd ed. Vancouver: Applied Therapeutics;1992:1–42.

9. Leme PR et al. Kinetic model for the disposition and metabolism of moderate and high-dose methotrexate (NSC-740) in man. Cancer Chemother Rep. 1975;59:811.

10. Pratt CB et al. High-dose methotrexate used alone and in combination for measurable primary or metastatic osteosarcoma. Cancer Treat Rep. 1980;64:11.

11. Evans WE, Pratt CB. Effect of pleural effusion on high-dose methotrexate kinetics. Clin Pharmacol Ther. 1978;23:68.

12. Isacoff WH et al. Pharmacokinetics of high-dose methotrexate with citrovorum factor rescue. Cancer Treat Rep. 1977;61:1665.

13. Stoller RG et al. Pharmacokinetics of high-dose methotrexate (NSC-740). Cancer Chemother Rep. 1975(Pt. III);6:19.

14. Liegler DG et al. The effect of organic acids on renal clearance of methotrexate in man. Clin Pharmacol Ther. 1969;10:849.

15. Cadman EC et al. Systemic methotrexate toxicity. Arch Intern Med. 1976;136:1321.

16. Ahmad S et al. Methotrexate-induced renal failure and ineffectiveness of peritoneal dialysis. Arch Intern Med. 1978;138:1146.

17. Ellison NM, Servi RJ. Acute renal failure and death following sequential intermediate-dose methotrexate and 5-FU: a possible adverse effect due to concomitant indomethacin administration. Cancer Treat Rep. 1985;69:342.

18. Thyss A et al. Clinical and pharmacokinetic evidence of a life-threatening interaction between methotrexate and ketoprofen. Lancet. 1986;1:256.

19. Bleyer WA. Clinical pharmacology of intrathecal methotrexate. II. An improved dosage regimen derived from age-related pharmacokinetics. Cancer Treat Rep. 1977;61:1419.

20. Bonati M et al. Clinical pharmacokinetics of cerebrospinal fluid. Clin Pharmacokinet. 1982;7:312.

21. Bleyer WA et al. Neurotoxicity and elevated cerebrospinal fluid methotrexate concentration in meningeal leukemia. N Engl J Med. 1973; 289:770.

22. Duffner PK et al. CT abnormalities and altered methotrexate clearance in children with CNS leukemia. Neurology. 1984;34:229.

23. Solimando DA, Wilson JT. Prevention of accidental intrathecal administration of vincristine sulfate. Hosp Pharm. 1982;17:540.

Phenobarbital   9

Phenobarbital is a long-acting barbiturate used in the treatment of seizure disorders, insomnia, and anxiety. It is most commonly administered orally, but it may be administered intramuscularly and intravenously as well.

The usual adult maintenance dose of 2 mg/kg/day produces a steady-state plasma concentration of approximately 20 mg/L. Phenobarbital has a half-life of five days; therefore, therapeutic plasma concentrations are not achieved for two to three weeks following the initiation of a maintenance regimen. When therapeutic levels of 20 mg/L are required immediately, a loading dose of 15 mg/kg can be administered, usually in three divided doses of 5 mg/kg.

Therapeutic and Toxic Concentrations

In adults, phenobarbital concentrations of 10 to 30 mg/L are required for seizure control.[1] The upper end of the therapeutic range is limited by the appearance of side effects such as central nervous system (CNS) depression and ataxia.[2] Occasionally, patients exhibit no symptoms of toxicity even when phenobarbital concentrations exceed 40 mg/L.[3] Phenobarbital concentrations in excess of 100 to 150 mg/L are considered potentially lethal, although patients with much higher concentrations have survived.[3-5] Many patients develop excessive sedation when plasma phenobarbital concentrations are rapidly pushed into the therapeutic range. For this reason, many clinicians (if given the option) prefer to start patients on about 25% of the target maintenance dose for the first week of therapy, and then increase the maintenance dose by another 25% for each of the subsequent three weeks; a full maintenance dose regimen is achieved on the fourth week of therapy. This technique of slowly increasing the maintenance dose allows many patients to adjust to their phenobarbital concentrations; however, it does prolong the time required to achieve concentrations in the usually accepted therapeutic range.[6]

Bioavailability (F)

While it has not been well studied, the available data indicate that at least 80% and probably >90% of phenobarbital administered orally is absorbed. Complete bioavailability (F = 1.0) is supported by the observation that similar plasma concentrations are observed when the same dose of phenobarbital is given orally and parenterally.

Key Parameters

Therapeutic Plasma Concentrations	10–30 mg/L
Bioavailability (F)	>0.9
S (for Na salt)	0.9
Vd	0.6–0.7 L/kg
Cl[a]	
Children	8 mL/kg/hr (0.2 L/kg/day)
Adults	4 mL/kg/hr (0.1 L/kg/day)
t½	
Children	2.5 days
Adults	5 days
Fraction Free (α)	0.5

[a] Primarily metabolized by the liver, 20% cleared renally. Clearance in children >1 year of age is approximately twice the adult value.

Phenobarbital is frequently administered as the sodium salt which is approximately 91% phenobarbital acid (S = 0.91); however, a correction for the salt form is seldom made since the degree of error is small and the therapeutic range is relatively broad. When phenobarbital is administered parenterally, it is usually administered at a rate of no more than 50 mg/min to avoid toxicities associated with the propylene glycol diluent.[7]

Volume of Distribution (Vd)

The volume of distribution for phenobarbital is approximately 0.7 L/kg.[8,9]

Clearance (Cl)

Phenobarbital is primarily metabolized by the liver; <20% is eliminated by the renal route.[10] The average total plasma clearance for phenobarbital is ≈4 mL/kg/hr or 0.1 L/kg/day. This clearance value of approximately 0.1 L/kg/day results in the following clinical observation:

for every 1 mg/kg/day of phenobarbital administered, a steady-state phenobarbital level of about 10 mg/L is achieved. (Equation 35.)

$$\text{Cpss ave} = \frac{(S)(F)(\text{Dose}/\tau)}{Cl}$$

$$= \frac{(0.9)(1 \text{ mg/kg/day})}{0.1 \text{ L/kg/day}}$$

$$= 9 \text{ mg/L} \quad or \quad \approx 10 \text{ mg/L}$$

This clinical guideline suggests that in adult patients, maintenance doses of 2 mg/day/kg should result in steady-state concentrations of ≈20 mg/L. The clearance in children 1 to 18 years of age is approximately twice the average adult clearance.[11,12] Therefore, they generally require maintenance doses of phenobarbital that are about twice those of the average adult, or a maintenance dose of 4 to 5 mg/kg/day will be needed to achieve steady-state plasma concentrations of 20 mg/L.

Half-Life (t½)

The plasma half-life of phenobarbital is five days in most adult patients, but may be as short as two to three days in some individuals, especially children.

Time to Sample

Phenobarbital has a half-life of approximately five days; as a result, plasma samples obtained within the first one to two weeks of therapy yield relatively little information about the eventual steady-state concentrations. For this reason, routine plasma phenobarbital concentrations should be monitored two to three weeks after the initiation or a change in the phenobarbital regimen. Plasma samples obtained before this time should be used either to determine whether an additional loading dose is needed (e.g., when plasma concentrations are much lower than desired), or whether the maintenance dose should be withheld (e.g., phenobarbital concentrations are much greater than desired).

Once steady state has been achieved, the time of sampling within a dosing interval of phenobarbital is not critical; plasma concentrations can be obtained at almost any time relative to the phenobarbital dose. As a matter of consistency, however, trough concentrations are generally recommended and if phenobarbital is being administered by the intravenous route, care should be taken to sample at least one hour after the end of the infusion to avoid the distribution phase.

Question #1. W.R., a 39-year-old, 70 kg male, developed generalized seizures several months after an automobile accident in which he sustained head injuries. Phenobarbital is to be initiated. Calculate a loading dose of phenobarbital that will produce a plasma level of 20 mg/L.

Since this is a loading dose problem and there is no existing initial drug concentration, Equation 11 should be used:

$$\text{Loading Dose} = \frac{(Vd)(Cp)}{(S)(F)}$$

If F and S are assumed to be 1.0 and the volume of distribution is assumed to be 0.7 L/kg (see Phenobarbital Key Parameters on page 290) or 49 L, the calculated loading dose will be 980 mg or approximately 1 gm as shown below.

$$\text{Loading Dose} = \frac{(49 \text{ L})(20 \text{ mg/L})}{(1.0)(1.0)}$$
$$= 980 \text{ mg} \quad or \quad \approx 1 \text{ gm}$$

This 1 gm dose is very close to the usual loading dose of 15 mg/kg. It may be administered orally, intramuscularly, or intravenously.

Generally, the loading dose is divided into three or more portions and administered over several hours. The necessity for dividing the loading dose when administered orally or intramuscularly is not clear. It is probably done as a precaution against toxicity should a two-compartmental distribution exist or to avoid cardiovascular toxicity from the propylene glycol diluent in the injectable dosage form (also see Section 10: Phenytoin on page 312).

Question #2. **Calculate an oral maintenance dose for W.R. which will maintain a phenobarbital concentration of 20 mg/L. How should the dose be administered?**

Since clearance is the major determinant of the maintenance dose, this parameter must be estimated for W.R. While there is some intersubject variability, the average clearance of phenobarbital in adults is 4 mL/kg/hr or 0.1 L/kg/day. Thus, the expected clearance for W.R., who is 70 kg, is 7 L/day:

$$\text{Clearance Phenobarbital} = (0.1 \text{ L/kg/day})(\text{Weight in kg})$$

Eq. 9.1

$$= (0.1 \text{ L/kg/day})(70 \text{ kg})$$
$$= 7.0 \text{ L/day}$$

If S and F are assumed to be 1.0, the maintenance dose of phenobarbital can be calculated using Equation 16:

$$\text{Maintenance Dose} = \frac{(\text{Cl})(\text{Cpss ave})(\tau)}{(\text{S})(\text{F})}$$
$$= \frac{(7 \text{ L/day})(20 \text{ mg/L})(1 \text{ day})}{(1.0)(1.0)}$$
$$= 140 \text{ mg}$$

In practice, the daily dose is usually divided into two or more portions; however, with a half-life of five days (Equation 32), once daily dosing should suffice:[8]

$$t\frac{1}{2} = \frac{(0.693)(\text{Vd})}{\text{Cl}}$$
$$= \frac{(0.693)(49 \text{ L})}{7.0 \text{ L/day}}$$
$$= 4.85 \text{ days } or \approx 5 \text{ days}$$

Interestingly, the calculated dose corresponds to an empiric clinical guideline which has been used for many years: The phenobarbital steady-state level produced by a maintenance dose will be approximately equal to ten times the daily dose in mg/kg:

$$\frac{\text{W.R.'s Maintenance}}{\text{Dose (mg/kg)}} = \frac{140 \text{ mg}}{70 \text{ kg}}$$

$$= 2 \text{ mg/kg}$$

According to the clinical guideline, the level in mg/L produced by this dose will be 20 mg/L (2 × 10).

***Question #3.* If W.R. does not receive a loading dose, how long will it take to achieve a minimum therapeutic level of 10 mg/L following the initiation of the maintenance dose? How long will it take to achieve a steady-state level of 20 mg/L?**

To answer a question involving time, knowledge of the half-life is required. The half-life for phenobarbital in W.R. is approximately five days as calculated in Question 2. If it takes three to five half-lives to approach steady state, approximately 15 to 20 days will be required to achieve the final plateau concentration of 20 mg/L. Because the minimum therapeutic concentration of 10 mg/L is one-half of the predicted steady-state concentration of 20 mg/L, one half-life or five days will be required for the phenobarbital concentration to accumulate to 10 mg/L.

$$Kd = \frac{0.693}{t\tfrac{1}{2}} \qquad \text{(Eq. 8.4)}$$

$$= \frac{0.693}{5 \text{ days}}$$

$$= 0.139 \text{ days}^{-1}$$

$$Cp_1 = \frac{(S)(F)(\text{Dose}/\tau)}{Cl}(1 - e^{-Kdt_1}) \qquad \text{(Eq. 37)}$$

$$= (20 \text{ mg/L})(1 - e^{-(0.139)(5 \text{ days})})$$

$$= (20 \text{ mg/L})(0.5)$$

$$= 10 \text{ mg/L}$$

Question #4. K.P., a 62-year-old, 57 kg female, was admitted for poor seizure control. Prior to admission she had been receiving an unknown dose of phenobarbital. On admission, the phenobarbital concentration was 5 mg/L, and she was started on 60 mg of phenobarbital Q 8 hr (180 mg/day). Five days later, the phenobarbital concentration was measured and reported as 17 mg/L. Calculate her final steady-state concentration on the present regimen.

There are several ways of approaching this problem. Since Cpss ave is defined by clearance, one could use the average clearance for phenobarbital (0.1 L/kg/day × 57 kg = 5.7 L/day) and insert this value into Equation 35:

$$Cpss\ ave = \frac{(S)(F)(Dose/\tau)}{Cl}$$
$$= \frac{(1)(1)(180\ mg/day)}{5.7\ L/day}$$
$$= 31.6\ mg/L$$

Another method could be used to estimate the steady-state value. The concentration of 17 mg/L reported on the fifth day is assumed to represent the sum of the fraction of the initial concentration (5 mg/L) remaining at this point in time plus the accumulated concentration resulting from five daily doses of 180 mg. If K.P.'s half-life for phenobarbital is five days, the fraction of the initial concentration remaining after one half-life will be 0.5 and contribution to the reported concentration at five days will be 2.5 mg/L. The remaining portion of the reported concentration (14.5 mg/L) represents 50% of the steady-state level which will be produced by the 180 mg/day dose. Therefore, the predicted Cpss ave would be 29 mg/L (2 × 14.5 mg/L).

One also could use the empiric clinical guideline discussed in Question 3 regarding the prediction of Cpss ave from the mg/kg dose of phenobarbital. In this case the mg/kg dose would be 180 mg/57 kg or 3.16 mg/kg. The predicted Cpss ave would be 31.6 mg/L (3.16 × 10).

All of these estimates are based upon the assumption that K.P.'s pharmacokinetic parameters for phenobarbital are similar to those reported in the literature. Since the estimates for Cpss ave are at the high end of the therapeutic range, it would be reasonable to obtain another plasma concentration 15 to 20 days after the initiation of the maintenance dose. Also, because the repeat concentration will be obtained after more than two half-lives have passed, K.P.'s clearance for phenobarbital can be estimated more reliably. (See Part I: Interpretation of Plasma Drug Concentrations on page 73.)

Question #5. N.P., a 35-year-old, 80 kg male, is being treated for a seizure disorder secondary to a motor vehicle accident. He has been receiving 200 mg/day of phenobarbital (100 mg BID) for the past 15 days. The phenobarbital serum concentration just before the morning dose on Day 16 (i.e., at the trough of the 30th and just prior to the 31st dose) was reported to be 29 mg/L. Calculate the phenobarbital concentration you would have predicted on that day if N.P. has average pharmacokinetic parameters for phenobarbital.

The average pharmacokinetic parameters for N.P. are as follows: $Cl = 8$ L/day (0.1 L/kg/day $\times$ 80 kg); $Vd = 56$ L (0.7 L/kg $\times$ 80 kg); $Kd = 0.143$ days^{-1}; and $t\frac{1}{2} = 4.9$ days.

$$Kd = \frac{Cl}{Vd} \qquad \text{(Eq. 27)}$$

$$= \frac{8 \text{ L/day}}{56 \text{ L/day}}$$

$$= 0.143 \text{ day}^{-1}$$

$$t\frac{1}{2} = \frac{0.693}{Kd} \qquad \text{(Eq. 31)}$$

$$= \frac{0.693}{0.143 \text{ day}^{-1}}$$

$$= 4.85 \text{ days}$$

Since N.P. has been receiving his phenobarbital maintenance dose for 15 days or approximately three half-lives, the phenobarbital concentration is assumed to be a steady-state level. Equation 47 can be used to predict the trough concentration at steady state. Using the previously calculated parameters, the steady state trough level should be approximately 24 mg/L based upon the calculation below.

$$Cpss\ min = \frac{\frac{(S)(F)(Dose)}{Vd}}{(1 - e^{-Kd\tau})} (e^{-Kd\tau})$$

$$= \frac{\frac{(1)(1)(100\ mg)}{56\ L}}{(1 - e^{-(0.143\ day^{-1})(0.5\ days)})} (e^{-(0.143)(0.5\ days)})$$

$$= \left[\frac{1.78\ mg/L}{0.069} \right] [0.93]$$

$$= [25.9][0.93]$$

$$= 24\ mg/L$$

Question #6. Considering the measured phenobarbital concentration of 29 mg/L in N.P., what method is most appropriately used to adjust his pharmacokinetic parameters? Do these patient-specific parameters suggest that a maintenance dose adjustment is necessary if the goal is to maintain the phenobarbital concentration at $\approx$25 mg/L?

The measured trough concentration of phenobarbital is greater than the predicted concentration; therefore, N.P.'s phenobarbital clearance is likely to be lower than expected. (See Equation 32 below.) If this is true, then his phenobarbital half-life is likely to be longer than five days, and a non-steady-state approach will have to be used to revise his clearance value.

$$\uparrow t_{1/2} = \frac{(0.693)(Vd)}{\downarrow Cl}$$

Although there are a number of models, Equation 55 which describes the concentration (Cp_2) following the Nth dose, fits this situation nicely: (See Part I: Selecting the Appropriate Equation: Series of Individual Doses on page 66.)

$$Cp_2 = \frac{\frac{(S)(F)(Dose)}{Vd}}{(1 - e^{-Kd\tau})} (1 - e^{-Kd(N)\tau})(e^{-Kdt_2})$$

Tau (τ) is the dosing interval of 0.5 days, N is the number of doses administered (30), and t_2 is the time elapsed since the last dose (0.5 days). In order to calculate the concentration at the time of sampling (Cp_2), the elimination rate constant will have to be adjusted first by reducing the expected clearance value in Equation 27.

$$Kd = \frac{Cl}{Vd}$$

Unfortunately, there is not a direct solution to this problem, and a trial and error method must be used to find the clearance value which will predict the observed phenobarbital concentration of 29 mg/L. For example, if a phenobarbital clearance of 6 L/day is used in Equation 27, an elimination rate constant of 0.107 days^{-1} is calculated. This elimination rate constant, when placed in Equation 55, results in an expected phenobarbital concentration of approximately 26 mg/L.

$$Kd = \frac{Cl}{Vd}$$

$$= \frac{6 \text{ L/day}}{56 \text{ L}}$$

$$= 0.107 \text{ day}^{-1}$$

$$Cp_2 = \frac{\frac{(S)(F)(Dose)}{Vd}}{(1 - e^{-Kd\tau})} (1 - e^{-Kd(N)\tau})(e^{-Kdt_2})$$

$$= \frac{\frac{(1)(1)(100 \text{ mg})}{56 \text{ L}}}{(1 - e^{-(0.107 \text{ days}^{-1})(0.5 \text{ days})})} (1 - e^{-(0.107 \text{ days}^{-1})(30)(0.5 \text{ days})})$$

$$(e^{-(0.107 \text{ days}^{-1})(0.5 \text{ days})})$$

$$= \frac{1.78 \text{ mg/L}}{(0.052)} (1 - 0.2)(0.948)$$

$$= 25.9 \text{ mg/L } \textit{or} \approx 26 \text{ mg/L}$$

Further decreasing the phenobarbital clearance to 5 L/day results in an elimination rate constant of 0.0893 days^{-1} and when this elimination rate constant is used in Equation 55, a phenobarbital concentration of 28.7 mg/L is calculated.

$$Kd = \frac{Cl}{Vd}$$

$$= \frac{5 \text{ L/day}}{56 \text{ L}}$$

$$= 0.0893 \text{ days}^{-1}$$

$$Cp_2 = \frac{\dfrac{(S)(F)(Dose)}{Vd}}{(1 - e^{-Kd\tau})}(1 - e^{-Kd(N)\tau})(e^{-Kdt_2})$$

$$= \frac{\dfrac{(1)(1)(100 \text{ mg})}{56 \text{ L}}}{(1 - e^{-(0.0893 \text{ days}^{-1})(0.5 \text{ days})})}(1 - e^{-(0.0893 \text{ days}^{-1})(30)(0.5 \text{ days})})$$

$$(e^{-(0.0893 \text{ days}^{-1})(0.5 \text{ days})})$$

$$= \frac{1.78 \text{ mg/L}}{(0.0437)}(0.738)(0.956)$$

$$= 28.7 \text{ mg/L } or \approx 29 \text{ mg/L}$$

The convergence of the predicted and observed plasma concentration suggests that N.P.'s phenobarbital clearance is approximately 5 L/day. Assuming that this clearance is reasonably accurate, the predicted steady-state phenobarbital concentration (Equation 35) would then be approximately 40 mg/L on the current dosing regimen of 200 mg/day as calculated below.

$$Cpss \text{ ave} = \frac{(S)(F)(Dose/\tau)}{Cl}$$

$$= \frac{(1)(1)(200 \text{ mg/1 day})}{5 \text{ L/day}}$$

$$= 40 \text{ mg/L}$$

If a steady-state concentration of approximately 25 mg/L is desired, a reduction in the maintenance dose to approximately 125 mg/day would be necessary as shown below (Equation 16).

$$\text{Maintenance Dose} = \frac{(Cl)(Cpss\ ave)(\tau)}{(S)(F)}$$
$$= \frac{(5\ L/day)(25\ mg/L)}{(1)(1)}$$
$$= 125\ mg/day$$

Since N.P.'s revised phenobarbital clearance is based upon a measured drug level obtained at less than two half-lives (i.e., 15 days) after therapy was initiated, the revision and expected steady-state concentration must be considered somewhat uncertain.

$$t\tfrac{1}{2} = \frac{(0.693)(Vd)}{Cl}$$
$$= \frac{(0.693)(56\ L)}{5\ L/day}$$
$$= 7.8\ days$$

While it may be appropriate to reduce the phenobarbital dose, additional plasma level monitoring will be necessary in 24 to 40 days to ensure that the steady-state concentration is actually about 25 mg/L on a daily dose of 125 mg.

Question #7. **Calculate a revised plasma concentration for N.P. using a non-steady state continuous infusion model.**

A continuous infusion model is usually satisfactory when predicting steady-state phenobarbital plasma concentrations (Equation 35) because of the relatively long half-life and short dosing interval for phenobarbital. In this case Equation 37 will have to be used because the phenobarbital concentration was obtained before steady state had been achieved. (See Figure 9.1 and Part I: Figure 31 on pages 302 and 78, respectively.)

$$Cp_1 = \frac{(S)(F)(Dose/\tau)}{Cl}(1 - e^{-Kdt_1})$$

An important check in using Equation 37 is to multiply the duration of the infusion (t_1) by the infusion rate (dose divided by τ). This product should equal the total amount of drug which has been administered to the patient. For example, in N.P. the infusion rate of 100 mg divided by 0.5 days times duration of the infusion of 15 days results in a total administered dose of 3000 mg.

$$\text{Total Amount of Drug Administered} = (\text{Dose}/\tau)(t_1)$$

Eq. 9.2

$$= (100 \text{ mg}/0.5 \text{ days})(15 \text{ days})$$
$$= 3000 \text{ mg}$$

This amount (3000 mg) is equal to the total amount of phenobarbital actually administered (i.e., 100 mg × 30 doses). Early in a regimen, the total amount of drug administered and the duration of the theoretical infusion are somewhat disparate. For example, immediately after the administration of the second phenobarbital dose, a total of 200 mg has been administered, while the total time elapsed is only one-half day. However, use of Equation 9.2 suggests that only 100 mg has been administered. While this problem is most apparent early in therapy, it is seldom an issue after multiple doses have been administered. This is because a variation in one dosing interval represents a relatively small percentage error with respect to the total amount of drug administered.

Using Equation 37, the previously calculated clearance of 5 L/day, and the corresponding elimination rate constant of 0.0893 day^{-1}, a phenobarbital concentration of 29.6 mg/L is calculated.

$$Cp_1 = \frac{(1)(1)(100 \text{ mg}/0.5 \text{ days})}{5 \text{ L}/\text{day}}(1 - e^{-(0.0893 \text{ days}^{-1})(15 \text{ days})})$$
$$= 40 \text{ mg/L}(0.74)$$
$$= 29.6 \text{ mg/L}$$

The similarities between the predicted phenobarbital concentration using the continuous infusion and the intermittent bolus model suggest that either model could be used, with the continuous infusion model requiring fewer computations.

Question #8. J.R., an epileptic male who has been managed chronically on phenobarbital 120 mg/day, has recently-

$$Cp_1 = \frac{(S)(F)(Dose/\tau)}{Cl}(1 - e^{-Kdt_1}) \qquad \text{(Eq. 37)}$$

$$Cp_2 = \frac{\frac{(S)(F)(Dose)}{Vd}}{(1 - e^{-Kd\tau})}(1 - e^{-Kd(N)\tau})(e^{-Kdt_2}) \qquad \text{(Eq. 55)}$$

Figure 9.1. Plasma Concentration-Time Curve for the Accumulation and Eventual Attainment of Steady State for a Drug Administered With a Dosing Interval That is Much Shorter Than the Elimination Half-Life. The solid smooth line represents the accumulation pattern during a continuous input model as expressed in Equation 37, and the saw-toothed pattern indicates the accumulation pattern for a drug administered intermittently, as in Equation 55. Note that the plasma concentrations predicted by the intermittent input model are very similar to the accumulation pattern of the continuous input model.

developed hypoalbuminemia secondary to nephrotic syndrome. Will his phenobarbital concentration be affected by decreases in his albumin concentration or renal function?

Only 40% to 50% of phenobarbital is bound to plasma proteins; therefore, alpha (the fraction of phenobarbital that is free) is 0.5 to 0.6.[13,14] The concentration of a drug that is bound to protein to the extent of 50% or less is not likely to be significantly affected by changes in plasma protein concentrations or protein binding affinity.

The renal clearance for phenobarbital is probably <20% of the total clearance in patients with normal renal function and an uncontrolled urine pH (e.g., the urine pH is not intentionally adjusted).[10] Therefore, it is unlikely that patients with renal failure will require significant adjustments in their phenobarbital dosage regimens.

To summarize, J.R.'s phenobarbital concentrations are not likely to be significantly affected by his hypoalbuminemia or poor renal function.

Question #9. R.T. is a 25-year-old, 70 kg male with chronic renal failure and a seizure disorder. He has been maintained on 60 mg of phenobarbital BID and has steady-state concentrations of 20 mg/L. Over the past three months, his renal function has progressively worsened and he is to be started on four hours of hemodialysis three times weekly. Will he require an adjustment of his maintenance regimen? (See Part I: Dialysis of Drugs on page 104.)

To determine whether a significant amount of drug is lost during each dialysis period, the three steps outlined in Part I: Dialysis of Drugs should be examined. First, the apparent volume of distribution for unbound drug should be estimated using Equation 82. Using a volume of distribution of 0.7 L/kg or 49 L for this 70 kg patient and a free fraction or alpha of 0.5 for phenobarbital, the apparent unbound volume of distribution for phenobarbital in R.T. is approximately 98 L. Since this is less than the upper limit of 250 L for a dialyzable drug, dialysis possibly could remove a significant amount of phenobarbital.

$$\begin{aligned} \text{Unbound Volume} \atop \text{of Distribution} &= \frac{\text{Vd}}{\alpha} \\ &= \frac{49 \text{ L}}{0.5} \\ &= 98 \text{ L} \end{aligned}$$

R.T.'s clearance of phenobarbital must be estimated next. The usual clearance of 0.1 L/kg/day, or 7 L/day for the 70 kg patient, represents a total body clearance of approximately 5 mL/min. This value is low enough (i.e., <500 to 800 mL/min) that dialysis could significantly increase the total clearance.

$$\begin{aligned} \text{Clearance} \atop \text{(mL/min)} &= [7 \text{ L/day}] \left[\frac{1000 \text{ mL/L}}{1440 \text{ min/day}} \right] \\ &= 4.9 \text{ mL/min } \textit{or} \approx 5 \text{ mL/min} \end{aligned}$$

Finally, estimate the drug's half-life using Equation 32. The apparent half-life for phenobarbital of approximately five days is much longer than the lower limit of one to two hours set in Criterion 3 (i.e., hemodialysis is unlikely to significantly alter the dosing regimen if the drug half-life is very short).

$$\begin{aligned} t\tfrac{1}{2} &= \frac{(0.693)(\text{Vd})}{\text{Cl}} \\ &= \frac{(0.693)(49 \text{ L})}{7 \text{ L/day}} \\ &= 4.9 \text{ days} \end{aligned}$$

Since the unbound volume of distribution and phenobarbital clearance of R.T. are relatively small, and the half-life is much greater than the lower limit of one to two hours, a significant amount of phenobarbital could be cleared during a dialysis period. For this reason, the actual clearance of phenobarbital during hemodialysis will have to be determined.

The clearance of phenobarbital by hemodialysis has not been studied extensively; however, the use of hemodialysis in the treatment of two phenobarbital overdoses indicates that the clearance of phenobarbital by hemodialysis is approximately 3 L/hr.[5,15] If this value is inserted into Equation 76 along with the patient's calculated clearance (Cl_{pat}) of 0.25 L/hr,

$$Cl = \frac{(S)(F)(Dose/\tau)}{Cpss\ ave} \qquad \text{(Eq. 15)}$$

$$= \frac{(1)(1)(60\ mg/0.5\ day)}{20\ mg/L}$$

$$= 6\ L/day\ or\ 0.25\ L/hr$$

a dialysis replacement dose can be calculated. Equation 76 was selected to calculate the replacement dose because of the long half-life and relatively short dosing interval for phenobarbital (see Part I: Dialysis of Drugs on page 104 and Figure 33 on page 106).

$$\text{Post Dialysis Replacement Dose} = (Vd)(Cpss\ ave)\left(1 - e^{-\left(\frac{(Cl_{pat}\ +\ Cl_{dial})}{Vd}\right)(T_d)}\right)$$

$$= [49\ L][20\ mg/L]\left[1 - e^{-\left(\frac{0.25\ L/hr\ +\ 3.0\ L/hr}{49\ L}\right)(4\ hr)}\right]$$

$$= (980\ mg)(1 - e^{-(0.0666\ hr^{-1})(4\ hr)})$$

$$= (980\ mg)(1 - 0.77)$$

$$= (980\ mg)(0.23)$$

$$= 225.4\ mg$$

This replacement dose of approximately 225 mg represents the amount of drug eliminated from the body during the dialysis period by both metabolic and dialysis clearance. The vast majority of the drug eliminated during the four-hour dialysis period represents drug eliminated by the dialysis route. For this reason, the total daily phenobarbital dose on days of dialysis would be 120 mg (maintenance dose) plus the postdialysis dose of ≈200 mg.

Standard replacement doses of phenobarbital after dialysis are frequently in the range of 200 to 300 mg. While this replacement dose appears to be large when compared to the maintenance dose, it is not unusual. If there is concern about the size of the postdialysis replacement dose, one could administer a smaller dose of 100 to 200 mg after dialysis and continue to monitor the patient during subsequent dialysis periods to ensure that the phenobarbital concentration does not continue to decline due to additional elimination by the dialysis route.

Question #10. H.P., a 5-year-old, 20 kg male, is to be started on phenobarbital for his seizure disorder. Calculate the maintenance dose of sodium phenobarbital that will produce a steady-state concentration of ≈20 mg/L.

In order to calculate H.P.'s phenobarbital maintenance dose, one would first assume his clearance to be ≈2 L/day (0.2 L/kg/day × 10 kg). This clearance value, while larger than the usual adult value, is consistent for children. Using Equation 16 with a target concentration of 20 mg/L, and a salt form (S) fraction of 0.9, a daily maintenance dose of ≈40 mg can be calculated.

$$\text{Maintenance Dose} = \frac{(\text{Cl})(\text{Cpss ave})(\tau)}{(\text{S})(\text{F})}$$

$$= \frac{(2 \text{ L/day})(20 \text{ mg/L})(1 \text{ day})}{(0.9)(1)}$$

$$= 44.4 \;\; or \;\; \approx 40 \text{ mg}$$

Depending upon the clinical situation, one could administer a loading dose to rapidly achieve therapeutic concentrations or start the patient on his maintenance dose without a loading dose. In the latter situation, the urgency of the clinical situation will determine whether the initial maintenance dose should be 40 mg/day or one quarter of the target maintenance dose (10 mg/day) for the first week, increased by 10 mg/day weekly until the final maintenance dose of 40 mg/day is being administered. As noted previously, excessive sedation can be a consequence of starting the patient on the full maintenance dose. H.P. should be monitored for both therapeutic and potential side effects during this period of dose titration.

Question #11. **S.M., a 45-year-old, 60 kg female, was recently placed on 120 mg/day of phenobarbital. Ten days ago her concentration was 15 mg/L and today her phenobarbital concentration is 24 mg/L. Based on the data provided, what would you calculate her steady-state phenobarbital concentration to be?**

In order to calculate S.M.'s phenobarbital concentration, one will first have to determine her clearance. Unfortunately, because phenobarbital has a long half-life, it is unlikely that the present level of 24 mg/L represents steady state. Therefore some type of iterative search or indirect procedure must be used to extract clearance. One method is to combine Equations 26 and 37 where C^o is the initial phenobarbital concentration of 15 mg/L and, in Equation 37, the infusion rate is essentially represented by the daily dose of 120 mg/day. In both Equations 26 and 37, t would be ten days, or the time interval between C^o and the current plasma concentration of 24 mg/L.

$$Cp_1 = C^o(e^{-Kdt}) + \frac{(S)(F)(Dose/\tau)}{Cl}(1 - e^{-Kdt_1})$$

$$24 \text{ mg/L} = (15 \text{ mg/L})(e^{(-Kd)(10 \text{ days})}) +$$
$$\left[\frac{(1)(1)(120 \text{ mg/day})}{Cl}(1 - e^{(-Kd)(10 \text{ days})})\right]$$

Unfortunately, the resolution to this problem first requires assuming S.M.'s volume of distribution (0.7 L/kg × 60 kg or ≈42 L) and then iteratively solving for the clearance (Cl) and Kd (Cl/Vd = Cl/42 L) until the result is a calculated concentration equal to the observed Cp_1 of 24 mg/L. As discussed previously, this is a sometimes laborious procedure and an alternative approach that could be of use is the mass balance equation (Equation 58).

$$Cl = \frac{SFD/\tau - \dfrac{(Cp_2 - Cp_1)\ Vd}{t}}{Cp\ ave}$$

In the above equation, if one substitutes S.M.'s maintenance dose of phenobarbital, the corresponding Cp_1 of 15 mg/L and Cp_2 of 24 mg/L and assumes that the Cp ave is $\approx$19.5 mg/L, or halfway between the initial and present phenobarbital concentrations, a clearance of $\approx$4.2 L/day is calculated.

$$Cl = \frac{(1)(1)(120\ mg/day) - \dfrac{(24\ mg/L - 15\ mg/L)(42\ L)}{10\ days}}{19.5\ mg/L}$$

$$= \frac{120\ mg/day - \dfrac{378\ mg}{10\ days}}{19.5\ mg/L}$$

$$= \frac{82.2\ mg/day}{19.5\ mg/L}$$

$$= 4.2\ L/day$$

This clearance value of 4.2 L/day corresponds to a half-life of approximately 7 days (Equation 32).

$$t^{1/2} = \frac{(0.693)(Vd)}{Cl}$$

$$= \frac{(0.693)(42\ L)}{4.2\ L/day}$$

$$= 6.9\ days$$

$$Kd = \frac{0.693}{t^{1/2}} \tag{Eq. 8.4}$$

$$= \frac{0.693}{6.9 \text{ days}}$$

$$= 0.1 \text{ day}^{-1}$$

As discussed in Part I, there are several conditions that should be met if the prediction calculated by use of the mass balance equation is to be reasonably accurate. First, the time between the first and second plasma concentrations should be at least one but no longer than two drug half-lives. Second, if plasma concentrations are rising, Cp_2 should be less than twice Cp_1. Third, the rate of drug administration should be reasonably regular and smooth. By examining the drug half-life, the change in plasma concentrations, and the dosing regimen, it is clear that we have met all three of these conditions; therefore, one would anticipate that the clearance value predicted should be reasonably accurate.

If there was concern about the validity of the revised clearance, derived from the mass balance equation, the clearance value of 4.2 L/day along with the corresponding elimination rate constant of 0.1 days^{-1} could be used in Equations 26 and 37 to confirm that both the iterative search and mass balance equations generate essentially the same answer.

$$Cp_1 = C^o(e^{-Kdt}) + \frac{(S)(F)(Dose/\tau)}{Cl}(1 - e^{-Kdt_1})$$

$$= (15 \text{ mg/L})(e^{-(0.1)(10 \text{ days})}) + \left[\frac{(1)(1)(120 \text{ mg/day})}{4.2 \text{ L/day}}(1 - e^{-(0.1)(10 \text{ days})})\right]$$

$$= 15 \text{ mg/L } (0.368) + [(28.57 \text{ mg/L})(1 - 0.368)]$$

$$= 5.52 \text{ mg/L} + 18 \text{ mg/L}$$

$$= 23.54 \text{ mg/L}$$

As can be seen from this calculation, the predicted concentration using the exponential equations results in a value very close to the observed concentration. This comparison is useful when there is concern that the assumptions implicit in the mass balance equation have oversimplified a more complex problem. Our comparison indicates both approaches are equivalent.

In order to calculate the expected steady-state plasma concentration of approximately 29 mg/L, Equation 35 would be used in conjunction with our revised phenobarbital clearance of 4.2 L/day.

$$Cpss \ ave = \frac{(S)(F)(Dose/\tau)}{Cl}$$

$$= \frac{(1)(1)(120 \ mg/day)}{4.2 \ L/day}$$

$$= 28.57 \ or \ \approx 29 \ mg/L$$

References

1. Buchthal F et al. Relation of EEG and seizures to phenobarbital in serum. Arch Neurol. 1968;19:567.

2. Plass GL, Hine CH. Hydantoin and barbiturate blood levels observed in epileptics. Arch Int Pharmacodyn Ther. 1960;128:375.

3. Sushine I. Chemical evidence of tolerance to phenobarbital. J Lab Clin Med. 1957;50:127.

4. Baselt RC et al. Therapeutic and toxic concentrations of more than 100 toxicologically significant drugs in blood, plasma, or serum: a tabulation. Clin Chem. 1975;21:44.

5. Kennedy AC et al. Successful treatment of three cases of very severe barbiturate poisoning. Lancet. 1969;1:995.

6. Levy RE et al. Carbamazepine, valproic acid, phenobarbital and ethosuximide. In: Evans WE et al. eds. Applied Pharmacokinetics: Principles of Therapeutic Drug Monitoring. 3rd edition. Vancouver: Applied Therapeutics, Inc., 1992.

7. Gal P. Phenobarbital and primidone. In: Taylor WJ, Diers-Caviness MH, eds. A Text Book for the Clinical Application of Therapeutic Drug Monitoring. Irving: Abbot Laboratories Diagnostics Division; 1986; 237–52.

8. Havidberg E, Dam M. Clinical pharmacokinetics of anticonvulsants. Clin Pharmacokinet. 1976;1:151.

9. Alvin J et al. The effect of liver disease in man on the disposition of phenobarbital. J Pharmacol Exp Ther. 1975;192:224.

10. Linton AL et al. Methods of forced diuresis and its application in barbiturate poisoning. Lancet. 1967;2:377.

11. Heimann G, Gladtke E. Pharmacokinetics of phenobarbital in childhood. Eur J Clin Pharmacol. 1977;12:305.

12. Painter MJ et al. Phenobarbital and diphenylhydantoin levels in neonates with seizures. J Pediatr. 1978;92:315.

13. Waddell WJ, Butler TC. The distribution of phenobarbital. J. Clin Invest. 1957;36:1217.

14. Houghton GW et al. Brain concentrations of phenytoin, phenobarbitone, and primidone in epileptic patients. Eur J Clin Pharmacol. 1975;9:73.

15. Henderson LW, Merrill JP. Treatment of barbiturate intoxication. Ann Intern Med. 1966;64:876.

Phenytoin 10

Phenytoin is primarily used as an anticonvulsant and is occasionally used in the treatment of certain types of cardiac arrhythmias.[1] It is usually administered orally in single or divided doses of 200 to 400 mg/day. When a rapid therapeutic effect is required, a loading dose of 15 mg/kg can be administered by the oral or intravenous route. Although phenytoin can be administered intramuscularly, this route should be avoided because of slow and erratic absorption.

Individualizing the dose of phenytoin is beset by two major problems. First, binding of phenytoin to plasma proteins is decreased in patients with renal failure or hypoalbuminemia. Second, the metabolic capacity for phenytoin is limited; therefore, modest changes in the maintenance dose result in disproportionate changes in steady-state plasma concentrations. The capacity-limited metabolism of phenytoin also eliminates the clinical usefulness of half-life ($t\frac{1}{2}$) as a pharmacokinetic parameter and makes estimates of the time required to achieve steady state difficult.

Therapeutic and Toxic Plasma Concentrations

Phenytoin plasma concentrations of 10 to 20 mg/L are generally accepted as therapeutic.[2–4] Plasma concentrations in the range of 5 to 10 mg/L can be therapeutic for some patients, but concentrations <5 mg/L are not likely to be effective.[5]

A number of phenytoin side effects, such as gingival hyperplasia, folate deficiency, and peripheral neuropathy, do not appear to be related to plasma phenytoin concentrations. In contrast, central nervous system (CNS) side effects do correlate with plasma concentration. Far-lateral nystagmus usually occurs in patients with plasma phenytoin concentrations >20 mg/L. The concentration range associated with this effect, however, is broad with some patients showing symptoms at concentrations of 15 mg/L and others having no nystagmus at concentrations >30 mg/L. While far-lateral nystagmus is often used to monitor phenytoin therapy, it is seldom considered a true drug side effect or toxicity and is not a reason to reduce the phenytoin dose. Other CNS symptoms such as ataxia and diminished mental capacity are frequently observed in patients with concentrations exceeding 30 mg/L and 40 mg/L, respectively.[3] In addition, precautions should be taken when phenytoin is administered by the intravenous route because the propylene glycol diluent has cardiac depressant properties.[2]

Key Parameters

Therapeutic Plasma Concentration	10 to 20 mg/L
F	1.0
S[a]	0.92
Vd	0.65 L/kg
Cl	Concentration-dependent
Vm[b]	7 mg/kg/day
Km	4 mg/kg/day
t½[c]	Concentration-dependent
α(fraction free in plasma)	0.1

[a] Capsules and the injectable preparation; S = 1.0 for suspension and chewable tablet.
[b] Vm values are >7 mg/kg/day for children.
[c] See t½ section for time to steady state.

Alterations in Plasma Protein Binding. The usual phenytoin therapeutic range of 10 to 20 mg/L represents the total drug concentration which consists of unbound (or free) drug concentration plus phenytoin which is bound to plasma albumin. The usual alpha (α) or free fraction of phenytoin is $\approx$ 0.1. Therefore, approximately 90% of phenytoin in the plasma is bound to serum albumin; about 10% is unbound and free to equilibrate with the tissues where the pharmacologic effects and metabolism occur.

There are two approaches one can use to interpret phenytoin levels when protein binding is significantly altered. The first is to adjust all of the parameters (i.e., therapeutic range, volume of distribution, and "clearance") to those that would be observed in the presence of altered plasma binding. The second is to equate the measured or observed plasma concentration to that which would be observed under normal binding conditions ($Cp_{Normal\ Binding}$). In this instance, parameters associated with normal plasma protein binding would also be used. While either of these approaches is acceptable, it is the author's belief that the second method is least likely to result in calculation errors. Therefore, this latter approach will be used throughout the chapter when alterations in plasma binding are encountered.

The three factors which are known to significantly alter the plasma protein binding of phenytoin are: hypoalbuminemia, renal failure, and displacement by other drugs.

Hypoalbuminemia. In patients with a low serum albumin, Equation 8 can be used to determine the plasma concentration that would have been observed with a normal albumin concentration.

$$Cp_{\text{Normal Binding}} = \frac{Cp'}{(1 - \alpha)\left[\dfrac{P'}{P_{\text{NL}}}\right] + \alpha}$$

Cp' is the observed plasma concentration reported by the laboratory; α is the normal free fraction of phenytoin ($\alpha = 0.1$);[6-8] P' is the patient's serum albumin in units of gm/dL; P_{NL} is the normal serum albumin (4.4 gm/dL); and $Cp_{\text{Normal Binding}}$ is the plasma drug concentration that would have been observed if the patient's serum albumin concentration had been normal.

$$\text{Phenytoin } Cp_{\text{Normal Binding}} = \frac{Cp'}{\left((1 - 0.1)\dfrac{\text{Patient's Albumin}}{4.4 \text{ gm/dL}}\right) + 0.1}$$

Eq. 10.1

This equation is most useful when a patient has an unusual serum albumin concentration, but does not have significantly diminished renal function and is not taking other drugs known to displace phenytoin.

Renal Failure. In patients with end-stage renal disease, the free fraction of phenytoin increases from 0.1 to $\approx$0.2 to 0.35.[6,9,10-12] Some of this change in plasma binding is due to the decrease in serum albumin concentration known to be associated with end-stage renal disease, and some of the binding changes are due to a change in the binding affinity of phenytoin to serum albumin. When the creatinine clearance is >25 mL/min, the change in the binding affinity is minimal and no adjustment for renal function need be made. However, if the creatinine clearance is <10 mL/min and the patient is undergoing hemodialysis treatments, binding changes can be significant.[13]

In the latter circumstance, Equation 8 can be altered to accommodate changes in both the serum albumin concentration and the affinity of phenytoin for serum albumin.

$$Cp_{Normal\ Binding} = \frac{Cp'}{(0.48)(1-\alpha)\left[\dfrac{P'}{P_{NL}}\right] + \alpha}$$

Eq. 10.2

$$Phenytoin\ Cp_{Normal\ Binding} = \frac{Cp'}{\left((0.48)(1-0.1)\dfrac{Patient's\ Albumin}{4.4\ gm/dL}\right) + 0.1}$$

Eq. 10.3

The above equations should only be used in patients with end-stage renal disease receiving hemodialysis treatments because the factor which represents the decreased affinity (0.48) was derived from these types of patients. Note that in Equation 10.3 alpha is 0.1 because the phenytoin concentration (Phenytoin $Cp_{Normal\ Binding}$) calculated by the equation corrects for both serum albumin and renal dysfunction. In addition, it should be recognized that Equations 10.1 and 10.3 are only approximate estimates of normal phenytoin concentrations and there can be considerable variance among individual patients. The general concept, however, that phenytoin binding needs to be considered when evaluating phenytoin concentration is an important one to remember when using phenytoin concentrations to adjust a patient's dosing regimen. In patients with renal failure who are not undergoing intermittent hemodialysis, binding affinity is unpredictably altered when the creatinine clearance is between 10 to 25 mL/min. The plasma concentration of drugs cannot be interpreted accurately for this group of patients.[13]

Drug Displacement. Drugs also can displace phenytoin from plasma-protein binding sites. As explained in Part I: Desired Plasma Concentration on page 9, it is usually difficult to estimate the extent of drug displacement from protein-binding sites because the concentration of the displacing agent is seldom known. One exception to this rule is the situation when serum concentrations of both valproic acid and phenytoin are being monitored. When the serum valproic acid concentration is <35 mg/L, the displacement of phenytoin appears to be minimal and adjustment of the phenytoin concentration is probably not warranted. When the valproic acid concentration exceeds 50 mg/L, the extent of phenytoin displacement from plasma-protein binding sites increases; at valproic acid concentrations of ≈70 mg/L, phenytoin serum concentrations decrease by 40%.[14,15] (See 17: Valproic Acid on page 463.)

Bioavailability (F)

Phenytoin is completely absorbed (F = 1.0) from most currently available products;[16] however, there are different salt forms of phenytoin. The capsule and injectable preparations consist of the sodium salt (S = 0.92) of phenytoin, while the chewable tablet and suspension contain the acid form (S = 1.0) of phenytoin. The rate of phenytoin absorption following oral administration is slow because of the limited solubility of phenytoin. Serum concentrations of phenytoin peak 3 to 12 hours after oral administration.[17]

Phenytoin is absorbed slowly and the bioavailability could be less than 100% in patients with rapid gastrointestinal transit times.[18] Phenytoin concentrations are markedly decreased in patients receiving liquid dietary supplements (nasogastric feedings). Presumably, a change in gastrointestinal motility decreases the apparent bioavailability of phenytoin, although the specific mechanism has not been proven.[19] In some patients receiving nasogastric feedings, phenytoin doses of up to 1200 mg/day were required to achieve therapeutic concentrations. Discontinuation of the enteral feedings resulted in a marked increase in the phenytoin plasma concentrations.

The bioavailability of phenytoin is difficult to evaluate because of the drug's capacity-limited metabolism.[20] The slow absorption of phenytoin also tends to diminish the change in concentration following an oral dose. In most patients receiving oral phenytoin, the change in concentration (ΔCp) will be about half that observed when giving the drug by the intravenous route. The slow rate of absorption also results in delayed peak concentrations which occur between 3 and 12 hours with normal doses. When loading doses of 1 gm are administered orally, serum concentrations usually peak in about 24 hours; if the dose is increased to ≈1600 mg, the peak may be delayed as much as 30 hours.[21,22] While the absorption of phenytoin is almost certainly a very complex process, one approach the author has used is to assume an absorption rate of ≈50 mg/hr. This absorption rate is consistent with the observations stated above and is sometimes useful when estimating a time when the peak concentration will occur following oral administration. In addition, while it is common practice to divide large doses into 5 mg/kg increments administered every two hours, there are no studies documenting that this procedure is optimal in terms of the dose size or interval between doses.

Volume of Distribution (Vd)

The volume of distribution of phenytoin in patients with normal renal function and with normal serum albumin concentrations is ≈ 0.65 L/kg.[6,23,24] Although the volume of distribution for phenytoin is increased in patients with diminished plasma binding, the loading dose should not be changed because changes in the volume of distribution resulting from binding alterations are accompanied by equal and opposite changes in the desired phenytoin concentration. Also, the amount of phenytoin in the plasma represents only a small fraction of the total amount of phenytoin in the body. While one could adjust the apparent volume of distribution based upon alterations in binding, the approach taken in this chapter will be to correct any measured concentrations altered by binding to the concentration that would be observed under normal plasma binding conditions. Therefore, a volume of distribution of 0.65 L/kg, which represents normal plasma binding ($\alpha = 0.1$), should be used in all computations.

Capacity-Limited Metabolism

For most drugs, the rate of metabolism (and/or excretion) is proportional to the plasma concentration. Clearance is the volume of plasma which is completely cleared of drug per unit of time. [See Part I: Clearance (Cl) on page 26.] Clearance often can be viewed as the fixed proportionality constant that makes the steady-state plasma concentration equal to the rate of drug administration (R_A) as illustrated by Equation 14:

$$R_A = (Cl)(Cpss\ ave)$$

R_A is (S)(F)(Dose/τ). *This view of first-order pharmacokinetics, however, does not apply to phenytoin because the clearance of phenytoin decreases as Cpss ave increases.*

The clearance of phenytoin from plasma occurs primarily by metabolism, and the rate of phenytoin metabolism approaches its maximum at therapeutic concentrations. Thus, *the metabolism of phenytoin is described as being capacity-limited.*[3,24-28] Capacity-limited metabolism results in clearance values that decrease with increasing plasma concentrations. Therefore, when the maintenance dose is increased, the plasma concentration rises disproportionately.[25,29-34] (See Figure 10.1.) This disproportionate rise in the steady-state plasma level makes dosage adjustment difficult.

The model which appears to fit the metabolic pattern for phenytoin elimination is the one originally proposed by Michaelis and Menten. The velocity (v) or rate at which an enzyme system can metabolize a substrate (s) can be described by the following equation:

$$v = \frac{(Vm)(S)}{Km + S}$$

Eq. 10.4

Vm is the maximum metabolic capacity and Km is the substrate concentration at which v will be one-half of Vm. When the average steady-state phenytoin concentration (Cpss ave) is substituted for S and the daily dose or administration rate of phenytoin [R_A or (S)(F)(Dose/τ)] for v,[30,32-34] Equation 10.4 can be rewritten as:

$$(S)(F)(Dose/\tau) = \frac{(Vm)(Cpss\ ave)}{Km + Cpss\ ave}$$

Eq. 10.5

Equation 10.5 can also be rearranged as follows:

$$Cpss = \frac{(Km)[(S)(F)(Dose/\tau)]}{Vm - (S)(F)(Dose/\tau)}$$

Eq. 10.6

In accordance with the original definition of Vm and Km for Equation 10.4, Vm is the maximum rate of metabolism (metabolic capacity) and Km is the plasma concentration at which the rate of metabolism is one-half the maximum. The units for Vm and Km are mg/day and mg/L, respectively.

Figure 10.1. Changes in Steady-State Phenytoin Plasma Concentrations with Dose for Five Patients. For each patient the plasma phenytoin concentration at steady state increases disproportionately with an increase in the rate of administration. In all patients the daily dose required to achieve a steady-state concentration of 20 mg/L is not much greater than that required to achieve a value of 10 mg/L. The five patients were selected in this study because their dosage needed to be changed several times to control their epileptic seizures. From reference 52.

Equation 10.6 illustrates the sensitive relationship between the rate of phenytoin administration and Cpss ave when the rate of administration approaches Vm, the maximum metabolic capacity. The rate of phenytoin administration must be less than Vm or steady state will never be achieved. If Vm– (S)(F)(Dose/τ) were 0, Cpss would be infinity:

$$Cpss = \frac{Km\,[(S)(F)(Dose/\tau)]}{Vm\,-\,(S)(F)(Dose/\tau)}$$

$$= \frac{Km\,[(S)(F)(Dose/\tau)]}{0}$$

$$= [\infty]$$

If $(S)(F)(Dose/\tau)$ is greater than Vm, Cpss ave will be a negative number, indicating that steady state can never be achieved.

As can be seen from Equation 10.6, the relationship between steady-state phenytoin concentrations and the maintenance dose can be extremely sensitive. Understanding and being able to use pharmacokinetic parameters for phenytoin helps clinicians make initial dose adjustments; clinical guidelines also have been used for this purpose. For example, the following dose increments have been suggested using phenytoin concentrations as a guide: 100 mg when concentrations ≤ 7 mg/L; 50 mg when concentrations are 7 to <12 mg/L; and a maximum of 30 mg when concentrations are ≥ 12 mg/L. While these guidelines are consistent with the usual pharmacokinetic parameters, any increase in dose should be carefully considered in the context of patient compliance. One should also keep in mind the fact that adding 100 mg/day will cause a more dramatic rise in the steady-state phenytoin concentration in a patient taking 200 mg/day than in a patient taking 400 mg/day.[35]

Plasma concentrations which correspond to a metabolic rate that is one-half the maximum (Km) are usually between 1 and 20 mg/L.[29,31–33,36] The maximum metabolic capacity (Vm) appears to be between 5 and 15 mg/kg/day in most patients.[29,32,33] The relationship between Km and Vm is not clear, but if one of these parameters is low, the other is frequently also low.[29,30,33] The average values for Km and Vm are difficult to establish. It is the author's opinion that 4 mg/L for Km and 7 mg/kg/day for Vm are reasonable estimates for the average patient.

For pediatric patients, the Vm is usually larger than 7 mg/kg/day. Vm values are approximately 10 to 13 mg/kg/day for children six months through six years of age, and 8 to 10 mg/kg/day for children 7 through 16 years of age.[37–39] Km values for children vary considerably in the literature; some authors have suggested values of 2 to 3 mg/L,[38,40] while others have suggested that a Km value of 6 to 8 mg/L is more appropriate.[37,39] An average Km value of 7 mg/L, while uncertain, is not an unreasonable estimate for children between the ages of 6 months and 16 years of age.

Concentration-Dependent Clearance

The relationship between phenytoin clearance and phenytoin plasma concentration (Cpss ave) can be seen by studying Equation 10.5 and comparing it to the equivalent first-order equation (Equation 10.7, a rearrangement of Equation 15). If the term (Cl)(Cpss ave) in Equation 10.7 is substituted for (S)(F)(Dose/τ) in Equation 10.5, the term (Vm)/(Km + Cpss ave) represents phenytoin clearance in Equation 10.8.

$$(S)(F)(Dose/\tau) = \frac{(Vm)(Cpss\ ave)}{Km + Cpss\ ave}$$

$$(S)(F)(Dose/\tau) = (Cl)(Cpss\ ave)$$

Eq. 10.7

$$Cl_{Phenytoin} = \frac{Vm}{Km + Cpss\ ave}$$

Eq. 10.8

If Cpss ave is very small compared to Km, clearance will be a relatively constant value (Vm/Km) and the metabolism will appear to follow first-order pharmacokinetics. If Cpss ave approaches or exceeds Km, the apparent clearance will decrease and the metabolism will no longer appear to follow a first-order process. As clearance decreases with increasing phenytoin concentration, the velocity or metabolic rate will increase, but *not* in proportion to the increase in plasma concentration (see Figure 10.1). Since Km values are generally below the usual therapeutic range, nearly all patients will display capacity-limited metabolism.

Alterations in plasma binding will also alter the apparent Km value. However, the general approach taken in this chapter will be to adjust the measured concentration to that which would be observed under normal plasma binding conditions and to use pharmacokinetic parameters which are based on normal plasma binding.

Concentration-Dependent Half-Life

The usual reported half-life (t½) for phenytoin is ≈22 hours;[26] however, the t½ is not a constant value because the clearance of phenytoin changes with the plasma concentration. If Equation 10.8 (the clearance equation for phenytoin) is substituted into Equation 32 (the usual equation for half-life), the half-life of phenytoin can be derived:

$$Cl_{Phenytoin} = \frac{Vm}{Km + Cpss\ ave}$$

$$t\frac{1}{2} = \frac{(0.693)(Vd)}{Cl}$$

$$t\frac{1}{2}_{Phenytoin} = \frac{(0.693)(Vd)}{Vm}(Km + Cpss\ ave)$$

Eq. 10.9

Based on Equation 10.9 it can be predicted that the half-life of phenytoin will increase as the plasma concentration increases, an observation that has been confirmed.[27]

Limited Utility of Half-Life. The clinical usefulness of the phenytoin half-life is limited because the time required to achieve steady state can be much longer than the usual three to four times the apparent half-life. Likewise, the time required for a plasma concentration to decay following discontinuation of the maintenance dose will be less than predicted by the apparent half-life.

The problems associated with capacity-limited metabolism can best be explained by first examining the relationship between the rate of drug administration and elimination for a first-order drug. For a first-order drug, when the rate of administration (R_A) exceeds the rate of drug elimination from the body (R_E) the amount of drug in the body per unit of time will increase and the drug will accumulate. If the rate of elimination exceeds the rate of drug administration, the amount of drug in the body per unit of time will decrease, and there will be a net loss of drug from the body.

$$R_A - R_E = \frac{\Delta\ Amount}{t}$$

Eq. 10.10

The rate of drug elimination for a first-order drug is the product of clearance (Cl) and plasma concentration (Cp). When the pharmacokinetic parameters clearance and plasma concentration are substituted into Equation 10.10, the change in the amount of drug in the body (Δ amount) per unit of time is small when the product of Cl and Cp approaches the rate of drug administration. When the change in amount of drug in the body is small, the plasma concentration must be approaching steady state (i.e., $R_A \approx R_E$).

$$R_A - (Cl)(Cp) = \frac{\Delta\ Amount}{t}$$

Eq. 10.11

For capacity-limited drugs, however, clearance (Vm/(Km + Cp)) is not a constant factor. This expression for clearance is inserted into Equation 10.11 below to form Equation 10.12.

$$R_A - \frac{(Vm)}{(Km + Cp)}(Cp) = \frac{\Delta\ Amount}{t}$$

Eq. 10.12

As Cp exceeds Km, the rate of drug elimination approaches Vm. (See Phenytoin: Capacity-Limited Metabolism on page 317.) In such cases, it may be possible to have a rate of elimination which is very close to the rate of drug administration, resulting in very small changes in amount of drug in the body per unit of time. This situation may continue for prolonged periods under certain conditions. When R_A is greater than Vm, accumulation could continue forever or at least until the patient becomes toxic. Capacity-limited accumulation problems are most dramatic when the plasma concentration greatly exceeds the Km value.

Time to Reach Steady State. The time required to achieve 90% of steady state can be calculated as follows:[41]

$$t_{90\%} = \frac{(Km)(Vd)}{[Vm - (S)(F)(Dose/day)]^2}[(2.3\ Vm) - (0.9)(S)(F)(Dose/day)]$$

Eq. 10.13

The $t_{90\%}$ is the time required for a patient to achieve 90% of the steady-state plasma concentration on a dosing regimen, given the Km, Vd and Vm. The units are mg/L for Km; L for Vd; and mg/day for Vm and dose.

Equation 10.13 assumes that the initial plasma concentrations are zero. If the initial plasma concentration is between zero and the steady-state concentration, 90% of steady state will be achieved sooner than predicted by Equation 10.13. Nevertheless, it is still appropriate to use Equation 10.13 to predict the time to achieve steady-state concentrations even when the initial plasma concentration is greater than zero. When therapy with phenytoin is initiated, at first the drug accumulates rapidly so that initial plasma concentrations do not, in most cases, significantly reduce the time required to achieve 90% of steady state. Equation 10.13 should not be used, however, when the initial plasma concentration is greater than the desired steady-state concentration.

When Does a Concentration Represent a Steady-State Value?
When a phenytoin plasma concentration is measured, there is frequently a question as to whether the concentration represents a steady-state level. This question can be answered by the use of Equation 10.14:

$$90\% \ t = \frac{[115 + (35)(Cp)][Cp]}{(S)(F)(Dose)}$$

Eq. 10.14

Cp is in mg/L and the dose is in mg/day normalized for a 70 kg patient. The 90% t value which is calculated by this equation represents the minimum amount of time the patient must have been receiving the maintenance regimen before it can be assumed that the measured Cp is at steady state. Equation 10.14 is relatively conservative in that in its derivation, a Km value of 2 mg/L has been assumed; therefore, the 90% t value is longer than would be required if the Km value were actually greater than 2 mg/L. Therefore, steady state may already have been achieved in a patient who has been receiving the maintenance regimen for a shorter time period than calculated in Equation 10.14. Also note that the Cp in Equation 10.14 must reflect normal plasma protein binding for the calculated 90% t to be valid.

Rate of Decline: Phenytoin Levels. The decline of the phenytoin concentration after discontinuation of therapy can be described by Equation 10.15:

$$t = \frac{\left[(Km)\left(\ln \frac{Cp^o}{Cp_t}\right)\right] + (Cp^o - Cp_t)}{\dfrac{Vm}{Vd}}$$

Eq. 10.15

Cp^o is the initial plasma concentration and Cp_t is the plasma concentration at the end of the time interval t. When both Cp^o and Cp_t are much greater than Km, the time required to decline from Cp^o to Cp_t is primarily controlled by the maximum rate of metabolism (or Vm) and the apparent volume of distribution.

This equation is most frequently used to estimate the Vm value in a patient who has either intentionally or accidentally received excessive phenytoin doses. In this instance, a decline in the phenytoin concentration can be observed over several days. Care should be taken, however, to ensure that no further drug is being administered to the patient. One must also consider that absorption of phenytoin may continue for several days after an acute overdose or following discontinuation of an oral maintenance regimen.[22,42]

Time to Sample

Depending on the disease state being treated and the clinical condition of the patient, the time of sampling for phenytoin can vary greatly. In patients requiring rapid achievement and maintenance of therapeutic phenytoin concentrations, it is usually wise to monitor phenytoin concentrations within two to three days of therapy initiation. This is to ensure that the patient's metabolism is not remarkably different from that which would be predicted by average literature-derived pharmacokinetic parameters. A second phenytoin concentration would normally be obtained in six to seven days; subsequent doses of phenytoin can then be adjusted. If the plasma phenytoin concentrations have not changed over a three to five day period, the monitoring interval can usually be increased to once weekly in the acute clinical setting. In stable patients requiring long-term therapy, phenytoin plasma concentrations are generally monitored at 3- to 12-month intervals.

The time required to achieve steady state with phenytoin can be prolonged. Therefore, plasma levels of phenytoin should be monitored before steady state to avoid sustained periods of low or high phenytoin concentrations. Nevertheless, these early phenytoin concentrations must be used cautiously in the design of new dosing regimens.

In patients receiving divided daily doses of phenytoin by the oral route, the time of sampling is not critical, because the slow absorption of phenytoin minimizes the fluctuations between peak and trough concentrations. Trough concentrations are generally recommended, however, for routine monitoring. In patients who are receiving phenytoin doses intravenously, trough concentrations can be adjusted by Equation 10.16 to calculate the average plasma concentration of phenytoin.

$$\text{Cpss ave} = [\text{Cpss min}] + \left[(0.5)\frac{(S)(F)(Dose)}{Vd} \right]$$

Eq. 10.16

This equation assumes that the Cpss ave is approximately halfway between the trough and peak concentrations.

In patients receiving phenytoin orally, the average concentration can be approximated by multiplying the change in concentration anticipated with the intravenous dose by 0.25. This 0.25 factor assumes that the fluctuation in plasma concentrations following oral administration is approximately half of that which would be expected if the drug were administered intravenously. It also assumes that the average concentration lies approximately halfway between the peak and trough concentrations.

$$\text{Cpss ave} = [\text{Cpss min}] + \left[(0.25)\frac{(S)(F)(Dose)}{Vd} \right]$$

Eq. 10.17

Use of Equation 10.17 is most appropriate when patients are receiving single daily doses of >5 mg/kg and when the phenytoin concentration is <5 mg/L. In patients with phenytoin concentrations >5 mg/L or in those receiving their phenytoin in divided daily doses, use of Equation 10.17 is less critical.

Question #1. **Calculate the phenytoin loading dose required to achieve a plasma concentration of 20 mg/L in B.F., a 70 kg male. Describe how this loading dose should be administered by both the oral and intravenous routes.**

Equation 11 can be used to estimate the loading dose that will produce a plasma concentration of 20 mg/L. If the volume of distribution for phenytoin is assumed to be 0.65 L/kg (see Phenytoin Key Parameters on page 313), the volume of distribution for B.F. would be 45.5 L (70 kg × 0.65 L/kg). The salt factor (S) is 0.92 for the oral or injectable phenytoin dosage forms since the sodium salt is used, and the bioavailability is 100% (F = 1.0).

$$\text{Loading Dose} = \frac{(Vd)(Cp)}{(S)(F)}$$

$$= \frac{(45.5 \text{ L})(20 \text{ mg/L})}{(0.92)(1.0)}$$

$$= 989 \text{ mg}$$

This loading dose of 989 mg is reasonably close to the usual, recommended loading dose of 1000 mg or 15 mg/kg.

If this loading dose is administered intravenously, it should be administered slowly to avoid the cardiovascular toxicities associated with the propylene glycol diluent.[2] A maximum rate of 50 mg/min or 100 mg every five minutes should be used until the entire loading dose is administered or toxicities are encountered.[1]

If the 1000 mg loading dose is to be given orally, a 400 mg dose followed by two 300 mg doses (≈5 mg/kg) at two-hour intervals is recommended so that the entire loading dose is administered over four hours. The oral loading dose is divided into three separate doses to decrease the possibility of nausea and vomiting which may be associated with a single large dose.[21] When the loading dose is administered orally, slow absorption causes the peak concentration to be delayed and lower than the expected 20 mg/L.[21,22] It is usually about one-half of the value calculated by the IV bolus dose model.

$$\Delta Cp = (0.5)\left(\frac{(S)(F)(Dose)}{Vd}\right)$$

Eq. 10.18

Question #2. S.B. is a 37-year-old, 70 kg male with a seizure disorder that has only partially been controlled with 300 mg/day of phenytoin. His plasma phenytoin concentration has been measured twice over the past year and both times it was reported to be 8 mg/L. Calculate a dose which will achieve a steady-state concentration of 15 mg/L.

To establish the new daily dose, it is necessary to assume a Vm or Km for S.B. and then to rearrange Equation 10.5 to calculate the other parameter. The following represents a rearrangement of Equation 10.5 to solve for Vm:

$$(S)(F)(Dose/\tau) = \frac{(Vm)(Cpss\ ave)}{Km + Cpss\ ave}$$

$$Vm = \frac{(S)(F)(Dose/\tau)(Km + Cpss\ ave)}{Cpss\ ave}$$

Eq. 10.19

If Km is assumed to be 4 mg/L, S to be 0.92 (capsules contain the sodium salt), and F to be 1.0, then Vm would be:

$$Vm = \frac{(0.92)(1.0)(300\ mg/day)(4\ mg/L + 8\ mg/L)}{8\ mg/L}$$

$$= \frac{(276\ mg/day)(12\ mg/L)}{8\ mg/L}$$

$$= 414\ mg/day$$

To calculate the dose required to achieve a steady-state concentration of 15 mg/L, Equation 10.5 can be rearranged as follows:

$$(S)(F)(Dose/\tau) = \frac{(Vm)(Cpss\ ave)}{Km + Cpss\ ave}$$

$$Dose = \frac{(Vm)(Cpss\ ave)(\tau)}{(Km + Cpss\ ave)(S)(F)}$$

Eq. 10.20

Using the assumed Km of 4 mg/L and the calculated Vm of 414 mg/day, the daily dose required to achieve a steady-state concentration of 15 mg/L would be:

$$Dose = \frac{(414\ mg/day)(15\ mg/L)(1\ day)}{(4\ mg/L + 15\ mg/L)(0.92)(1.0)}$$
$$= 355\ mg$$

This 18% dosage adjustment should result in a nearly 100% increase in the steady-state plasma level if the assumed Km of 4 mg/L is correct. A daily dose of 355 mg would be difficult to administer; therefore, this initial dosing estimate would probably be rounded off to 350 mg/day and doses of 300 and 400 mg could be prescribed for alternate days.

An alternative approach is illustrated in Figure 10.2. This method allows one to estimate the most probable Km and Vm values for a patient, given the current dosing regimen and measured average steady-state phenytoin concentration.

If the steps outlined in Figure 10.2 are followed, a Km value of 5 mg/L and a Vm value of 6.4 mg/kg/day (451 mg/day for this 70 kg patient) can be determined. When these values are used in Equation 10.17 (or when Figure 10.2 is used), a new dose of ≈350 mg/day is calculated. This second method which uses the "orbit graph" is perhaps slightly superior to the first in which a Km value of 4 mg/L was assumed. This method attempts to define the most likely set of Km and Vm values for the patient given the dosing history and measured phenytoin concentration.

Figure 10.2 can only be used for adult patients, and the phenytoin concentrations used in plotting lines A and B must represent those which would be expected when plasma protein binding conditions are normal. Figure 10.2 also requires that the phenytoin concentration used be an average steady-state value.

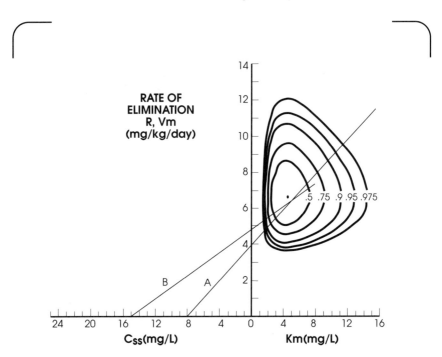

Figure 10.2. Orbit Graph. The most probable values of V_{max} and Km for a patient may be estimated using a single steady-state phenytoin concentration and a known dosing regimen. The eccentric circles or "orbits" represent the fraction of the sample patient population whose Km and V_{max} values are within that orbit. 1) Plot the daily dose of phenytoin (mg/kg/day) on the vertical line (rate of elimination). 2) Plot the steady-state concentration (C_{ss}) on the horizontal line. 3) Draw a straight line connecting C_{ss} and daily dose through the orbits (line A). 4) The coordinates of the midpoint of the line crossing the innermost orbit through which the line passes are the most probable values for the patient's Vm and Km. 5) To calculate a new maintenance dose, draw a line from the point determined in Step 4 to the new desired $C_{ss'}$ (line B). The point at which line B crosses the vertical line (rate of elimination) is the new maintenance dose (mg/kg/day). The line A represents a C_{ss} of 8 mg/L on 276 mg/day of phenytoin acid (300 mg/day of sodium phenytoin) for a 70 kg steady-state concentration was 15 mg/L (µg/mL). From reference 53. The original figure is modified so that R and V_{max} are in mg/kg/day of phenytoin acid. Reprinted from Applied Pharmacokinetics: Principles of Therapeutic Drug Monitoring, 3rd ed., 1992, published by Applied Therapeutics, Inc.

Question #3. Calculate a loading dose that would rapidly increase S.B.'s plasma phenytoin concentration from 8 to 15 mg/L.

Equation 12 can be used to calculate an incremental loading dose. If the Vd is 45.5 L (70 kg × 0.65 L/kg), S = 0.92, and F = 1.0, the loading dose required to increase S.B.'s plasma concentration from 8 to 15 mg/L would be:

$$\frac{\text{Incremental}}{\text{Loading Dose}} = \frac{(\text{Vd})(\text{Cp desired} - \text{Cp initial})}{(S)(F)}$$

$$= \frac{(45.5 \text{ L})(15 \text{ mg/L} - 8 \text{ mg/L})}{(0.92)(1.0)}$$

$$= 346 \text{ mg}$$

This loading dose should be given in addition to the new maintenance dose of 350 mg/day.

Administration of the loading dose will allow more rapid evaluation of the new maintenance dose. If the plasma concentration is <14 mg/L after one week, the dosage can be adjusted a second time. If a loading dose is not given and if at the end of one week the plasma concentration is <14 mg/L, one will be unable to determine whether steady state has been achieved. The plasma levels may remain low or continued administration of 350 mg/day may eventually result in a Cpss ave of ≈15 mg/L.

Question #4. L.C., a 40-year-old, 80 kg male who has been receiving 300 mg/day of phenytoin for the past three weeks (21 days), has a phenytoin level of 14 mg/L. Why is the reported phenytoin level of 14 mg/L not likely to represent a steady-state concentration?

If phenytoin was eliminated according to first-order pharmacokinetics, 21 days would have been more than enough time for steady state to have been achieved based upon a half-life of 15 to 24 hours.

Phenytoin, however, exhibits capacity-limited metabolism; therefore, the time required to achieve steady state is frequently much longer than one would estimate using first-order pharmacokinetic principles. Equation 10.14 should be used to calculate the minimum number of days phenytoin must be administered before it can be safely assumed that the measured concentration represents a steady-state level. First, the daily dose of phenytoin should be normalized to 70 kg:

$$\left[\frac{300 \text{ mg}}{80 \text{ kg}}\right][70 \text{ kg}] = 262.5 \text{ mg}$$

When this value is placed into Equation 10.14 along with an assumed F of 1.0 and an S of 0.92, the 90% t value can be calculated.

$$
\begin{aligned}
90\% \text{ t} &= \frac{[115 + (35)(Cp)][Cp]}{(S)(F)(Dose)} \\
&= \frac{[115 + (35)(14)](14)}{(0.92)(1)(262.5)} \\
&= \frac{(115 + 490)(14)}{241.5} \\
&= 35 \text{ days}
\end{aligned}
$$

The calculated 90% t value of 35 days is longer than the actual duration of therapy (21 days), suggesting that steady state may not yet have been achieved. If an additional loading dose was administered within the first 21 days of therapy, or if the Km value is >2 mg/L, then the plasma level obtained at 21 days may actually represent a steady-state concentration. Due to this uncertainty, additional phenytoin plasma concentrations should be monitored to detect possible accumulation of phenytoin into a potentially toxic concentration range.

Question #5. **A.P., a 52-year-old, 60 kg female, received a 1000 mg loading dose of phenytoin followed by a daily maintenance regimen of 300 mg. Eight days following the initial loading dose, A.P.'s plasma phenytoin level was 11**

mg/L. Should her dose be adjusted at this time to achieve the desired phenytoin concentration of 10 to 20 mg/L?

A 1 gm loading dose should produce an initial concentration of 23.5 mg/L in A.P. according to Equation 49 below. Therefore, the plasma concentration of 11 mg/L eight days later probably represents a plasma concentration that is declining and will continue to decline if the maintenance regimen remains at 300 mg/day.

$$Cp° = \frac{(S)(F)(\text{Loading Dose})}{Vd}$$

$$= \frac{(0.92)(1)(1000 \text{ mg})}{(0.65 \text{ L/kg})(60 \text{ kg})}$$

$$= \frac{920 \text{ mg}}{39 \text{ L}}$$

$$= 23.5 \text{ mg/L}$$

The first step in calculating the new maintenance dose would be to estimate the rate at which the body had been eliminating phenytoin as it declined from the initial concentration of 23.5 mg/L to the observed concentration of 11 mg/L. The Amount Eliminated/t can be calculated by using Equation 10.21, which considers the rate of phenytoin administration $(S)(F)(\text{Dose})/(\tau)$ and the net change in the amount of phenytoin in the body $(Cp_2 - Cp_1)(Vd)/t$.

$$\frac{\text{Amount Eliminated}}{t} = (S)(F)(\text{Dose}/\tau) - \left[\frac{(Cp_2 - Cp_1)(Vd)}{t}\right]$$

Eq. 10.21

In the above equation, Cp_1 is the initial phenytoin concentration which is either predicted or measured, and Cp_2 is the second phenytoin concentration; "t" is the time interval between Cp_1 and Cp_2. It should be pointed out that Cp_1 and Cp_2 phenytoin concentrations should represent the same plasma protein binding circumstances as Vd in Equation 10.1. As suggested in the initial part of the chapter, the author recommends calculating a plasma concentration under normal binding conditions rather than correcting the volume of distribution for the altered plasma binding. Using this approach for A.P., the elimination rate for phenytoin during this eight-day interval would be 337 mg/day of acid phenytoin, which corresponds to ≈366 mg/day of sodium phenytoin.

$$\frac{\text{Amount Eliminated}}{t} = (S)(F)(Dose/\tau) - \left[\frac{(Cp_2 - Cp_1)(Vd)}{t}\right]$$

$$= [(0.92)(1)(300\ mg/day)] - \left[\frac{(11\ mg/L - 23.5\ mg/L)(39\ L)}{8\ days}\right]$$

$$= 276\ mg/day + 61\ mg/day$$

$$= 337\ mg/day\ of\ acid\ phenytoin,\ or$$

$$366\ mg/day\ of\ sodium\ phenytoin\ (337/0.92)$$

This elimination rate represents an average of A.P.'s actual elimination rate (which was >366 mg/day when her phenytoin concentration was 23 mg/L and is <366 mg/day when her phenytoin concentration is 11 mg/L). Therefore, a dose of ≈360 mg/day should maintain an average phenytoin concentration somewhere between 23 and 11 mg/L.

If the desired steady-state phenytoin concentration is not between Cp_1 and Cp_2, additional steps are required to estimate the new maintenance dose. In this case, the amount eliminated per unit of time and the average of Cp_1 and Cp_2 can be placed in the following equation to approximate the patient's Vm.

$$Vm = \frac{\left[\frac{\text{Amount Eliminated}}{t}\right]\left[Km + \left(\frac{Cp_1 + Cp_2}{2}\right)\right]}{\left(\frac{Cp_1 + Cp_2}{2}\right)}$$

Eq. 10.22

This new Vm and assumed Km value would then be used in Equation 10.20 to calculate the new phenytoin maintenance dose.

$$\text{Dose} = \frac{(Vm)(Cpss\ ave)(\tau)}{(Km + Cpss\ ave)(S)(F)}$$

This approach is more uncertain, however, because a Km value had to be assumed in Equation 10.22 to estimate the Vm value used in Equation 10.20.

If the following three rules are not met, the chances that Equations 10.21 and 10.22 will accurately predict the patient's pharmacokinetic parameters and subsequent maintenance doses are substantially diminished.

1) The time between Cp_1 and Cp_2 should be ≥ 3 days.

2) If plasma concentrations are rising, Cp_2 should be $\leq 2 \times Cp_1$. If plasma concentrations are declining, Cp_2 should be $\geq \frac{1}{2}$ of Cp_1.

3) The phenytoin dose, dosage form and route should be consistent.

If any of the three rules above are broken, Equations 10.21 and 10.22 do not become necessarily invalid, but their accuracy is usually less than the usual uncertainties associated with phenytoin dose adjustments.

Question #6. R.M., a 32-year-old, 80 kg male, had been taking 300 mg/day of phenytoin; however, his dose was increased to 350 mg/day because his seizures were poorly controlled and because his plasma concentration was only 8 mg/L. Now he complains of minor CNS side effects and his reported plasma phenytoin concentration is 20 mg/L. Renal and hepatic function are normal. Assume that both of the reported plasma concentrations represent steady-state levels and that R.M. has complied with the prescribed dosing regimens. Calculate R.M.'s apparent Vm and Km and a new daily dose of phenytoin that will result in a steady-state level of about 15 mg/L.

The relationship between daily dose and Cpss can be made linear by plotting daily dose (rate in) versus daily dose divided by Cpss (clearance) for at least two steady-state plasma levels. The graph for R.M. is plotted in Figure 10.3, where the rate-in intercept (390 mg/day) is Vm and the slope of the line (-2.5 mg/L) is the negative value of Km.

Using these values, the daily dose of phenytoin which will achieve a steady-state level of 15 mg/L can be calculated using Equation 10.20:

$$
\begin{aligned}
\text{Dose} &= \frac{(\text{Vm})(\text{Cpss ave})(\tau)}{(\text{Km} + \text{Cpss ave})(\text{S})(\text{F})} \\
&= \frac{(390 \text{ mg/day})(15 \text{ mg/L})(1 \text{ day})}{(2.5 \text{ mg/L} + 15 \text{ mg/L})(1.0)(1.0)} \\
&= 334 \text{ mg}
\end{aligned}
$$

The most convenient dose to the calculated value of 334 mg/day would be 330 mg/day, which could be administered as three 100 mg capsules and one 30 mg capsule.

S was assumed to be 1.0 in the above equation, despite the fact that R.M. is taking phenytoin capsules which contain the sodium salt. Compensation for salt form would be inappropriate because the actual doses of phenytoin sodium were plotted in Figure 10.3. If the doses had been plotted as phenytoin acid, the Vm would have been slightly lower, Km would have been unchanged, and an S of 0.92 would have been used in Equation 10.20 to calculate the daily dose required to achieve a steady-state concentration of 15 mg/L.

An alternate approach to plotting the data for R.M. would be to calculate the negative value of Km by use of Equation 10.23:

$$
-\text{Km} = \frac{R_1 - R_2}{\left(\dfrac{R_1}{\text{Cpss}_1}\right) - \left(\dfrac{R_2}{\text{Cpss}_2}\right)}
$$

Eq. 10.23

$$\text{Slope} = \frac{R_1 - R_2}{\left(\dfrac{R_1}{Cpss_1}\right) - \left(\dfrac{R_2}{Cpss_2}\right)}$$

Figure 10.3. The Rate of Administration (R) or the Daily Dose of Phenytoin (mg/day) Versus the Clearance of Phenytoin (R/Cpss, L/day) Is Plotted for Two or More Different Daily Doses of Phenytoin. A straight line of the best fit is drawn through the points plotted. The intercept on the rate of administration axis is Vm (mg/day) and the slope of the line is the negative value of Km.

where R_1 and R_2 represent the initial and new maintenance doses, respectively. $Cpss_1$ and $Cpss_2$ represent the steady-state concentrations produced by these doses. Again, assuming S and F to be 1.0, a value of -2.5 mg/L is calculated.

$$
\begin{aligned}
-Km &= \frac{(300 \text{ mg/day} - 350 \text{ mg/day})}{\left(\dfrac{300 \text{ mg/day}}{8 \text{ mg/L}}\right) - \left(\dfrac{350 \text{ mg/day}}{20 \text{ mg/L}}\right)} \\[2mm]
&= \frac{-50 \text{ mg/day}}{37.5 \text{ L/day} - 17.5 \text{ L/day}} \\[2mm]
&= -2.5 \text{ mg/L}
\end{aligned}
$$

The value of 2.5 mg/L can then be used in Equation 10.19 with either of the maintenance doses and the corresponding steady-state levels to calculate the Vm:

$$Vm = \frac{(S)(F)(Dose/\tau)(Km + Cpss\ ave)}{Cpss\ ave}$$

$$= \frac{(1)(1)(300\ mg/day)(2.5\ mg/L + 8\ mg/L)}{8\ mg/L}$$

$$= 393.75\ or\ \approx 390\ mg/day$$

The calculated and graphically-determined values for Km and Vm should be exactly the same. Small differences sometimes occur, however, because of differences in mechanical drawing skills.

Question #7. If R.M.'s doses are withheld, how long will it take for the phenytoin concentration of 20 mg/L to decline to 15 mg/L?

The phenytoin half-life will be of little value in predicting the time required for the plasma concentration to decay because the apparent half-life will change as the plasma concentration changes.

The time required for the phenytoin plasma concentration to fall from an initial concentration (Cp^o) to a lower concentration (Cp_t) can be calculated using Equation 10.15. For R.M., who has a volume of distribution of 52 L (0.65 L/kg × 80 kg), a Vm of 390 mg/day, and a Km of 2.5 mg/L, the time required for the initial plasma concentration of 20 mg/L to decline to 15 mg/L will be about 0.76 days:

$$t = \frac{\left[(Km)\left(\ln\frac{Cp^o}{Cp_t}\right)\right] + (Cp^o - Cp_t)}{\dfrac{Vm}{Vd}}$$

$$= \frac{\left[(2.5\ mg/L)\left(\ln\frac{20}{15}\right)\right] + [20\ mg/L - 15\ mg/L]}{\dfrac{390\ mg/day}{52\ L}}$$

$$= 0.76\ days$$

This rate of decline assumes that phenytoin will not continue to be absorbed from the gastrointestinal tract for a significant period following discontinuation of the drug. In the author's experience, however, the initial rate of decline for one to three days is slower than expected because of prolonged absorption.[22,42]

Question #8. E.W., a 56-year-old, 60 kg female, has chronic renal failure and a seizure disorder. She undergoes hemodialysis treatments three times a week, has a serum albumin of 3.3 gm/dL, and takes 300 mg/day of phenytoin. Her reported steady-state plasma phenytoin concentration is 5 mg/L. Should her daily phenytoin dose be increased? What would be her phenytoin concentration if she had a normal serum albumin concentration and normal renal function?

It is critical to carefully evaluate measured phenytoin plasma concentrations in uremic patients because plasma protein binding is altered in these individuals. In patients with normal renal function, about 90% of the measured plasma phenytoin concentration is bound to albumin and 10% is free (α NL = 0.1).[6–8,13] Because binding affinity and albumin concentrations are decreased in uremic patients, the fraction of the total phenytoin concentration that is free in patients with very poor renal function increases from 0.1 to the range of 0.2 to 0.35.[6,9–13] In patients with renal failure who have normal serum albumin levels, the fraction free is $\approx$0.2.[6,10] (Also see Part I: Figures 3 through 5 and Desired Plasma Concentration.)

Since the fraction free (α) for phenytoin is increased in uremic individuals, lower plasma concentrations will produce pharmacologic effects which are equivalent to those produced by higher levels in nonuremic individuals. E.W.'s case can be used as an illustration.

Using E.W.'s serum albumin of 3.3 gm/dL and her phenytoin concentration of 5 mg/L (Cp') in Equation 10.3, a phenytoin concentration of 11.9 mg/L is calculated:

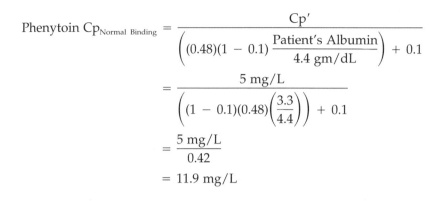

$$\text{Phenytoin Cp}_{\text{Normal Binding}} = \cfrac{\text{Cp}'}{\left((0.48)(1 - 0.1)\cfrac{\text{Patient's Albumin}}{4.4 \text{ gm/dL}}\right) + 0.1}$$

$$= \cfrac{5 \text{ mg/L}}{\left((1 - 0.1)(0.48)\left(\cfrac{3.3}{4.4}\right)\right) + 0.1}$$

$$= \cfrac{5 \text{ mg/L}}{0.42}$$

$$= 11.9 \text{ mg/L}$$

Therefore, E.W.'s measured plasma phenytoin concentration of 5 mg/L is comparable to a concentration of 12 mg/L in a patient with normal plasma binding. The usually accepted therapeutic range for phenytoin in nonuremic patients is 10 to 20 µg/mL, and E.W.'s free plasma concentration corresponds to the low end of this range. If E.W.'s seizure disorder is well controlled, no adjustment in the maintenance dose is necessary. However, if seizures are poorly controlled and phenytoin doses must be adjusted, the comparable plasma concentration for a patient with normal plasma binding (12 mg/L) should be used in all calculations since the values for Km reported in the literature were determined in patients with normal plasma protein binding.

Phenytoin is not dialyzed to a significant extent, and dialysis does not change the protein binding characteristics in uremia.[9,10] Therefore, doses should not be adjusted for E.W. on the basis of dialysis. Changes in plasma protein binding occur within a few days after the development of acute renal failure.[43] Conversely, there is some evidence that following a renal transplant, the plasma protein binding of phenytoin increases rapidly over the first two to four postoperative days and is almost normal two weeks following a successful transplant.[11]

Question #9. **Since phenytoin is bound to plasma protein to a significant extent, will a substantial amount of drug be lost during plasmapheresis or plasma exchange?**

Although 90% of the phenytoin in the serum is bound to albumin, the vascular space represents only a small fraction of the total volume of distribution for phenytoin. Of the total amount of drug in the body, only 5% is within the vascular space. Since most of the phenytoin is actually in the tissue compartments, plasmapheresis or plasma volume exchange should not result in a significant loss of phenytoin from the body. Most studies indicate that somewhere between 5% and 10% of phenytoin is lost from the body during plasmapheresis.[44]

Question #10. S.T. is a 47-year-old, 60 kg male with glomerular nephritis. His creatinine clearance is reasonably good, but he has a serum albumin concentration of 2.0 gm/dL. S.T. is receiving 300 mg/day of phenytoin and has a steady-state phenytoin concentration of 6 mg/L. What would his phenytoin concentration be if his serum albumin were normal? (Assume a normal albumin concentration is 4.4 gm/dL.)

The fraction of a drug concentration which is bound to plasma proteins is a function of the drug's affinity for the binding sites on the plasma protein and the number of binding sites available. The number of binding sites is proportional to the amount or concentration of plasma protein to which the drug is bound. Phenytoin is an acidic drug and appears to be bound primarily to albumin.[7] The relationship between a phenytoin concentration which is observed (Cp') when a patient has a low serum albumin (P') relative to the phenytoin concentration (Cp$_{Normal\ Binding}$) that would be observed if the serum albumin were normal (P) is described by Equation 8 (see Part I: Desired Plasma Concentration on page 9 and Figures 3, 4, and 5) and Equation 10.1:

$$Cp_{Normal\ Binding} = \frac{Cp'}{(1 - \alpha)\left[\dfrac{P'}{P_{NL}}\right] + \alpha}$$

$$Phenytoin\ Cp_{Normal\ Binding} = \frac{Cp'}{\left((1 - 0.1)\dfrac{Patient's\ Albumin}{4.4\ gm/dL}\right) + 0.1}$$

The plasma phenytoin concentration that corresponds to a normal albumin concentration in S.T. can be calculated as follows:

$$Cp_{\text{Normal Binding}} = \frac{6 \text{ mg/L}}{\left(\left(1 - 0.1\right)\left(\dfrac{2.0 \text{ gm/dL}}{4.4 \text{ gm/dL}}\right)\right) + 0.1}$$

$$= \frac{6 \text{ mg/L}}{(0.9)(0.45) + 0.1}$$

$$= 11.8 \text{ mg/L}$$

$Cp_{\text{Normal Binding}}$ should be used in any calculations requiring Km, as described previously.

Question #11. A.R., a 66-year-old, 60 kg male, was admitted to the hospital because of poor seizure control. He had been receiving 350 mg/day of phenytoin acid as an outpatient and on admission had a phenytoin plasma concentration of 3 mg/L. Noncompliance was suspected, and a dose of 350 mg/day as sodium phenytoin was ordered. Five days after administration a second phenytoin level was reported as 18 mg/L. Has steady state been achieved? Is it reasonable to assume that A.R.'s Vm is close to the average values reported in the literature (i.e., 7 mg/kg/day)?

The usual guideline of three to four half-lives as the time required to achieve steady state does not hold true for phenytoin because its metabolism is capacity-limited. The rate of phenytoin accumulation is the difference between the rate of metabolism and the rate of administration. However, unlike drugs following first-order elimination, the rate of elimination is not proportionate to the plasma concentration. Therefore, the time required to reach steady state can be prolonged. This will be especially true when the plasma concentrations are much greater than Km. After the daily dose of 350 mg for this 60 kg patient is corrected to 408.3 mg/day for a 70 kg patient, Equation 10.14 can be used to calculate a 90% t value of 35.7 days.

$$90\% \text{ t} = \frac{[(115) + (35)(Cp)][Cp]}{(S)(F)(Dose)}$$

$$= \frac{[(115) + (35)(18)][18]}{(0.92)(1)(408.3)}$$

$$= \frac{(745)(18)}{375.7}$$

$$= 35.7 \text{ days}$$

A.R. has been on this maintenance regimen for only five days; therefore, the plasma concentration of 18 mg/L does not represent a steady-state condition. Equation 10.21 can be used to estimate the amount of drug eliminated per day:

$$\frac{\text{Amount Eliminated}}{t} = (S)(F)(Dose/\tau) - \left[\frac{(Cp_2 - Cp_1)(Vd)}{t}\right]$$

$$= (0.92)(1)(350 \text{ mg/day}) - \left[\frac{(18 \text{ mg/L} - 3 \text{ mg/L})(0.65 \text{ L/kg} \times 60 \text{ kg})}{5 \text{ days}}\right]$$

$$= 322 \text{ mg/day} - \left[\frac{(15 \text{ mg/L})(39 \text{ L})}{5 \text{ days}}\right]$$

$$= 205 \text{ mg/day}$$

If a Km of 4 mg/L is assumed, a Vm of $\approx$283 mg/day or 4.7 mg/kg/day is calculated for A.R. using Equation 10.22:

$$Vm = \frac{\left[\dfrac{\text{Amount Eliminated}}{t}\right]\left[Km + \left(\dfrac{Cp_1 + Cp_2}{2}\right)\right]}{\left(\dfrac{Cp_1 + Cp_2}{2}\right)}$$

$$= \frac{(205 \text{ mg/day})\left[4 \text{ mg/L} + \left(\dfrac{3 \text{ mg/L} + 18 \text{ mg/L}}{2}\right)\right]}{\left(\dfrac{3 \text{ mg/L} + 18 \text{ mg/L}}{2}\right)}$$

$$= \frac{(205)(4 \text{ mg/L} + 10.5 \text{ mg/L})}{10.5 \text{ mg/L}}$$

$$= 283 \text{ mg/day} \quad or \quad \frac{283 \text{ mg/day}}{60 \text{ kg}}$$

$$= 4.7 \text{ mg/kg/day}$$

This Vm value of $\approx$4.7 mg/kg/day is somewhat less than the average value of 7 mg/kg/day but is not unreasonable. It can be used to approximate a new maintenance dose. Note that even though Cp_2 was not $\leq 2 \times Cp_1$ the mass balance approach can be used as an initial adjustment.

Question #12. Why does changing from oral to intramuscular phenytoin result in a sudden and dramatic decrease in phenytoin levels?

Phenytoin is a relatively insoluble compound which crystallizes within the muscle following intramuscular administration.[45] The phenytoin crystals are slowly absorbed and the absorption rate is decreased initially. The subsequent decrease in the plasma concentration of phenytoin will be more than proportional to the reduction in absorption from the intramuscular injection because phenytoin metabolism is capacity-limited. In one study,[46] a change from oral to intramuscular administration resulted in an initial 40% to 60% decrease in the phenytoin plasma level, while the metabolite elimination decreased by only 16% to 20%. Therefore, the intramuscular route of administration for phenytoin should be avoided.

Question #13. What effect does phenobarbital have on steady-state phenytoin concentrations? What other drugs might interact with phenytoin?

Clinically, the addition of phenobarbital does not change steady-state phenytoin concentrations.[47] Phenobarbital, however, may induce the metabolism of phenytoin and, thereby, increase the metabolic capacity of phenytoin (i.e., increase Vm). Furthermore, competition between phenobarbital and phenytoin for the same metabolic enzymes would have the effect of increasing Km. If Vm is increased, phenytoin clearance will increase and the phenytoin concentration will decrease. Increasing Km will have the opposite effect; therefore, there may be no net effect on the phenytoin concentration. See Equation 10.6:

$$Cpss = \frac{(Km)[(S)(F)(Dose/\tau)]}{Vm - (S)(F)(Dose/\tau)}$$

Similar problems exist in evaluating the mechanism for the increased phenytoin concentrations associated with drugs such as isoniazid, chloramphenicol, and cimetidine.[48–50] In the case of isoniazid, animal data suggest that there is noncompetitive inhibition of metabolic enzymes which reduces the Vm.[51] The interaction appears to be more significant in patients who are phenotypically slow acetylators of isoniazid.[51]

Valproic acid, phenylbutazone, and salicylates reportedly displace phenytoin from albumin.[52] This protein displacement would decrease the total phenytoin concentration, but not the free or unbound concentration. The result is an increased α and a decreased therapeutic range.

References

1. Bigger JT et al. Relationship between the plasma level of diphenylhydantoin sodium and its cardiac antiarrhythmic effects. Circulation. 1968;38:363.

2. Louis S et al. The cardiocirculatory changes caused by intravenous Dilantin and its solvent. Am Heart J. 1967;74:523.

3. Kutt H et al. Diphenylhydantoin metabolism, blood levels and toxicity. Arch Neurol. 1964;11:642.

4. Lund L. Effects of phenytoin in patients with epilepsy in relation to its concentration in plasma. In: David DS, Prichard NBC, eds. Biological Effects of Drugs in Relation to Their Concentration in Plasma. Baltimore: University Park Press; 1972:227.

5. Lascelles PT et al. The distribution of plasma phenytoin levels in epileptic patients. J Neurol Neurosurg Psychiatry. 1970;33:501.

6. Odar-Cederlof I et al. Kinetics of diphenylhydantoin in uremic patients: consequence of decreased protein binding. Eur J Clin Pharmacol. 1974;7:31.

7. Koch-Weser J, Sellers EM. Binding of drugs to serum albumin. N Engl J Med. 1976;294:311.

8. Lund L et al. Plasma protein binding of diphenylhydantoin in patients with epilepsy. Clin Pharmacol Ther. 1972;13:196.

9. Adler DS et al. Hemodialysis of phenytoin in a uremic patient. Clin Pharmacol Ther. 1975;18:65.

10. Reidenberg MM et al. Protein binding of diphenylhydantoin and desmethylimipramine in plasma from patients with poor renal function. N Engl J Med. 1971;285:264.

11. Odar-Cederlof I. Plasma protein binding of phenytoin and warfarin in patients undergoing renal transplantation. Clin Pharmacokinet. 1977;2:147.

12. Reidenberg MM. The binding of drugs to plasma proteins and the interpretation of measurements of plasma concentrations of drugs in patients with poor renal function. Am J Med. 1977;62:466.

13. Liponi DL et al. Renal function and therapeutic concentrations of phenytoin. Neurology. 1984;34:395.

14. Mattson RH et al. Valproic acid in epilepsy; clinical and pharmacological effects. Neurology. 1978;3:20.

15. Monks A, Richens A. Effect of single dose of sodium valproate on serum phenytoin levels and protein binding in epileptic patients. Clin Pharm Ther. 1980;27:89.

16. Jusko WJ et al. Nonlinear assessment of phenytoin bioavailability. J Pharmacokinet Biopharm. 1976;4:327.

17. Gugler R et al. Phenytoin: pharmacokinetics and bioavailablility. Clin Pharmacol Ther. 1976;19:135.

18. Cacek AT. Review of alterations in oral phenytoin bioavailablility associated with formulation, antacids, and food. Ther Drug Monit. 1986;8:166.

19. Bauer LA. Interference of oral phenytoin absorption by continuous nasogastric feedings. Neurology. 1982;32:570.

20. Neuvonen PJ. Bioavailablility of phenytoin; clinical pharmacokinetic and therapeutic implications. Clin Pharmacokinet. 1978;3:20.

21. Wilder BJ et al. Plasma diphenylhydantoin levels after loading and maintenance doses. Clin Pharmacol Ther. 1973;14:797.

22. Jung D et al. Effect of dose on phenytoin absorption. Clin Pharm Ther. 1980;28:479.

23. Havidberg E, Dam M. Clinical pharmacokinetics of anticonvulsants. Clin Pharmacokinet. 1976;1:151.

24. Glazko AJ et al. Metabolic disposition of diphenylhydantoin in normal human subjects following intravenous administration. Clin Pharmacol Ther. 1969;10:498.

25. Bochner F et al. Effects of dosage increments on blood phenytoin concentrations. J Neurol Neurosurg Psychiatry. 1972;35:873.

26. Arnold K et al. The rate of decline of diphenylhydantoin in human plasma. Clin Pharmacol Ther. 1970;11:121.

27. Houghton GW, Richens A. Rate of elimination of tracer doses of phenytoin at different steady state serum phenytoin concentrations in epileptic patients. Br J Clin Pharmacol. 1974;1:155.

28. Lund L et al. Pharmacokinetics of single and multiple doses of phenytoin in man. Eur J Clin Pharmacol. 1974;7:81.

29. Mawer GE et al. Phenytoin dose adjustments in epileptic patients. Br J Clin Pharmacol. 1974;1:163.

30. Lambie DG et al. Therapeutic and pharmacokinetic effects of increasing phenytoin in chronic epileptics on multiple drug therapy. Lancet. 1976;2:386.

31. Richens A. A study of the pharmacokinetics of phenytoin (diphenylhydantoin) in epileptic patients, and the development of a nomogram for making dose increments. Epilepsia. 1975;16:627.

32. Ludden TM et al. Individualization of phenytoin dosage regimens. Clin Pharmacol Ther. 1977;21:287.

33. Martin E et al. The clinical pharmacokinetics of phenytoin. J Pharmacokinet Biopharm. 1977;5:579.

34. Mullen PW. Optimal phenytoin therapy: a new technique for individualizing dosage. Clin Pharmacol Ther. 1978;23:228.

35. Privitera MD. Clinical rules for phenytoin dosing. Ann Pharmacother. 1993;27:1169–73.

36. Atkinson AJ, Shaw JM. Pharmacokinetic study of a patient with diphenylhydantoin toxicity. Clin Pharmacol Ther. 1973;14:521.

37. Bauer LA, Blouin RA. Phenytoin Michaelis-Menten pharmacokinetics in caucasian pediatric patients. Clin Pharmacokinet. 1983;8:545.

38. Grasela TH et al. Steady state pharmacokinetics of phenytoin from routinely collected patient data. Clin Pharmacokinet. 1983;8:355.

39. Dodson WE. Nonlinear kinetics of phenytoin in children. Neurology. 1982;32:42–8.

40. Chiba et al. Michaelis-Menten pharmacokinetics of diphenylhydantoin: an application in the pediatric age patient. J Pediatr. 1980;96:479.

41. Tozer TN, Winter ME. Phenytoin. In: Evans WE et al, eds. Applied Pharmacokinetics: Principles of Therapeutic Drug Monitoring, 3rd ed. Vancouver: Applied Therapeutics; 1992:1.

42. Wilder BJ et al. Correlation of acute diphenylhydantoin intoxication with plasma levels and metabolite excretion. Neurology. 1973;23:1329.

43. Andreasen F, Jakobsen P. Determination of furosemide in blood and its binding to proteins in normal plasma and in plasma from patients with acute renal failure. Acta Pharmacol Toxicol (Copenh). 1974;35:49.

44. Matzke GR. Editorial: does plasma exchange alter drug therapy? Clin Pharm. 1984;3:421.

45. Wilensky AJ et al. Inadequate serum levels after intramuscular administration of diphenylhydantoin. Neurology. 1973;23:318.

46. Wilder BJ et al. A method for shifting from oral to intramuscular diphenylhydantoin administration. Clin Pharmacol Ther. 1974;16:507.

47. Morselli PL et al. Interaction between phenobarbital and DPH in animals and epileptic patients. Ann NY Acad Sci. 1971;169:88.

48. Kutt H et al. Depression of parahydroxylation of diphenylhydantoin by antituberculosis chemotherapy. Neurology. 1966;16:594.

49. Rose JQ et al. Intoxication caused by interaction of chloramphenicol and phenytoin. JAMA. 1977;237:2630.

50. Bartle WR et al. Dose-dependent effect of cimetidine on phenytoin kinetics. Clin Pharmacol Ther. 1983;33:649.

51. Kutt H et al. Inhibition of diphenylhydantoin metabolism in rats and in rat liver microsomes by antitubercular drugs. Neurology. 1968;18:706.

52. Richens A, Dunlop A. Serum phenytoin levels in the management of epilepsy. Lancet. 1975;2:247.

53. Vozeh S et al. Predicting individual phenytoin dosage. J Pharmacokinet Biopharm. 1981;9:131.

Primidone   11

Primidone (Mysoline) is an effective agent in the treatment of generalized and complex partial seizures. Although primidone has anticonvulsant activity of its own, much of the anticonvulsant activity stems from the conversion of primidone to its active metabolite, phenobarbital. Primidone is available as 50 and 250 mg tablets, as well as a 250 mg/5 mL suspension. Primidone is primarily metabolized to phenylethylmalonamide (PEMA) and phenobarbital; approximately 15% to 25% of primidone is excreted unchanged in the urine. Plasma concentrations of PEMA usually are not monitored because its activity is relatively minor. The concomitant use of primidone and phenobarbital is generally unwarranted since excessive concentrations of phenobarbital are likely to develop.

The daily recommended dose of primidone for adults is approximately 10 to 20 mg/kg and 15 to 30 mg/kg for children. These doses are approximately five times the usual dose of phenobarbital; approximately ⅕ of primidone is converted to phenobarbital.

Therapeutic and Toxic Plasma Concentrations

The range of therapeutic plasma concentrations for primidone is 5 to 12 mg/L;[1,2] side effects are common at concentrations exceeding 15 mg/L.[3] The most common side effects associated with primidone are similar to those of phenobarbital, and include sedation, confusion, dizziness, and ataxia.

Bioavailability (F)

Since parenteral formulations of primidone are unavailable, bioavailability data for this drug are incomplete. Nevertheless, primidone appears to be rapidly absorbed (plasma concentrations peak one to three hours following ingestion) and it appears to be 100% bioavailable (F = 1.0). Primidone is labeled in terms of the milligrams of acid compound; therefore, it has a salt factor (S) of 1.0.

Volume of Distribution (Vd)

Data on primidone are limited and the specific characteristics of its disposition are uncertain. An apparent volume of distribution of about 0.6 L/kg appears to be consistent with the available data.[1,4]

Key Parameters

Therapeutic Plasma Concentrations	5–12 mg/L
F	100%
S	1.0
Vd	0.6 L/kg
Cl	
total	0.06 L/kg/hr
to phenobarbital	0.012 L/kg/hr
$t\frac{1}{2}$	7 hr

Clearance (Cl)

Primidone has a clearance value of ≈0.06 L/kg/hr.[4,5] About 20% of primidone is converted to phenobarbital, which would represent a clearance to phenobarbital of ≈0.012 L/kg/hr.[5] Approximately 25% of primidone appears to be eliminated unchanged in the urine, corresponding to a renal clearance of ≈0.015 L/kg/hr.

Half-Life (t½)

The apparent half-life for primidone is approximately eight hours, with a range of 4 to 15 hours.[2] This relatively short half-life suggests that primidone as a parent compound may require relatively frequent dosing at intervals of 6 to 12 hours. Primidone should accumulate relatively rapidly, with plateau concentrations being achieved within 24 hours.

Time to Sample

The sampling time of primidone should be consistent within the dosing interval because of its relatively short half-life. As with other drugs, trough concentrations (i.e., those obtained just before a dose) of primidone are probably the most reproducible and most convenient. Several weeks, however, must elapse before primidone anticonvulsant effects are fully stabilized because of the long phenobarbital half-life. (See Figure 11.1.) In addition, phenobarbital serum concentrations should be monitored because a significant amount of primidone is metabolized to phenobarbital.

Doses must be altered with caution in patients who have been receiving primidone for less than three to four weeks because of the time needed for phenobarbital to reach a steady-state concentration.[6]

> **Question #1.** D.M., a 65 kg, 25-year-old male, has been taking 250 mg of primidone Q 6 hr for approximately three months. What would be the calculated trough concentration of primidone?

To calculate the anticipated trough primidone concentration, one must first estimate a clearance and volume of distribution for D.M. as shown on the next page:

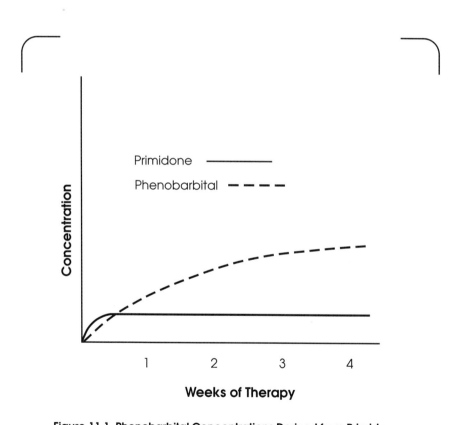

Figure 11.1. Phenobarbital Concentrations Derived from Primidone.
During the first few days to weeks after starting primidone therapy, primidone and phenobarbital plasma concentrations are similar. As steady state is approached, the phenobarbital level is approximately two to four times greater than the primidone concentration. (See text.)

$$\text{Primidone Cl} = (0.06 \text{ L/kg/hr})(65 \text{ kg})$$
$$= 3.9 \text{ L/hr}$$

$$\text{Primidone Vd} = (0.6 \text{ L/kg})(65 \text{ kg})$$
$$= 39 \text{ L}$$

The elimination rate constant and half-life can then be calculated using Equations 27 and 31, respectively.

$$\text{Kd} = \frac{\text{Cl}}{\text{Vd}}$$
$$= \frac{3.9 \text{ L/hr}}{39 \text{ L}}$$
$$= 0.1 \text{ hr}^{-1}$$

$$t^{1/2} = \frac{0.693}{\text{Kd}}$$
$$= \frac{0.693}{0.1 \text{ hr}^{-1}}$$
$$= 6.9 \text{ hr}$$

The elimination rate constant of 0.1 hr^{-1}, an assumed salt form (S) of 1.0, and a bioavailability (F) of 1.0 can then be used in Equation 47 to calculate the trough concentration.

$$\text{Cpss min} = \frac{\dfrac{(S)(F)(\text{Dose})}{\text{Vd}}}{(1 - e^{-\text{Kd}\tau})} (e^{-\text{Kd}\tau})$$

$$= \frac{\dfrac{(1)(1)(250 \text{ mg})}{39 \text{ L}}}{(1 - e^{-(0.1 \text{ hr}^{-1})(6 \text{ hr})})} (e^{-(0.1 \text{ hr}^{-1})(6 \text{ hr})})$$

$$= \left[\frac{6.4 \text{ mg/L}}{0.45}\right][0.55]$$

$$= [14.2 \text{ mg/L}][0.55]$$

$$= 7.8 \text{ mg/L}$$

This expected trough concentration of ≈8 mg/L is within the usual therapeutic range. Also, as can be seen from the calculation above, the expected peak concentration (Cpss max) of 14.2 mg/L does not appear to be excessive.

Question #2. Calculate the expected steady-state pheno-barbital concentration which would be produced by D.M.'s primidone regimen.

A number of approaches could be taken to calculate D.M.'s phenobarbital concentration. One approach would be to first calculate the average steady-state level of primidone by using Equation 35 and the appropriate values for the salt form, bioavailability, dosing interval, and clearance.

$$
\begin{aligned}
\text{Cpss ave} &= \frac{(S)(F)(\text{Dose}/\tau)}{Cl} \\
&= \frac{(1)(1)(250 \text{ mg}/6 \text{ hr})}{3.9 \text{ L/hr}} \\
&= \frac{41.7 \text{ mg/hr}}{3.9 \text{ L/hr}} \\
&= 10.7 \text{ mg/L}
\end{aligned}
$$

This average steady-state plasma concentration of primidone could then be used along with the expected clearance of primidone to phenobarbital of 0.78 L/hr (0.012 L/kg/hr × 65 kg) to calculate the rate at which primidone is being converted to phenobarbital (R_A). This is illustrated below using Equation 14:

$$
\begin{aligned}
R_A &= (Cl)(\text{Cpss ave}) \\
&= (0.78 \text{ L/hr})(10.7 \text{ mg/L}) \\
&= 8.3 \text{ mg/hr}
\end{aligned}
$$

An administration rate of 8.3 mg/hr is equivalent to a daily phenobarbital dose of ≈200 mg (8.3 mg/hr × 24 hr). This daily administration rate of 200 mg would correspond to (S)(F)(Dose/τ) in Equation 35. The expected phenobarbital clearance of 6.5

L/day (0.1 L/kg/day × 65 kg) can then be used in Equation 35 below to predict the steady-state phenobarbital concentration as follows:

$$\text{Cpss ave} = \frac{(S)(F)(Dose/\tau)}{Cl}$$

$$= \frac{200 \text{ mg/day}}{6.5 \text{ L/day}}$$

$$= 31 \text{ mg/L}$$

This phenobarbital concentration of 31 mg/L is approximately three times the average expected primidone level and approximately four times the trough primidone concentration. The actual ratio of primidone to phenobarbital will vary depending upon the time of sampling within the primidone dosing interval. Alterations in the primidone to phenobarbital plasma ratio are usually due primarily to changes in primidone concentrations within the 5 to 12 hour dosing interval. Within this time interval, the serum concentration of phenobarbital will not decrease dramatically because phenobarbital has an intrinsically long half-life and primidone is continually being converted to phenobarbital.

An alternate approach to calculating the steady-state phenobarbital level is to recognize that approximately 20% of the primidone dose will be converted to phenobarbital; that is, ≈200 mg/day (0.2 × 1000 mg/day). This value could be inserted in Equation 35 to calculate the expected steady-state phenobarbital level of 31 mg/L. This approach avoids the necessity of calculating the expected average steady-state concentration of primidone.

Question #3. R.O., a 12-year-old, 35 kg female, is admitted to the hospital for observation because of poor seizure control. Her current drug regimen includes 200 mg/day of phenytoin and 750 mg/day of primidone. The day after admission, R.O.'s serum drug concentrations were reported to be 3 mg/L for phenytoin, 6 mg/L for primidone, and 8 mg/L for phenobarbital. What are possible explanations for the unusual ratio of phenobarbital to primidone?

Although only ⅕ of primidone is converted to phenobarbital, one generally observes an average steady-state phenobarbital level that is approximately two to four times greater than the average primidone level because of the marked differences in the clearance for these two compounds. Phenobarbital to primidone concentration ratios which are lower than this may represent one of three possibilities.

First, R.O. may have only recently been started on primidone and insufficient time may have elapsed for phenobarbital to accumulate to steady-state concentrations (phenobarbital t½ is four to five days). Primidone plasma concentrations usually plateau within 24 hours, while phenobarbital levels rise slowly over several weeks (see Figure 11.1 on page 351). A second possibility is patient noncompliance with the primidone regimen. A third possibility is that the patient converts very small amounts of primidone to phenobarbital or has an unusually high phenobarbital clearance.

In most cases, an unusually low phenobarbital to primidone ratio represents noncompliance; however, the other two possibilities should be explored. It would be difficult to evaluate unusual conversion or elimination of phenobarbital unless R.O. could be observed under a controlled environment where compliance could be guaranteed. Another option is to change R.O. from primidone therapy to phenobarbital and observe her phenobarbital disposition characteristics.

References

1. Kutt H. Pharmacodynamic and pharmacokinetic measurements of anti-epileptic drugs. Clin Pharmacol Ther. 1974;16:243.

2. Gallagher BB et al. The relationship of the anticonvulsant properties of primidone to phenobarbital. Epilepsia. 1970;11:293.

3. Booker HE. Primidone: toxicity. In: Woodbury DM et al, eds. Antiepileptic drugs. New York: Raven Press;1972:377–83.

4. Kauffman RE et al. Kinetics of primidone metabolism and excretion in children. Clin Pharmacol Ther. 1977;22:200.

5. Bogan J, Smith H. The relation between primidone and phenobarbitone blood levels. J Pharm Pharmacol. 1968;20:64.

6. Olesen OV, Dam M. The metabolic conversion of primidone to phenobarbitone in patients under long-term treatment. Acta Neurol Scand. 1967;43:348.

Procainamide 12

Procainamide is used to treat ventricular tachyarrhythmias, and is administered orally, intramuscularly, and intravenously. A loading dose of ≈1000 mg (15 mg/kg) is generally followed by a maintenance dose of 250 to 500 mg every three to four hours. The short plasma half-life of procainamide dictates the use of three- to four-hour dosing intervals unless sustained-release drug products are used. Long-term administration has been associated with immunologic reactions.

Pharmacokinetic predictions are complicated because procainamide is cleared renally as well as metabolically. Procainamide is metabolized to an active metabolite, N-acetylprocainamide (NAPA), which is an antiarrhythmic agent in its own right. The activity of the NAPA metabolite is limited, but monitoring NAPA plasma concentrations may be appropriate in patients with diminished renal function because it is primarily eliminated by the kidneys.

Therapeutic and Toxic Plasma Concentrations

Procainamide plasma concentrations of 4 to 8 mg/L are usually considered therapeutic.[1,2] Minor toxicities such as gastrointestinal disturbances, weakness, mild hypotension, and changes in the electrocardiogram (10% to 30% prolongation of the PR, QT, or QRS intervals) usually do not occur at plasma concentrations <8 mg/L. Toxicities may develop in as many as 30% of patients when plasma concentrations exceed 12 to 13 mg/L.[2] Plasma concentrations in the range of 15 to 20 mg/L, however, may be appropriate in some patients.[3–5] Patients in whom unusually high target procainamide concentrations were needed suffered from severe arrhythmias that were difficult to control with conventional therapy. While the therapeutic range of procainamide is undergoing re-evaluation, care should be taken to carefully evaluate the risk versus benefit of therapy in any patient with plasma concentrations above the usual therapeutic range.

Bioavailability (F)

The bioavailability of orally administered procainamide is approximately 85% (F = 0.85).[6] Absorption is usually rapid, and plasma concentrations peak one to two hours after administration. Considerable variation in absorption can occur,[6] and absorption can be very slow and possibly incomplete in patients with congestive heart failure (CHF).[1]

Key Parameters

Therapeutic Plasma Concentration	4–8 mg/L
F	0.85
S	0.87
Vd^a	2 L/kg
Cl^b	
Cl_{renal}	$[3][Cl_{Cr}]^c$
$Cl_{acetylation}$ (average)	0.13 L/kg/hr
Fast	0.19 L/kg/hr
Slow	0.07 L/kg/hr
$t\frac{1}{2}$	
α	5 min
β^d	3 hr
S (HCl salt)	0.87

[a] Decreased by 25% in patients with low cardiac output.
[b] Decreased by 25% to 50% in patients with low cardiac output.
[c] Units of Cl_{Cr} must be appropriate when Cl_{renal} is added to $Cl_{acetylation}$ and Cl_{other} (i.e., L/hr or L/kg/hr).
[d] Half-life increased in patients with renal and/or cardiac dysfunction.

While not well-studied, the sustained-release procainamide products appear to be completely absorbed over approximately three to four hours.[7,8] This absorption period limits the dosing interval for the sustained-release products to six hours in the majority of patients. Only in patients with a low clearance and prolonged elimination half-life can the dosing interval be extended beyond six hours. Although there have been reports of intact sustained-release tablets in the stool, these actually represent the inert matrix which remains after complete absorption of the drug.[9]

Volume of Distribution (Vd)

The volume of distribution of procainamide is $\approx$2 L/kg.[2,10] This volume is unchanged by renal failure,[10] but is decreased by about 25% in patients with decreased cardiac output.[2] In obese patients, the volume of distribution appears to correlate best with ideal body weight (IBW).[11]

Like lidocaine, procainamide distributes into an initial volume of distribution (Vi).[1,2,12] Since the myocardium responds as though it were located in the initial volume of distribution, loading doses (which are calculated based on a volume of distribution of 2 L/kg) should be given in increments small enough to avoid excessive plasma concentrations in Vi. (See Question 2.)

Clearance (Cl)

The clearance of procainamide in an average 70 kg patient with reasonably good renal function is ≈550 mL/min. In these patients, about one-half of the dose is cleared by metabolism, and the other one-half is cleared renally.[1] The clearance of procainamide can be broken down into three primary components: a renal clearance (Cl_{renal}), which is approximately three times creatinine clearance;[1,6,13,14] acetylation clearance ($Cl_{acetylation}$) which is based upon acetylation phenotype; and a non-renal, non-acetylated metabolic clearance, which will be referred to as clearance "other" (Cl_{other}). Clearance by acetylation is approximately 0.19 L/kg/hr in fast acetylators, and 0.07 L/kg/hr in slow acetylators; Cl_{other} is ≈0.1 L/kg/hr.

Although subjects with excellent renal function and cardiac output may have procainamide clearances >30 L/hr,[6,12,13] clearances of one-half this value are common in patients with diminished renal function or cardiac output.[2,3] It is difficult to know the degree to which each of the clearance pathways is affected by congestive heart failure. One approach that can be used in patients with CHF is to decrease the total calculated clearance (which has been based on renal function and body weight) to approximately 50% of the original value.

The clearance of procainamide in obese subjects is increased relative to their ideal body weight.[11] This appears to be due to increased renal clearance. Therefore, in obese subjects the renal clearance of procainamide should be based on total body weight (TBW) and the metabolic clearance on the patient's ideal body weight (see Question 8).

Half-Life (t½)

The apparent distribution half-life (α t½) is about five minutes.[2,6,12] The elimination half-life (β t½) of procainamide is a function of its volume of distribution and clearance. For a 70 kg patient with an average volume of distribution of 2 L/kg (140 L) and a clearance of 33 L/hr, the calculated elimination half-life (using Equation 32) is approximately three hours.

$$t\frac{1}{2} = \frac{(0.693)(Vd)}{Cl}$$

$$= \frac{(0.693)(140\ L)}{33\ L/hr}$$

$$= 3\ hr$$

This half-life is short, and frequent dosing will be necessary unless a continuous intravenous infusion or a sustained-release oral product is used.

The absorption time for the sustained-release procainamide drug products is somewhat short and probably in the range of four hours. This suggests that, depending upon the patient's procainamide half-life and the dosing interval chosen for the sustained-release drug product, the intermittent infusion model (Equation 57) is most appropriate for calculating procainamide trough concentrations.

$$Cpss_2 = \frac{\frac{(S)(F)(Dose/t_{in})}{Cl}(1\ -\ e^{-Kdt_{in}})}{1\ -\ e^{-Kd\tau}}\ (e^{-Kdt_2})$$

Note that for the trough concentration t_2 is the time interval (in hours) from the end of absorption to the next procainamide dose (i.e., $\tau\ -\ t_{in}$). This is the time over which the procainamide concentration will decay. As previously discussed, if t_2 is $\leq \frac{1}{3}$ t½, a continuous infusion model (Equation 35) can be used.

$$Cpss\ ave = \frac{(S)(F)(Dose/\tau)}{Cl}$$

For most patients receiving sustained-release procainamide products every six hours, Equation 35 is probably reasonable, even if one suspects that the value of t_2 is longer than $\frac{1}{3}$ of the half-life. This is because there is some variation in both the onset and the duration of absorption from sustained-release products. Therefore, the complexity of Equation 57 is probably not warranted in clinical practice unless the procainamide dosing intervals are 8 or 12 hours and the procainamide half-life is short.

N-Acetylprocainamide (NAPA)

Therapeutic and Toxic Plasma Concentrations. The exact relationship between plasma N-acetylprocainamide concentrations and antiarrhythmic activity has not been clearly established. Some researchers have observed that NAPA's activity is similar to that of procainamide when equal plasma concentrations are compared;[15–17] however, others have found that plasma concentrations of approximately 10 to 20 mg/L are required for partial suppression of ventricular contractions.[18,19] Little additional antiarrhythmic effects are observed when NAPA concentrations exceed 30 mg/L.[19]

Interestingly, when the therapeutic levels of 4 to 8 mg/L were established for procainamide,[1,2] NAPA concentrations were not considered, even though plasma NAPA concentrations are approximately equal to procainamide concentrations in many patients.[20,21] Although the activity of NAPA as an antiarrhythmic is in question, therapeutic and/or toxic effects are possible in some patients.[22] This may be related to elevated NAPA concentrations or an unusual sensitivity to the compound. Therefore, monitoring plasma NAPA concentrations may be useful, although in the majority of patients, knowledge of the plasma NAPA concentration does not alter the course of procainamide therapy.

Animal studies suggest that NAPA may be less toxic than procainamide. Although significant cardiac toxicity has not been observed with NAPA concentrations as high as 40 mg/L,[19,23] NAPA may have resulted in serious cardiac toxicity in isolated individuals when NAPA levels exceeded 30 mg/L.[22] In addition, systemic lupus erythematosus may be less likely to be associated with NAPA than with procainamide.[17]

NAPA Production. The rate of NAPA production depends upon the plasma concentration of procainamide and its clearance by acetylation, which is genetically determined. About 50% of blacks and Caucasians are rapid acetylators, and approximately 80% to 90% of Asians are rapid acetylators. Rapid acetylators convert ≈30% of an administered dose of procainamide to NAPA, while slow acetylators convert ≈15%.[24] This percentage conversion is based upon the acetylation clearance, which is approximately 0.19 L/hr/kg for a rapid acetylator and 0.07 L/hr/kg for a slow acetylator. The percentage conversion increases in patients with diminished renal function because a greater percentage of procainamide is cleared by the acetylation pathway.[10,14] This is illustrated by Equation 12.1.

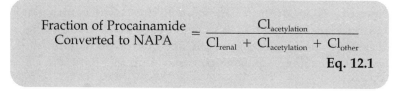

$$\frac{\text{Fraction of Procainamide}}{\text{Converted to NAPA}} = \frac{Cl_{acetylation}}{Cl_{renal} + Cl_{acetylation} + Cl_{other}}$$

Eq. 12.1

Volume of Distribution (Vd). The volume of distribution for NAPA appears to be about 1.5 L/kg.[25,26]

Clearance (Cl). NAPA has a renal clearance that is approximately 1.6 times creatinine clearance and a metabolic or non-renal clearance that is ≈0.025 L/hr/kg.[25]

Half-Life (t½). The usual half-life of NAPA in patients with normal renal function is approximately six hours. However, the half-life may increase to 30 hours or more in patients with poor renal function.[10,13]

Time to Sample (Procainamide and NAPA)

Since procainamide has a relatively short half-life (three hours), steady-state concentrations are achieved within 12 to 24 hours after therapy has begun. Although steady state is achieved quickly, the sampling time must be selected carefully within the dosing interval. When standard dosage forms of procainamide are administered on a regular, intermittent basis, trough plasma concentrations are probably more reproducible than peak concentrations. With sustained-release procainamide, however, the sampling time becomes relatively less important. Nevertheless, when dosing intervals exceed six hours, significant peak to trough variations may occur in patients with short procainamide half-lives, since the duration of absorption for procainamide from sustained-release drug products is probably about four hours.

Procainamide concentrations are most appropriately monitored within the first 24 to 48 hours of therapy, although additional plasma concentrations may be required later if significant changes in the patient's clinical status are observed. The half-life for NAPA is twice as long as that for procainamide and steady state will not be achieved for at least 24 hours in patients with good renal function; as long as one week may be required for patients with significantly decreased renal function.

Question #1. A.L., a 62-year-old, 70 kg male, was admitted to the coronary care unit with a diagnosis of acute myocardial infarction. A.L. has a history of mild chronic renal failure, a serum creatinine of 1.3 mg/dL, and a creatinine clearance of ≈50 mL/min. A.L. developed premature ventricular contractions (PVCs) which were unresponsive to lidocaine. Calculate a parenteral loading dose of procainamide designed to achieve a plasma concentration of ≈8 mg/L.

To calculate the loading dose required to achieve a procainamide plasma concentration of 8 mg/L, the volume of distribution must be estimated. Assuming A.L. does not have significant heart failure, the expected volume of distribution would be 140 L (2 L/kg × 70 kg). Using Equation 11 and assuming F to be 1.0 for parenteral administration and S to be 0.87 for the hydrochloride salt, the loading dose of procainamide would be:

$$\text{Loading Dose} = \frac{(Vd)(Cp)}{(S)(F)}$$

$$= \frac{(140 \text{ L})(8 \text{ mg/L})}{(0.87)(1)}$$

$$= 1287 \text{ mg } or \approx 1300 \text{ mg}$$

This calculated loading dose is reasonably close to the usual loading dose of 1000 mg.[27] If the patient had CHF, the volume of distribution and, therefore, the loading dose would have been decreased by about 25%.[2]

Question #2. If the loading dose of 1300 mg is to be given intravenously, how should it be administered?

Since procainamide is administered into an initial volume of distribution (Vi)[1,2,12] and the myocardium responds as though it were located in this initial volume,[2,12,27] it should be given in divided doses. If the entire loading dose is given as a single bolus, the initial plasma concentration will greatly exceed the desired 8 mg/L and toxicities may occur.

The apparent initial volume of distribution is approximately one-third of the total Vd. Therefore, as much as one-third of the total loading dose may be given as the first bolus. In this case, 300 to 400 mg could be administered initially as a slow infusion, followed by doses of 150 mg (one-half the original dose) every five minutes. Since the apparent distribution half-life is about five minutes,[2,12] each of the doses should be separated by at least five minutes to avoid accumulation in Vi. In most clinical situations, 100 mg is given every 5 minutes until the arrhythmia is abolished, toxicities are observed, or the total loading dose is administered.[27] Others have recommended infusing a total loading dose at a rate of ≈50 mg/min to achieve therapeutic concentrations rapidly while avoiding excessive accumulation in the first compartment.[13]

The patient should be closely monitored throughout the loading dose period for side effects, such as hypotension and rhythm disturbances, that may be related to excessive concentrations of procainamide.

***Question #3.* Calculate an infusion rate in mg/min that will maintain an average plasma procainamide concentration of 6 mg/L for A.L., the patient described in Question 1.**

Determine Clearance. Since the maintenance dose is determined by the patient's clearance, this parameter must be estimated before the infusion rate can be calculated. Using A.L.'s creatinine clearance (Cl_{Cr}) of 3 L/hr (50 mL/min), an average acetylation clearance of 0.13 L/kg/hr and a Cl_{other} of 0.1 L/kg/hr, a total clearance of ≈25 L/hr is calculated.

$$Cl_{renal} = (3)(Cl_{Cr})$$
$$= (3)(3 \text{ L/hr})$$
$$= 9 \text{ L/hr}$$

$$Cl_{acetylation} \atop (Average) = (0.13 \text{ L/kg/hr})(70 \text{ kg})$$
$$= 9.1 \text{ L/hr}$$

$$Cl_{other} = (0.1 \text{ L/kg/hr})(70 \text{ kg})$$
$$= 7 \text{ L/hr}$$

$$Cl_{total} = Cl_{renal} + Cl_{acetylation} + Cl_{other}$$

Eq. 12.2

$$= 9 \text{ L/hr} + 9.1 \text{ L/hr} + 7 \text{ L/hr}$$
$$= 25.1 \text{ L/hr}$$

Calculate a Maintenance Infusion. Using this clearance value of 25 L/hr and assuming S to be 0.87 and F to be 1.0, Equation 16 can be used to calculate a maintenance infusion of 172 mg/hr.

$$\text{Maintenance Dose} = \frac{(Cl)(Cpss \text{ ave})(\tau)}{(S)(F)}$$

$$= \frac{(25 \text{ L/hr})(6 \text{ mg/L})(1 \text{ hr})}{(0.87)(1)}$$

$$= 172 \text{ mg}$$

This infusion rate of 172 mg/hr is ≈2.9 mg/min and within the usual guidelines for procainamide infusions (1 to 3 mg/min).

Question #4. A.B., a 70 kg male with a Cl_{Cr} of 30 mL/min, has been receiving a constant procainamide infusion of 100 mg/hr. This infusion rate has resulted in a steady-state plasma procainamide concentration of 5 mg/L. Calculate an oral dosing regimen that will maintain his plasma procainamide concentrations between 4 and 8 mg/L.

Determine the Dosing Interval. Trough concentrations of procainamide should not be less than one-half of the peak concentrations; thus, the dosing interval should not exceed the half-life. The half-life of procainamide for A.B. can be estimated if the volume of distribution and clearance are known. If A.B. does not have significant congestive heart failure, the average volume of distribution (140 L based upon 2 L/kg) can be used. His procainamide clearance can be determined by use of Equation 15 since a steady-state procainamide plasma concentration resulting from a given maintenance infusion dose is known. An S of 0.87 and an F of 1.0 can be assumed:

$$Cl = \frac{(S)(F)(Dose/\tau)}{Cpss\ ave}$$

$$= \frac{(0.87)(1)(100\ mg/hr)}{5\ mg/L}$$

$$= 17.4\ L/hr$$

Using this clearance (17.4 L/hr) and the expected volume of distribution of 140 L, Equation 32 can be used to calculate A.B.'s half-life.

$$t^{1/2} = \frac{(0.693)(Vd)}{Cl}$$

$$= \frac{(0.693)(140\ L)}{17.4\ L/hr}$$

$$= 5.6\ hr$$

Based upon this half-life, a dosing interval of four to six hours should be used.

Calculate the Oral Maintenance Dose. The oral maintenance dose can be calculated in a number of ways. One method is to first select a dosing interval. Then, using the steady-state equation, a maintenance dose which will achieve an average concentration that is halfway between the desired peak and trough levels can be calculated. For example, using a desired average steady-state concentration of 6 mg/L, a dosing interval of four hours, the calculated clearance of 17.4 L/hr, an S of 0.87, and an F of 0.85, a maintenance dose of ≈565 mg every four hours is calculated using Equation 16.

$$Maintenance\ Dose = \frac{(Cl)(Cpss\ ave)(\tau)}{(S)(F)}$$

$$= \frac{(17.4\ L/hr)(6\ mg/L)(4\ hr)}{(0.87)(0.85)}$$

$$= 565\ mg\ Q\ 4\ hr$$

As a general rule, the dosing interval should be equal to or less than the drug half-life when the desired peak is less than or equal to twice the trough concentration. Procainamide is available in 250, 375, and 500 mg dosage forms; therefore, a dose of 500 mg every 4 hours might be selected. The peak and trough concentrations from this dose can be calculated using Equations 43 and 46, respectively.

$$\text{Cpss max} = \frac{\dfrac{(S)(F)(Dose)}{Vd}}{(1 - e^{-Kd\tau})}$$

$$\text{Cpss min} = (\text{Cpss max})(e^{-Kd\tau})$$

To solve the above equations, the elimination rate constant (Kd) must first be calculated. It can be determined from the half-life (5.6 hours) using Equation 8.4:

$$Kd = \frac{0.693}{t^{1/2}}$$

$$= \frac{0.693}{5.6 \text{ hr}}$$

$$= 0.124 \text{ hr}^{-1}$$

Then, a Cpss max of 6.8 mg/L can be calculated:

$$\text{Cpss max} = \frac{\dfrac{(S)(F)(Dose)}{Vd}}{(1 - e^{-Kd\tau})}$$

$$= \frac{\dfrac{(0.87)(0.85)(500 \text{ mg})}{140 \text{ L}}}{(1 - e^{-(0.124 \text{ hr}^{-1})(4 \text{ hr})})}$$

$$= \frac{2.64 \text{ mg/L}}{1 - 0.61}$$

$$= \frac{2.64 \text{ mg/L}}{0.39}$$

$$= 6.8 \text{ mg/L}$$

Once Cpss max is known, a Cpss min of 4.1 mg/L can also be calculated:

$$\text{Cpss min} = (\text{Cpss max})(e^{-Kd\tau})$$
$$= 6.8 \text{ mg/L } (e^{-(0.124 \text{ hr}^{-1})(4 \text{ hr})})$$
$$= (6.8 \text{ mg/L})(0.61)$$
$$= 4.1 \text{ mg/L}$$

The predicted peak and trough plasma concentrations of 6.8 mg/L and 4.1 mg/L, respectively, were based upon the assumption that absorption occurs rapidly. The dampening effect of absorption will produce peak concentrations that are slightly lower and trough concentrations that are slightly higher than predicted by the IV bolus model. One should recall that absorption rates vary considerably among patients,[6] especially those with congestive heart failure.[1]

If a sustained-release procainamide were to be used, one could first determine the daily dose of the infusion using Equation 3.

$$\begin{array}{l} \text{Amount of Drug Absorbed} \\ \text{or Amount Reaching the} \\ \text{Systemic Circulation} \end{array} = (S)(F)(\text{Dose})$$

$$= (0.87)(1.0)(100 \text{ mg/hr})(24 \text{ hr/day})$$
$$= 2088 \text{ mg/day}$$

Then, Equation 4 could be used to adjust for the difference in oral bioavailability.

$$\frac{\text{Dose of New}}{\text{Dosage Form}} = \frac{\begin{array}{c}\text{Amount of Drug Absorbed}\\\text{from Current Dosage Form}\end{array}}{(S)(F) \text{ of New Dosage Form}}$$
$$= \frac{2088 \text{ mg/day}}{(0.87)(0.85)}$$
$$= 2824 \text{ mg/day}$$

If this new dose were to be given every six hours (four times daily), then the individual doses given every six hours would be essentially equivalent to A.B.'s IV infusion rate of 100 mg/hr.

$$\frac{2824 \text{ mg}}{4} = 706 \text{ mg Q 6 hr}$$

Because the sustained-release procainamide products are available as 250, 500, 750, and 1000 mg tablets, the dosage form closest to the calculated dose is 750 mg. To confirm that 750 mg every six hours will produce a concentration similar to that achieved with the 100 mg/hr infusion, Equation 35 can be used to estimate the steady-state procainamide concentration.

$$\text{Cpss ave} = \frac{(S)(F)(\text{Dose}/\tau)}{Cl}$$
$$= \frac{(0.87)(0.85)(750 \text{ mg}/6 \text{ hr})}{17.4 \text{ L/hr}}$$
$$= 5.3 \text{ mg/L}$$

As discussed earlier, using a continuous infusion model for sustained-release procainamide products administered every six hours is probably reasonable given the minimal fluctuation in plasma concentration anticipated within the dosing interval. If a dosing interval of eight hours had been chosen instead, the continuous infusion model would be a little more problematic given the expected half-life of ≈5.6 hours. The decay time might result in significant fluctuations of the plasma concentration within the dosing interval. (See Question 5.)

Question #5. Using A.B.'s pharmacokinetic parameters, calculate the expected peak and trough concentrations from a sustained-release procainamide product when dosed 1000 mg Q 8 hr.

To calculate the steady-state peak and trough concentrations produced by a sustained-release drug product, one of two models can be used. In the first model, an average steady-state concentration is calculated on the assumption that procainamide plasma concentrations will fluctuate minimally during a dosing interval because absorption is prolonged. Using Equation 35 to make this calculation, an average concentration of $\approx$5.3 mg/L is predicted.

$$
\begin{aligned}
\text{Cpss ave} &= \frac{(S)(F)(\text{Dose}/\tau)}{Cl} \\
&= \frac{(0.87)(0.85)(1000\ \text{mg}/8\ \text{hr})}{17.4\ \text{L/hr}} \\
&= \frac{92\ \text{mg/hr}}{17.4\ \text{L/hr}} \\
&= 5.3\ \text{mg/L}
\end{aligned}
$$

As an alternative, Equation 57, which describes an intermittent steady-state infusion model, can be used. The term t_2 is the time interval between the end of the infusion and the time at which the concentration is measured. (Also see Part I: Selecting the Appropriate Equation on page 57.) When calculating the peak concentration with a dosing interval of 8 hours, t_{in} is assumed to be four hours, and t_2 to be zero hours. When calculating the trough concentration, t_2 in Equation 57 is assumed to be four hours. When the previously calculated parameters for clearance, elimination rate constant, S, and F are used, a peak concentration of 6.6 mg/L and a trough concentration of 4 mg/L can be calculated as shown below.

$$
\begin{aligned}
\text{Cpss}_2 &= \frac{\dfrac{(S)(F)(\text{Dose}/t_{in})}{Cl}\,(1 - e^{-Kdt_{in}})}{(1 - e^{-Kd\tau})}\,(e^{-Kdt_2}) \\[2mm]
&= \frac{\dfrac{(0.87)(0.85)(1000\ \text{mg}/4\ \text{hr})}{17.4\ \text{L/hr}}\,(1 - e^{-(0.124\ \text{hr}^{-1})(4\ \text{hr})})}{(1 - e^{-(0.124\ \text{hr}^{-1})(8\ \text{hr})})}\,[e^{-(0.124\ \text{hr}^{-1})(0\ \text{hr})}] \\[2mm]
&= \frac{(10.6\ \text{mg/L})(1 - 0.61)}{(1 - 0.37)}\,(1) \\[2mm]
&= 6.6\ \text{mg/L}
\end{aligned}
$$

$$\begin{array}{r}\text{Cpss}_2\\(\text{Trough})\end{array} = [6.6 \text{ mg/L}][e^{-\text{Kdt}_2}]$$

$$= (6.6 \text{ mg/L})(e^{-(0.124 \text{ hr}^{-1})(4 \text{ hr})})$$

$$= (6.6 \text{ mg/L})(0.61)$$

$$= 4.0 \text{ mg/L}$$

If the absorption time for a dosage form is substantially different than four hours, t_{in} should be adjusted accordingly.

Question #6. A.B., the patient described in Question 5, has a steady-state procainamide concentration of 5 mg/L. Estimate his plasma NAPA concentration.

The steady-state NAPA concentration (Cpss ave) can be determined from Equation 35 once the necessary parameters are derived. In this case it can be assumed that S and F are 1.0, since NAPA is produced directly from plasma procainamide. The rate of NAPA production (Dose/τ) can be calculated by multiplying the average steady-state procainamide concentration by the acetylation clearance of procainamide. If A.B. is phenotypically a rapid acetylator, the clearance to NAPA would be 0.19 L/kg/hr; if he is a slow acetylator, it would be 0.07 L/hr/kg. Assuming A.B. is a rapid acetylator, acetylation clearance would be 13.3 L/hr (0.19 L/kg/hr × 70 kg).

Using this clearance value of 13.3 L/hr and A.B.'s average procainamide concentration of 5 mg/L, the hourly NAPA production rate is 66.5 mg.

$$\text{Rate of Conversion to NAPA} = \left[\frac{\text{Cpss ave}}{(\text{Procainamide})}\right][\text{Cl}_{\text{acetylation}}]$$

Eq. 12.3

$$= (5 \text{ mg/L})(13.3 \text{ L/hr})$$

$$= 66.5 \text{ mg/hr}$$

This approach assumes that the molecular weight of procainamide and NAPA are not substantially different and that each milligram of procainamide converted to NAPA represents a milligram of NAPA. Once the rate of NAPA production (which is essentially the infusion rate of NAPA) and the clearance for NAPA are known, the average steady-state plasma concentration can be calculated from Equation 35, where the rate of conversion to NAPA equals $(S)(F)(Dose/\tau)$. If A.B. has a creatinine clearance of ≈1.8 L/hr (30 mL/min), his expected NAPA clearance would be 4.63 L/hr as shown below.

$$\text{NAPA } Cl_{total} = (1.6)(Cl_{Cr} \text{ in L/hr}) + (0.025 \text{ L/kg/hr})(\text{Weight in kg})$$

Eq. 12.4

$$= 2.88 \text{ L/hr} + 1.75 \text{ L/hr}$$
$$= 4.63 \text{ L/hr}$$

$$\text{NAPA } Cl_{renal} = (1.6)(Cl_{Cr})$$
$$= (1.6)(1.8 \text{ L/hr})$$
$$= 2.88 \text{ L/hr}$$

$$\text{NAPA } Cl_{metabolic} = (0.025 \text{ L/kg/hr})(\text{Weight in kg})$$
$$= (0.025 \text{ L/kg/hr})(70 \text{ kg})$$
$$= 1.75 \text{ L/hr}$$

Using this clearance value and the expected rate of conversion to NAPA of 66.5 mg/hr, a steady-state NAPA concentration of 14.4 mg/L can be calculated with Equation 35.

$$\text{Cpss ave} = \frac{(S)(F)(Dose/\tau)}{Cl}$$
$$= \frac{66.5 \text{ mg/hr}}{4.63 \text{ L/hr}}$$
$$= 14.4 \text{ mg/L}$$

Question #7. **What is the clinical significance of plasma NAPA concentrations? How might they alter the clinical**

use of procainamide and the interpretation of plasma procainamide concentrations?

Therapeutic plasma concentrations of procainamide were established before it was known that NAPA could be contributing to the therapeutic and, possibly, toxic effects of procainamide. The ratio of NAPA to procainamide concentrations is primarily a function of acetylation phenotype and renal function. Patients with poor renal function who are rapid acetylators will have the highest ratios of NAPA to procainamide concentrations.

Patients with high NAPA to procainamide ratios may experience therapeutic effects even when average or trough concen-

Creatinine Clearance, mL/min/70 Kg

Figure 12.1. Graphic Representation of The Expected Procainamide To NAPA Ratios At (Cpss ave) Versus Renal Function For Fast and Slow Acetylators. The graph was derived using average clearance values for rapid and slow acetylators and by adjusting NAPA clearance to renal function. Ratios of procainamide to NAPA concentrations which lie between the lines for fast and slow acetylators would be assigned to the closest adjacent line. Phenotype status is uncertain for patients with procainamide to NAPA concentration ratios that are intermediate.

trations of procainamide are below those usually associated with antiarrhythmic efficacy. The longer half-life of NAPA may also explain why many patients, especially those with renal failure, are well controlled on procainamide even though dosing intervals are longer than four to five hours; NAPA concentrations change relatively little when the procainamide dosing interval is six hours.

If NAPA is contributing to the antiarrhythmic effect, the full efficacy of a procainamide dosing regimen cannot be evaluated until NAPA concentrations have reached steady state. In patients with renal failure who have a NAPA half-life of 30 hours or longer, five days or more may be required before steady-state NAPA concentrations are achieved and maximal antiarrhythmic effects are observed. A similar situation will be encountered when procainamide is discontinued in patients with poor renal function. Within 24 to 36 hours after discontinuing the drug, procainamide levels will be essentially zero. However, one cannot ascertain whether or not the patient can be maintained without procainamide until several more days have elapsed and NAPA levels have declined substantially.

While it is not commonly used, the ratio of NAPA to procainamide concentrations could be evaluated to establish whether a patient is a rapid or slow acetylator. Since the rate of NAPA production equals the rate of NAPA elimination at steady state, the ratio of the average NAPA concentration to the average procainamide concentration at steady state should equal the total clearance of NAPA divided by procainamide's clearance by acetylation.

$$\text{Rate of NAPA Production} = \text{Rate of NAPA Elimination}$$

$$\frac{[\text{Cpss ave}][\text{Cl}_{acetylation}]}{(\text{Procainamide})} = \frac{[\text{Cpss ave}][\text{Cl}_{renal} + \text{Cl}_{metabolic}]}{(\text{NAPA})}$$

or

$$\frac{\text{Cpss ave (Procainamide)}}{\text{Cpss ave (NAPA)}} = \frac{\text{NAPA Cl}_{renal} + \text{NAPA Cl}_{metabolic}}{\text{Procainamide Cl}_{acetylation}}$$

This concept was applied to the development of Figure 12.1 which can be used as an aid to estimate whether a patient is a rapid or slow acetylator. To use this graph, measured NAPA and procainamide concentrations must be sampled under steady-state conditions and should approximate average concentrations within the dosing interval. The creatinine clearance is expressed in mL/min for a 70 kg individual; therefore, if a patient's weight varies significantly from 70 kg, the creatinine clearance should be normalized to the 70 kg weight.

Question #8. I.C., a 45-year-old, 100 kg, 5 foot 9 inch man with a serum creatinine of 1.5 mg/dL, has severe CHF and ventricular arrhythmias which are to be treated with oral procainamide. Recommend a dose of procainamide for this obese patient to achieve an average procainamide concentration of 5 mg/L.

Because I.C. is obese, one would first estimate his ideal body weight (IBW) using Equation 65.

$$\text{Ideal Body Weight For Males in kg} = 50 + 2.3(\text{Height in Inches} > 60)$$
$$= 50 + 2.3(9)$$
$$= 70.7 \text{ kg}$$

To calculate I.C.'s procainamide clearance, one would need to calculate his renal, acetylation and other clearance values. One could use Equation 63 and calculate his creatinine clearance in mL/kg/min by deleting the weight component of the equation.

$$\text{Cl}_{Cr} \text{ for Males (mL/min)} = \frac{(140 - \text{Age})(\text{Weight})}{(72)(\text{SrCr}_{ss})}$$

$$\text{Cl}_{Cr} \text{ for Males (mL/kg/min)} = \frac{(140 - \text{Age})}{(72)(\text{SrCr}_{ss})}$$
$$= \frac{(140 - 45)}{(72)(1.5 \text{ mg/dL})}$$
$$= 0.88 \text{ mL/kg/min}$$

$$\frac{\text{Cl}_{\text{Cr}}}{(\text{L/kg/hr})} = \left[\frac{\text{Cl}_{\text{Cr}}}{(\text{mL/kg/min})}\right]\left[\frac{60 \text{ min/hr}}{1000 \text{ mL/L}}\right]$$

$$= [0.88 \text{ mL/kg/min}]\left[\frac{60 \text{ min/hr}}{1000 \text{ mL/L}}\right]$$

$$= 0.0528 \text{ L/kg/hr}$$

Using this creatinine clearance of 0.0528 L/kg/hr, I.C.'s renal clearance of procainamide (based upon his total body weight) is ≈15.84 L/hr.

$$\text{Cl}_{\text{renal}} = (3)(\text{Cl}_{\text{Cr}})$$
$$= (3)(0.0528 \text{ L/kg/hr})(100 \text{ kg})$$
$$= 15.84 \text{ L/hr}$$

I.C.'s metabolic clearance can be estimated by assuming the average value for $\text{Cl}_{\text{acetylation}}$ and Cl_{other} and using I.C.'s ideal body weight. Ideal body weight was used here because procainamide's metabolic clearance appears to correlate more closely to I.C.'s non-obese weight. Combining the three clearance factors, I.C.'s total procainamide clearance can be calculated using Equation 12.2 (≈32.1 L/hr). Because I.C. has CHF, his total clearance should be reduced by about 50% to ≈16 L/hr.

$$\text{Cl}_{\text{acetylation}} = (0.13 \text{ L/kg/hr})(70.7 \text{ kg})$$
$$= 9.19 \text{ L/hr}$$

$$\text{Cl}_{\text{other}} = (0.1 \text{ L/kg/hr})(70.7 \text{ kg})$$
$$= 7.07 \text{ L/hr}$$

$$\text{Cl}_{\text{total}} = \text{Cl}_{\text{renal}} + \text{Cl}_{\text{acetylation}} + \text{Cl}_{\text{other}}$$
$$= 15.84 \text{ L/hr} + 9.19 \text{ L/hr} + 7.07 \text{ L/hr}$$
$$= 32.1 \text{ L/hr}$$

Reducing The Total Clearance By 0.5 For CHF:
$$= 32.1 \text{ L/hr} \times 0.5$$
$$= 16.05 \text{ L/hr}$$

To estimate I.C.'s elimination rate constant and half-life, his Vd must be calculated. Using ideal body weight and considering that CHF reduces the volume of distribution from about 2 L/kg to 1.5 L/kg, I.C.'s half-life is estimated to be ≈4.5 hours.

$$Vd = (1.5 \text{ L/kg})(70.7 \text{ kg})$$
$$= 106 \text{ L}$$

$$t^{1/2} = \frac{(0.693)(Vd)}{Cl}$$
$$= \frac{(0.693)(106 \text{ L})}{16 \text{ L/hr}}$$
$$= 4.59 \text{ hr}$$

Using Equation 16, a maintenance dose of approximately 650 mg every six hours is calculated.

$$\text{Maintenance Dose} = \frac{(Cl)(Cpss \text{ ave})(\tau)}{(S)(F)}$$
$$= \frac{(16 \text{ L/hr})(5 \text{ mg/L})(6 \text{ hr})}{(0.87)(0.85)}$$
$$= 649 \text{ mg (Q 6 hr)}$$

Assuming I.C.'s procainamide is to be given as a sustained-release drug product, one could choose to administer either 500 or 750 mg every six hours. Using Equation 35, average steady-state concentrations of approximately 3.9 and 5.8 mg/L can be calculated for each of these doses, respectively.

$$Cpss \text{ ave} = \frac{(S)(F)(Dose/\tau)}{Cl}$$
$$= \frac{(0.87)(0.85)(500 \text{ mg/6 hr})}{16 \text{ L/hr}}$$
$$= 3.85 \text{ mg/L}$$

or

$$= \frac{(0.87)(0.85)(750 \text{ mg/6 hr})}{16 \text{ L/hr}}$$
$$= 5.8 \text{ mg/L}$$

Either regimen would appear to be reasonable.

Because of the uncertainty in initial parameter estimates, I.C. should be carefully observed for both lack of efficacy and procainamide toxicity. While the clinical outcome is clearly the therapeutic goal, plasma concentrations may help to determine the optimal dose for I.C. that will control his arrhythmia while minimizing the possibility of adverse effects.

References

1. Koch-Weser J. Pharmacokinetics of procainamide in man. Ann NY Acad Sci. 1971;169:370.

2. Koch-Weser J, Klein SW. Procainamide dosage schedules, plasma concentrations and clinical effects. JAMA. 1971;215:1454.

3. Engel TR et al. Modification of ventricular tachycardia by procainamide in patients with coronary artery disease. Am J Cardiol. 1980;46:1033.

4. Giardina EV et al. Efficacy, plasma concentrations and adverse effects of a new sustained release procainamide preparation. Am J Cardiol. 1980;46:855.

5. Greenspan AM et al. Large dose procainamide therapy for ventricular tachyarrhythmia. Am J Cardiol. 1980;46:453.

6. Manion CV et al. Absorption kinetics of procainamide in humans. J Pharm Sci. 1977;66:981.

7. Smith TC, Kinkel AW. Plasma levels of procainamide after administration of conventional and sustained-release preparations. Curr Ther Res. 1980;27:217.

8. Vlasses PH et al. Immediate release and sustained-release procainamide: bioavailablility at steady-state in cardiac patients. Ann Intern Med. 1983;89:613.

9. Job ML et al. Carcass of a pill: no cause for alarm. N Engl J Med. 1981;305:231.

10. Gibson TP et al. Kinetics of procainamide and N-acetylprocainamide in renal failure. Kidney Int. 1977;12:422.

11. Christoff PV et al. Procainamide disposition in obesity. Drug Intell Clin Pharm. 1983;17:516.

12. Galeazzi RL et al. Relationship between the pharmacokinetics and pharmacodynamics of procainamide. Clin Pharmacol Ther. 1976;20:278.

13. Lima JJ et al. Pharmacokinetic approach to intravenous procainamide therapy. Eur J Clin Pharmacol. 1978;13:303.

14. Lima JJ et al. Clinical pharmacokinetics of procainamide infusions in relation to acetylator phenotype. J Pharmacokinet Biopharm. 1979; 7:69.

15. Elson J et al. Antiarrhythmic potency on N-acetylprocainamide. Clin Pharmacol Ther. 1975;17:134.

16. Bagwell EE et al. Correlation of the electrophysiological and antiarrhythmic properties of the N-acetyl metabolite of procainamide with plasma and tissue drug concentration in the dog. J Pharmacol Exp Ther. 1976;197:38.

17. Drayer DE et al. N-acetylprocainamide: an active metabolite of procainamide. Proc Soc Exp Biol Med. 1974;146:358.

18. Lee WK et al. Antiarrhythmic efficacy of N-acetylprocainamide in patients with premature ventricular contractions. Clin Pharmacol Ther. 1976;19:508.

19. Atkinson AJ Jr. et al. Dose ranging trial of N-acetylprocainamide in patients with premature ventricular contractions. Clin Pharmacol Ther. 1977;21:575.

20. Karlsson E et al. Acetylation of procainamide in man studied with a new gas chromatographic method. Br J Pharmacol. 1974;1:467.

21. Reidenburg MM et al. Polymorphic acetylation of procainamide in man. Clin Pharmacol Ther. 1975;17:722.

22. Vlasses PH et al. Lethal accumulations of procainamide metabolite in renal insufficiency. Drug Intell Clin Pharm. 1984;18:493. Abstract.

23. Bottorff MB et al. High-dose procainamide in chronic renal failure. Drug Intell Clin Pharm. 1983;17:279.

24. Gibson TP. Acetylation of Procainamide in man and its relationship to isonicotinic acid-hydrazide acetylation phenotype. Clin Pharmacol Ther. 1975;17:395.

25. Strong JM et al. Pharmacokinetics in man of the N-acetylated metabolite of procainamide. J Pharmacokinet Biopharm. 1975;3:223.

26. Strong JM et al. Absolute bioavailability in man of N-acetylprocainamide determined by a novel stable isotope method. Clin Pharmacol Ther. 1975;18:613.

27. Giardina EV, Heissenbuttel RH. Intermittent intravenous procainamide to treat ventricular arrhythmias. Ann Intern Med. 1973;78:183.

Quinidine   13

Quinidine is used to treat atrial fibrillation and other cardiac arrhythmias. It is administered orally as the sulfate, gluconate, or polygalacturonate salts and by slow intravenous infusions as the gluconate salt. Usual doses of quinidine are 200 to 300 mg orally three to four times a day.[1,2]

An assessment of the specificity of the assay used by the clinical laboratory is essential to the interpretation of quinidine plasma concentrations.[3] Likewise, congestive heart failure (CHF), liver disease, nephrotic syndrome, or recent stress can alter the protein binding and clearance of quinidine and thereby significantly influence the interpretation of plasma quinidine concentrations.

Therapeutic Plasma Concentrations

A number of quinidine assays of varying specificity have been used in the past. Each assay was associated with a different range of therapeutic plasma concentrations. The early quinidine assay procedures were less specific and tended to measure inactive metabolites, resulting in a therapeutic range for quinidine higher than the values currently used.[4-6] As assays became more specific and utilized extraction techniques to eliminate many of the polar metabolites, the therapeutic range for quinidine decreased.[7-9] Specific quinidine assays originally utilized either high performance liquid chromatography[10,11] or thin layer chromatography coupled with a florescence detection procedure.[12] Current assays used in clinical practice are almost always based upon some type of immunoassay technique. These are specific for quinidine and lead to a therapeutic range of 1 to 4 mg/L.[10,13,14]

Changes in *plasma protein binding* can alter the desired therapeutic concentrations of quinidine. Quinidine is a basic drug which is bound primarily to α_1-acid glycoprotein.[15,16] Although early studies suggested that quinidine was 80% to 90% bound to plasma proteins (i.e., α or fraction free = 0.2 to 0.1, respectively),[15,17] it is now known that the α or fraction free is ≈0.1 for most patients.[18] Since only the free or unbound drug is active, a change in the plasma protein binding could change the desired plasma concentration. (See Part I: Desired Plasma Concentrations on page 9.)

The plasma protein binding of quinidine is reduced in patients with chronic liver disease, presumably because the α_1-acid glycoprotein concentration is decreased.[11,19] Therefore, the α or fraction free is increased

Key Parameters[a]

Therapeutic Plasma Concentration		1–4 mg/L
Vd		
Normal		2.7 L/kg
Chronic Heart Failure		1.8 L/kg
Chronic Liver Disease		3.8 L/kg
Cl		
Normal		0.28 L/kg/hr
Congestive Heart Failure		0.17–0.23 L/kg/hr
Chronic Liver Disease		Decreased
Quinidine	S	F
Sulfate	0.82	0.7
Gluconate	0.62	0.7
Polygalacturonate	0.62	0.7

[a] Therapeutic range, Vd, and clearance are derived from specific quinidine assay procedures.

and the desired quinidine plasma concentrations for patients with chronic liver disease will be lower than usual. (See Part I: Figure 4 on page 11.) Although one would expect α to be increased in patients with nephrotic syndrome, studies have not been conducted in this type of patient. It is known, however, that nephrotic patients frequently have decreased α_1-acid glycoprotein concentrations in addition to hypoalbuminemia.[20] A decrease in plasma protein concentrations would result in lower therapeutic quinidine plasma concentrations. (See Part I: Figure 4 on page 11.)

The plasma protein binding of quinidine is increased following acute stress such as surgery.[15] Factors associated with alterations in α_1-acid glycoprotein concentrations appear to have in common tissue damage, wound healing, or an inflammatory response (see Table 13.1). Such events tend to increase the total drug concentration with relatively little change in the free drug levels. Since altered plasma binding may influence plasma quinidine concentrations, the relationship between the measured quinidine concentration (which represents both the bound and unbound drug) and clinical response should be assessed. For example, a patient with an unusually high quinidine concentration should be evaluated for the presence of clinical factors known to alter quinidine binding. One should also carefully assess the clinical response of the patient to ensure that it is consistent with the elevated plasma concentration [e.g., increased PR, QRS, or QT intervals on electrocardiogram (ECG)].

Bioavailability (F)

Quinidine is approximately 70% bioavailable (F = 0.7),[12,21–23] but a range of 47% to 96% has been reported.[11,12] It is rapidly absorbed and has a half-life of about seven hours. Some clinicians, therefore, prefer to use sustained-release quinidine formulations to minimize the need for frequent dosing. Quinidine is most commonly prescribed as the sulfate, gluconate, or polygalacturonate salt with corresponding S factors of approximately 0.82, 0.62, and 0.62, respectively. The bioavailability of these various quinidine preparations is similar; therefore, F is assumed to be 0.7.[23,25]

Volume of Distribution (Vd)

The initial volume of distribution of quinidine is 1.0 L/kg[26] and the apparent volume of distribution of quinidine is ≈2.7 L/kg.[11,26,27] The distribution half-life, however, is so brief (6 to 12 minutes) that the initial volume and associated two-compartment modeling is of no consequence

Table 13.1	Factors Known to Alter α_1-Acid Glycoprotein Concentrations[a]	
Increased	**Decreased**
Tumors	Pregnancy
Rheumatoid arthritis	Oral contraceptives
Rheumatic fever	Cirrhosis
Pulmonary tuberculosis	Nephritis
Acute infections	
Obstructive liver disease	
Inflammatory bowel disease	
Burns	
Fractures	
Trauma	
Surgery	
Myocardial infarction	

[a] From References 16,37,38

following oral administration.[11,26,27] Two-compartment modeling need only be considered if quinidine is to be given intravenously.

When intravenous (IV) administration of quinidine is necessary, a slow infusion is required in order to allow quinidine to equilibrate between the central volume of distribution and the tissue volume of distribution. Intravenous quinidine gluconate doses ≤6 mg/kg infused over 20 to 30 minutes are generally considered to be slow enough to allow equilibrium and avoid acute toxicities associated with the distribution phase.[28–30]

In patients with CHF, the volume of distribution of quinidine is decreased to about 1.8 L/kg.[11,27] In patients with chronic liver disease, the average volume of distribution of quinidine increases to about 3.8 L/kg[19] because the binding of quinidine to plasma proteins is decreased in these patients. A volume of distribution for quinidine as large as 9.7 L/kg has been observed in one patient.[11] Since decreased plasma protein binding is also expected in nephrotic patients,[20] they too will have larger volumes of distribution for quinidine. Although undocumented, one would also anticipate alterations in volume of distribution when any factor associated with a change in quinidine plasma binding is present. Factors associated with an increase in α_1-acid glycoprotein would be expected to decrease the volume of distribution, while factors associated with a decrease in the α_1-acid glycoprotein concentration would be associated with a larger volume of distribution for quinidine. (See Part I: Figure 6 on page 19 and Volume of Distribution (Vd) on page 18.)

When quinidine's volume of distribution is altered because of changes in plasma protein binding, the loading dose of quinidine will remain unchanged from that recommended for a patient with normal plasma protein binding. In this situation, the change in the apparent volume of distribution is due to a change in the protein-bound, rather than free, quinidine concentration. Therefore, the desired plasma concentration of quinidine will be lower and the volume of distribution larger whenever quinidine binding to plasma proteins is decreased. Conversely, quinidine levels will be higher whenever quinidine binding to plasma proteins is increased.[31] (See Part I: Desired Plasma Concentration on page 9.)

Clearance (Cl)

The average clearance for quinidine is 4.7 mL/kg/min or 0.28 mL/kg/hr.[11,26] Most of the clearance of quinidine is due to metabolism; only 20% of quinidine clearance is due to renal excretion.[11,26] The clearance of quinidine is decreased to 3.0 to 3.9 mL/kg/min or 0.17 to 0.23 L/kg/hr in patients with CHF, presumably because hepatic blood flow is diminished.[11,27]

Quinidine clearance is also decreased in patients with liver disease. Clearance values calculated from total plasma quinidine concentrations in patients with chronic liver disease may appear normal, but calculations that are based upon the increased free drug concentration in these patients reveal impaired metabolic capacity.[11,19] (See Part I: Clearance (Cl): Plasma Protein Binding on page 30.)

Several drugs affect the clearance of quinidine. The co-administration of nifedipine with quinidine may be associated with increased quinidine concentrations in some patients.[32] This nifedipine interaction is presumed to be due to a decrease in clearance secondary to a decrease in cardiac output. Amiodarone and cimetidine reduce the clearance of quinidine[33,34] through direct inhibition of microsomal metabolism. Anticonvulsant drugs such as phenytoin and phenobarbital reportedly increase quinidine clearance, presumably due to enzyme induction.[35]

In addition to the drug interactions, there is some evidence that quinidine exhibits dose-dependent or capacity-limited metabolism.[24,36] While non-linear pharmacokinetics for quinidine are not as significant as they are for phenytoin, some caution should be used when quinidine maintenance doses are increased to ensure that the final steady-state concentration is not excessive. (See Question 3.)

Elimination Half-Life

The usual half-life of quinidine is about seven hours.[11,26] The half-life is not affected by congestive heart failure because the volume of distribution and clearance are decreased by about the same proportion in patients with this condition.

$$t\frac{1}{2} = \frac{(0.693)(\downarrow Vd)}{\downarrow Cl}$$

The half-life is increased in patients with chronic liver disease because the metabolic capacity for quinidine is diminished and the volume of distribution is increased:

$$\uparrow t^{1}\!/_{2} = \frac{(0.693)(\uparrow Vd)}{\downarrow Cl}$$

In patients who exhibit plasma protein binding changes, but no alterations in the metabolism of the unbound or free quinidine, both the clearance and the volume of distribution should be altered proportionately and in the same direction. Consequently, there would be no change in the quinidine half-life.[31] Some disease states such as chronic liver disease, however, may be associated with a change in plasma protein binding as well as a diminished metabolic capacity.

Time to Sample

Since the half-life of quinidine is approximately seven hours and three to four half-lives are required to reach approximately 90% of steady state, the plasma concentration should, under normal circumstances, be evaluated after 24 hours of therapy. The best time to obtain a blood sample, for the purpose of measuring the plasma concentrations of both sustained-release and non-sustained release drugs, is just before the next scheduled dose (trough levels). This avoids many of the potential problems associated with delayed absorption and the uncertainty of when a peak concentration will occur following an oral dose (Part I: Interpretation of Plasma Drug Concentrations, Figure 29 on page 74).

If a patient develops symptoms of quinidine toxicity or is at very high risk for decreased quinidine clearance, a plasma sample should be evaluated even if the estimated time to steady state (i.e., 24 hours) has not elapsed. These early plasma concentrations may be useful in deciding whether to withhold further quinidine therapy or to reduce the dose. Plasma quinidine concentrations obtained before two half-lives yield relatively little information about the eventual steady-state concentration.

> **Question #1.** R.M., a 70 kg male with CHF and atrial fibrillation, is to be given quinidine sulfate 300 mg PO Q 6 hr. Should a plasma sample for quinidine concentration be obtained within 24 hours of starting therapy?

The half-life for quinidine is unlikely to be altered in a patient with CHF because both volume of distribution and clearance are decreased proportionately. Therefore, one would anticipate that

R.M. has a normal quinidine half-life (seven hours) and that steady-state samples could be obtained 21 to 35 hours after therapy is initiated.

Question #2. **What plasma concentration would be expected in R.M. if quinidine is assayed by a specific immunoassay? Is the prescribed quinidine sulfate regimen of 300 mg Q 6 hr likely to maintain his plasma quinidine concentrations within the therapeutic range?**

The plasma sample should be obtained immediately before the next dose of quinidine because plasma trough concentrations of drugs are more reproducible and can be predicted by using Equation 47:

$$\text{Cpss min} = \frac{\frac{(S)(F)(\text{Dose})}{Vd}}{(1 - e^{-Kd\tau})} (e^{-Kd\tau})$$

In this case, S will be 0.82 since 82% of quinidine sulfate is quinidine base. The following pharmacokinetic parameters can be used to calculate the trough concentration of quinidine for R.M. who has congestive heart failure: F = 0.7;[26] Cl = 3 mL/min/kg[27] or 12.6 L/hr; Vd = 1.8 L/kg[27] or 126 L; Dose = 300 mg; and τ = 6 hr. The elimination rate constant (Kd) can be determined from Equation 27:

$$Kd = \frac{Cl}{Vd}$$

$$= \frac{12.6 \text{ L/hr}}{126 \text{ L}}$$

$$= 0.1 \text{ hr}^{-1}$$

Assuming these values are correct for R.M., his predicted trough concentration of quinidine would be:

$$\text{Cpss min} = \frac{\dfrac{(S)(F)(Dose)}{Vd}}{(1 - e^{-Kd\tau})} (e^{-Kd\tau})$$

$$= \frac{\dfrac{(0.82)(0.7)(300 \text{ mg})}{126 \text{ L}}}{[1 - e^{-(0.1 \text{ hr}^{-1})(6 \text{ hr})}]} (e^{-(0.1 \text{ hr}^{-1})(6 \text{ hr})})$$

$$= \left[\frac{1.37 \text{ mg/L}}{(1 - e^{-0.6})}\right][e^{-0.6}]$$

$$= \left[\frac{1.37 \text{ mg/L}}{1 - 0.55}\right][0.55]$$

$$= \frac{1.37 \text{ mg/L}}{0.45} 0.55$$

$$= 1.67 \text{ mg/L } (\mu g/mL)$$

This plasma trough concentration of 1.67 mg/L is within the therapeutic range of 1 to 4 mg/L. The peak plasma quinidine concentration should also be estimated in R.M. to ensure that it does not exceed the upper limit of the therapeutic range. Equation 43 can be used to calculate the peak plasma concentration (Cpss max).

$$\text{Cpss max} = \frac{\dfrac{(S)(F)(Dose)}{Vd}}{(1 - e^{-Kd\tau})}$$

$$= \frac{\dfrac{(0.82)(0.7)(300 \text{ mg})}{126 \text{ L}}}{(1 - e^{-(0.1 \text{ hr}^{-1})(6 \text{ hr})})}$$

$$= \frac{1.37 \text{ mg/L}}{(1 - e^{-0.6})}$$

$$= \frac{1.37 \text{ mg/L}}{1 - 0.55}$$

$$= 3.04 \text{ mg/L } (\mu g/mL)$$

These calculations demonstrate that the prescribed regimen (i.e., quinidine sulfate 300 mg every six hours) should produce plasma concentrations that are within the usual therapeutic range. Since these calculations were based upon the assumption that quinidine was administered as intermittent IV boluses, oral administration should result in peak levels which are slightly lower and trough levels which are slightly higher than predicted. (See Part I: Figure 20 on page 51.)

Question #3. **The measured trough concentration of quinidine for R.M., 28 hours after the regimen was initiated, was 1.5 mg/L. Although this measured plasma trough concentration of quinidine approximates the calculated value and is within the therapeutic range, R.M. was not responding satisfactorily. The dose of quinidine was increased to 400 mg Q 6 hr and a second trough concentration obtained 15 days later was 3.0 mg/L. If possible errors in the sampling time or in the laboratory assay technique are ignored, what are the possible explanations for this disproportionate rise in the quinidine plasma level?**

The assumed values for the volume of distribution and clearance were based upon literature reports that may not be applicable to R.M. Furthermore, the true half-life of quinidine in R.M. may be longer than the expected seven hours. Since the quinidine plasma concentration was based upon a plasma sample that was obtained approximately 28 hours after starting the first regimen, the measured quinidine plasma concentration of 1.5 mg/L may not have represented a steady-state concentration if R.M.'s quinidine half-life is longer than seven hours. There is also the possibility that R.M.'s clinical status has changed. Perhaps his CHF worsened and decreased his quinidine clearance. R.M. also may have experienced an injury or a surgical procedure that could have increased his α_1-acid glycoprotein concentration; the latter would have increased his plasma protein binding of quinidine.[15]

In addition, quinidine may display some dose-dependent or capacity-limited metabolism. Bolme and Otto noted that when quinidine sulfate doses were increased 50%, from 600 mg/day to 900 mg/day, the steady-state quinidine concentration rose 94%. Furthermore, when the dose was increased another 33%, from 900 mg/day to 1200 mg/day, the steady-state plasma concentration rose 55%.[36]

Question #4. **What quinidine dosage adjustment is required for patients undergoing hemodialysis?**

Since quinidine is highly bound to plasma protein and has a relatively large volume of distribution, significant extraction of the drug from plasma would not be expected during dialysis. Nevertheless, to determine whether quinidine is likely to be dialyzed, one should follow the procedure outlined in Part I: Dialysis of Drugs on page 108. The first step in this determination focuses on the unbound volume of distribution for quinidine. Assuming a weight of 70 kg and an apparent volume of distribution of 2.7 L/kg, the size of the compartment necessary to account for the total amount of drug in the body would be $\approx$189 L (2.7 L/kg $\times$ 70 kg). Using Equation 82, it can be determined that this volume of distribution for quinidine corresponds to an unbound volume of distribution of 1890 L. This calculation assumes that the free fraction (α) for quinidine is 0.1.

$$\begin{aligned} \frac{\text{Unbound Volume}}{\text{of Distribution}} &= \frac{Vd}{\alpha} \\[6pt] &= \frac{189 \text{ L}}{0.1} \\[6pt] &= 1890 \end{aligned}$$

This volume of distribution for unbound quinidine (1890 L) is considerably larger than the upper limit of 250 L for dialyzable drugs. Therefore, significant amounts of quinidine are not removed by hemodialysis and doses do not need to be adjusted for patients with end-stage renal failure undergoing this procedure.[9,11] Removal of the more polar metabolites of quinidine by dialysis may decrease quinidine plasma concentrations measured by nonspecific assays.[11]

Question #5. S.F., a 52-year-old, 60 kg male with a long history of alcohol abuse and cirrhosis, developed premature ventricular contractions (PVCs) and CHF. Quinidine is to be administered to him. What is a reasonable starting dose for S.F.? What is a reasonable desired plasma quinidine concentration?

The pharmacokinetics of quinidine in S.F. are complex because of both CHF and liver disease. Patients with chronic liver disease have an increased free fraction of quinidine because their concentrations of α_1-acid glycoprotein are frequently low (see Part I: Figure 4 on page 11.) In fact, the free fraction of quinidine may be increased in S.F. by as much as two- or threefold. Therefore, if the goal is to achieve the same free or unbound concentration of quinidine, the desired plasma concentration of quinidine should be reduced to one-half or one-third the usual value of 1 to 4 mg/L.[11,19]

At first glance, it would seem reasonable to halve the usual quinidine maintenance dose of 200 mg every six hours. Then, the maximum and minimum quinidine plasma concentrations could be calculated based upon this reduced dosage regimen (100 mg every six hours). Although this approach seems reasonable, the pharmacokinetic parameters used to calculate the quinidine plasma concentrations that will be produced by this proposed new dosage regimen must also be adjusted for S.F.'s congestive heart failure and liver disease. For example, the volume of distribution will be decreased by the CHF, but it will be increased by the low protein concentration in proportion to the change in α.[11] (See Part I: Figure 6 on page 19.) Likewise, clearance would be increased by the decreased protein binding (See Part I: Figures 11 and 12 on page 32 and 33), but reduced by both CHF and chronic liver disease.[11]

The extent to which the clearance and volume of distribution for quinidine should be adjusted in S.F. cannot be quantified with accuracy, but doubling the apparent volume of distribution in patients with CHF (2×1.8 L/kg) and leaving the clearance unchanged at 0.28 L/hr/kg is not unreasonable. The clearance of quinidine in this situation need not be adjusted because the increase in the quinidine free fraction increases the clearance; however, this increased clearance is offset or balanced by S.F.'s liver disease and CHF which should decrease quinidine clearance.

The steady-state peak and trough concentrations which would be produced by a dose of 100 mg of quinidine sulfate every six hours can be calculated from Equations 43 and 47 assuming that: Vd is 3.6 L/kg (2×1.8 L/kg $= 3.6$ L/kg); Cl is 16.8 L/hr (0.28 L/kg/hr $\times 60$ kg $= 16.8$ L/hr); and Kd is 0.078 hr^{-1}. (See Equation 27.)

$$Kd = \frac{Cl}{Vd}$$

$$= \frac{16.8 \text{ L/hr}}{(3.6 \text{ L/kg})(60 \text{ kg})}$$

$$= \frac{16.8 \text{ L/hr}}{216 \text{ L}}$$

$$= 0.078 \text{ hr}^{-1}$$

$$Cpss \text{ max} = \frac{\frac{(S)(F)(Dose)}{Vd}}{(1 - e^{-Kd\tau})}$$

$$= \frac{\frac{(0.82)(0.7)(100 \text{ mg})}{216 \text{ L}}}{1 - e^{-(0.078 \text{ hr}^{-1})(6 \text{ hr})}}$$

$$= 0.71 \text{ mg/L}$$

$$Cpss \text{ min} = \frac{\frac{(S)(F)(Dose)}{Vd}}{(1 - e^{-Kd\tau})} (e^{-Kd\tau})$$

$$= [0.71 \text{ mg/L}][e^{-(0.078 \text{ hr}^{-1})(6 \text{ hr})}]$$

$$= 0.44 \text{ mg/L}$$

Although the calculated peak and trough levels of 0.71 mg/L and 0.44 mg/L are below the usual therapeutic range of 1 to 4 mg/L, the decreased plasma protein binding (i.e., increased alpha) should result in concentrations of free or unbound quinidine that are within the usual therapeutic range. That is, if α is increased two-fold in S.F., equivalent quinidine plasma concentrations in the presence of normal protein levels would be twice as high as those calculated (Cpss max = 1.42 mg/L and Cpss min = 0.88 mg/L). These plasma quinidine concentrations approach the therapeutic range of 1 to 4 mg/L. If subsequent measured concentrations of quinidine in plasma are significantly higher than the calculated values, two explanations must be considered: the intrinsic metabolic capability of the liver may be even worse than that assumed or the α_1-acid glycoprotein concentration may not be decreased by 50% in this patient with chronic liver disease. Since the degree to which quinidine binds to plasma protein is seldom known and since it is difficult to quantitate liver function, the clinical status of S.F. must be carefully evaluated before a change in the quinidine dosing regimen is considered.

Question #6. G.W., who has been receiving 200 mg of quinidine sulfate PO Q 6 hr, has been hospitalized and is now unable to take this medication orally. What intramuscular (IM) dose of quinidine gluconate would be equivalent to 200 mg quinidine sulfate PO Q 6 hr?

To determine a dose of IM quinidine gluconate that is equivalent to an oral dose of quinidine sulfate, the salt form (S) and bioavailability (F) of both dosage forms must be considered. A dose of quinidine sulfate contains only 82% quinidine (S $=$ 0.82) and a dose of quinidine gluconate contains only 62% quinidine (S $=$ 0.62). The bioavailability of quinidine from an oral dose of quinidine sulfate is about 70% (F $=$ 0.7) and the bioavailability of quinidine from an IM dose of quinidine gluconate is probably 100% (F $=$ 1.0). Equation 3 can be used to calculate the amount of quinidine reaching the systemic circulation following the administration of an oral quinidine sulfate dose.

$$\begin{array}{l} \text{Amount of Drug Absorbed} \\ \text{or Amount Reaching} \\ \text{the Systemic Circulation} \end{array} = (S)(F)(Dose)$$

$$= (0.82)(0.7)(200 \text{ mg})$$

$$= 114.8 \text{ mg}$$

Equation 4 can now be used to calculate the equivalent dose of IM quinidine gluconate:

$$\begin{array}{l} \text{Dose of New} \\ \text{Dosage Form} \end{array} = \dfrac{\begin{array}{c} \text{Amount of Drug Absorbed From} \\ \text{Current Dosage Form} \end{array}}{(S)(F) \text{ of New Dosage Form}}$$

$$= \dfrac{114.8 \text{ mg}}{(0.62)(1)}$$

$$= 185 \text{ mg } or \approx 200 \text{ mg}$$

As can be seen, the 200 mg oral dose of quinidine sulfate and the 200 mg intramuscular dose of quinidine gluconate are comparable due to the offsetting effects of their bioavailabilities and salt forms.

Question #7. How can quinidine gluconate be administered safely by the intravenous (IV) route?

Despite early reports of serious cardiovascular toxicities associated with the IV administration of quinidine, quinidine gluconate can be administered intravenously when diluted in 50 to 100 mL of IV fluid and infused over 20 to 30 minutes. Undue cardiovascular side effects associated with two-compartment modeling of quinidine can be avoided when quinidine is administered in this manner.[30] During the IV infusion of quinidine, the patient's blood pressure should be monitored. If the patient becomes hypotensive, the quinidine infusion should be discontinued and IV fluids should be administered.

Question #8. H.H., a 58-year-old, 60 kg male with CHF, has been receiving 300 mg of quinidine sulfate as a sustained-release (SR) dosage form Q 8 hr. Calculate the expected steady-state trough concentration.

The plasma concentration of quinidine fluctuates little within a dosing interval when sustained-release quinidine products are being used. Therefore, the expected steady-state trough concentration from a sustained-release quinidine formulation can be approximated using Equation 35 for Cpss ave:

$$\text{Cpss ave} = \frac{(S)(F)(\text{Dose}/\tau)}{Cl}$$

If the bioavailability (F) for the sustained-release quinidine is assumed to be 70% (F = 0.7); the salt form (S) of quinidine sulfate to be 82% of quinidine base (S = 0.82); the dosing interval (τ) to be eight hours; and the clearance to be 10.8 L/hr (0.18 L/kg/hr × 60 kg for H.H., who has CHF), a steady-state quinidine concentration can be calculated as follows:

$$Cpss\ ave = \frac{(0.82)(0.7)(300\ mg/8\ hr)}{10.8\ L/hr}$$

$$= \frac{21.5\ mg/hr}{10.8\ L/hr}$$

$$= 2.0\ mg/L\ (\mu g/mL)$$

References

1. Thompson GW. Quinidine as a cause of sudden death. Circulation. 1956;14:757.

2. Wetherbee DG et al. Ventricular tachycardia following the administration of quinidine. Am Heart J. 1952;43:89.

3. Guentert TW et al. Divergence in pharmacokinetic parameters of quinidine obtained by specific and non-specific assay methods. Pharmacokinet Biopharm. 1979;7:303.

4. Hartel G, Harjanne A. Comparisons of two methods for quinidine determination and chromatographic analysis of the difference. Clin Chem Acta. 1969;23:124.

5. Conn HL, Luchi RJ. Some cellular and metabolic considerations relating to the action of quinidine as a prototype antiarrhythmic agent. Am J Med. 1969;37:685.

6. Sokolow M, Ball RE. Factors influencing conversion of chronic atrial fibrillation with special reference to serum quinidine concentration. Circulation. 1956;14:568.

7. Di Bonna GF. Measurement of plasma quinidine. N Engl J Med. 1974;290:1325. (Letter).

8. Cramer G, Isakson B. Quantitative determination of quinidine in plasma. Scand J Clin Lab Invest. 1963;15:553.

9. Kessler KM et al. Quinidine elimination in patients with congestive heart failure or poor renal function. N Engl J Med. 1974;290:706.

10. Powers J, Sadee W. Determination of quinidine by high-performance liquid chromatography. Clin Chem. 1978;24:299.

11. Conrad KA et al. Pharmacokinetic studies of quinidine in patients with arrhythmias. Circulation. 1977;55:1.

12. Ueda CT et al. Absolute quinidine bioavailability. Clin Pharmacol Ther. 1976;20:260.

13. Drayer DE et al. Steady-state serum levels of quinidine and active metabolites in cardiac patients with varying degrees of renal function. Clin Pharmacol Ther. 1987;24:31–9.

14. Carliner NH et al. Relation of ventricular premature beat suppression to serum quinidine concentration determined by a new specific assay. Am Heart J. 1980;100:483–9.

15. Fremstad D et al. Increased plasma binding of quinidine after surgery. A preliminary report. Eur J Clin Pharmacol. 1976;10:441.

16. Piafsky KM. Disease-induced changes in the plasma binding of basic drugs. Clin Pharmacokinet. 1980;5:246.

17. Chow MS et al. Pharmacokinetic data and drug monitoring: antibiotics and antiarrhythmics. J Clin Pharmacol. 1975;15:405.

18. Kessler KM. Blood collection techniques; heparin, and quinidine protein binding. Clin Pharmacol Ther. 1979;23:204.

19. Kessler KM et al. Quinidine pharmacokinetics in patients with cirrhosis, or receiving propranolol. Am Heart J. 1978;96:627.

20. Staprans I, Felts JM. The effect of alpha-1 acid glycoprotein on triglyceride metabolism in nephrotic syndrome. Biochem Biophys Res Commun. 1977;79:1272.

21. Guentert TW et al. Gastrointestinal absorption of quinidine from some solutions and commercial tablets. J Pharmacokinet Biopharm. 1980; 8:243.

22. Covinsky JO et al. Relative bioavailablility of quinidine gluconate and quinidine sulfate in healthy volunteers. J Clin Pharmacol. 1979;19:261.

23. McGilveray IJ et al. Bioavailability of 11 quinidine formulations and pharmacokinetic variation in humans. J Pharm Sci. 1981;70:524.

24. Russo J et al. Assessment of quinidine gluconate for nonlinear kinetics following chronic dosing. J Clin Pharmacol. 1982;22:264–70.

25. Soeterbock AM, Vanthiel M. Serum quinidine levels after chronic administration of four different quinidine formulations. J Int Med Res. 1976;4:393–401.

26. Ueda CT et al. Disposition kinetics of quinidine. Clin Pharmacol Ther. 1976;19:30.

27. Ueda CT, Dzindzio BS. Quinidine kinetics in congestive failure. Clin Pharmacol Ther. 1978;23:158.

28. Woo E, Greenblatt DJ. A re-evaluation of intravenous quinidine. Am Heart J. 1978;96:829–32.

29. Hirschfeld DS et al. Clinical and electrophysiological effects of intravenous quinidine in man. Br Heart J. 1977;39:309–16.

30. Swerdlow CD. Safety and efficacy of intravenous quinidine. Am J Med. 1983;75:36.

31. Woo E, Greenblatt DJ. Pharmacokinetics and clinical implications of quinidine protein binding. J Pharm Sci. 1979;68:466.

32. Farringer JA et al. Nifedipine induced alteration in serum quinidine concentrations. Am Heart J. 1984;108:1570.

33. Saal AK et al. Effect of amiodarone on serum quinidine and procainamide levels. Am J Cardiol. 1984;53:1264.

34. Hardy BG et al. Effect of cimetidine on the pharmacokinetics and pharmacodynamics of quinidine. Am J Cardiol. 1983;52:172.

35. Data JL et al. Interactions of quinidine with anticonvulsant drugs. N Engl J Med. 1976;294:699.

36. Bolme P, Otto U. Dose-dependence of the pharmacokinetics of quinidine. Eur J Clin Pharmacol. 1977;12:73.

37. Pike E et al. Binding and displacement of basic drugs, acidic and neutral drugs in normal and orsomucoid deficient plasma. Clin Pharmacokinet. 1981;6:367.

38. Barre J et al. Problems in therapeutic drug monitoring: Free drug level monitoring. 1988;10:133–43.

Salicylates   14

Salicylates possess analgesic, anti-inflammatory, and antipyretic properties. Although salicylates have many uses, this chapter will focus on the analgesic and anti-inflammatory effects of these agents. Salicylates are available in parenteral, rectal, and oral dosage forms, but the oral dosage forms are used primarily in anti-inflammatory therapy. There are a number of ester and salt forms, as well as liquid, tablet, and capsule dosage forms of salicylates. Salicylates exhibit some capacity-limited plasma protein binding; therefore, serum albumin concentration is an important factor to consider when evaluating serum salicylate plasma levels.

Therapeutic and Toxic Plasma Concentrations

The therapeutic concentration of salicylic acid necessary for anti-inflammatory activity ranges from 100 to 300 mg/L (10 to 30 mg/dL). Salicylates can produce a variety of side effects, including tinnitus, which generally occurs at concentrations >200 mg/L. In the case of acute or chronic overdoses, serious acid-base imbalances can develop.[1,2] Other more common side effects include gastrointestinal bleeding, alterations in renal function, and decreased platelet activity. Some of these effects may be dose-related, but no clear relationship has been established between the salicylate plasma concentration and some of these adverse effects.

Bioavailability (F)

Salicylates are rapidly and completely absorbed when administered orally.[3] The salt form, however, should be considered when calculating the maintenance dose because the fraction of salicylic acid in a dose can range from 57% to almost 90%. (See Table 14.1.)

Volume of Distribution (Vd)

Salicylates have an average volume of distribution of ≈0.2 L/kg. This value, however, depends upon the degree of plasma protein binding. At low salicylate plasma concentrations, the volume of distribution is <0.2 L/kg, and at concentrations exceeding 200 mg/L, the volume of distribution is larger.[4,5] This change in the volume of distribution with increasing plasma concentrations is due to saturable plasma protein binding, which becomes significant as serum salicylate concentrations approach and then exceed 100 mg/L.[5,6] For practical therapeutic purposes,

Key Parameters

Therapeutic Range	100–300 mg/L or 10–30 mg/dL
F	100%
S	See Table 14.1
Vd[a]	0.2 L/kg
Cl[b]	0.012 L/kg/hr
t½[c]	10–24 hr
Free Fraction (α)	0.1–0.2 (See text)

[a] The capacity-limited plasma protein binding results in a volume of distribution which increases with dose. On average, the Vd is $\approx$0.2 L/kg at salicylate concentrations of 200 mg/L.

[b] The clearance of salicylates declines as the plasma concentrations increase from <5 to $\approx$100 mg/L, but remains relatively stable between 100 and 300 mg/L.

[c] The half-life of salicylates reflects a complex relationship between the apparent volume of distribution and clearance. In the therapeutic range, most patients have a half-life of approximately 10 to 15 hours.

a volume of distribution of $\approx$0.2 L/kg is probably a satisfactory assumption when serum salicylate concentrations are within the therapeutic range of 100 to 300 mg/L. Furthermore, the necessity for determining a more accurate volume of distribution is not usually important clinically because loading doses of salicylates are unnecessary.

Clearance (Cl)

Within the therapeutic range, salicylates have a plasma clearance of $\approx$0.012 L/kg/hr.[7] The primary route of salicylate elimination occurs through five pathways: a linear renal pathway, two linear metabolic pathways, and two capacity-limited metabolic pathways. Saturable plasma protein binding results in an unbound or free fraction of salicylic acid of $\approx$0.1 at concentrations of 100 mg/L, and $\approx$0.2 at concentrations of 300 mg/L.[7] The clearance for salicylates remains relatively linear over the therapeutic range of 100 to 300 mg/L because the two capacity-limited processes offset one another. Capacity-limited metabolism results in a decreased salicylate clearance, while capacity-limited plasma protein binding increases salicylate clearance at higher concentrations. (See Figure 14.1.)

Although a significant proportion of salicylate is cleared renally, dosage adjustments in renal failure generally are not considered. Large anti-inflammatory doses of salicylates are seldom used in patients with diminished renal function because gastrointestinal bleeding and coagulopathies can be potentiated in such individuals.

Antacids, which produce relatively minor increases in urinary pH, can significantly increase the urinary clearance of salicylates.[7] For this reason, patients on therapeutic anti-inflammatory doses of salicylates should be cautioned against the intermittent use of antacids. Subtherapeutic concentrations may result when antacids are added to therapy, or potentially toxic concentrations may occur if antacids are discontinued in a patient whose salicylate dose had been adjusted to compensate for the increased renal clearance.

Half-Life (t½)

The apparent half-life for salicylates is quite variable. It ranges from three hours or less at low concentrations to approximately 24 hours at salicylate concentrations of 100 to 300 mg/L.[8–10] The clinical application of salicylate half-life is limited, however, because of its capacity-limited metabolism. One would expect that a steady state would be achieved within three to four days when anti-inflammatory doses are used (e.g., when the plasma half-life is approximately 24 hours). Data suggest, however, that following a change in the maintenance dose of salicylate, approximately seven days are required for a new steady state to be achieved.[9] This time requirement, which is longer than the usual three to five half-life rule, is probably due (at least in part) to the capacity-limited metabolism of salicylates.

Table 14.1   Dosage Forms of Salicylates

Compound	Dosage Forms	Equivalents
Acetylsalicylic acid (Aspirin)	Capsules and plain, chewable, and enteric-coated tablets	77% SA[a]
Sodium salicylate	Tablets	86% SA
Choline salicylate	Liquid (870 mg/5 mL)	57% SA

[a] SA = Salicylic Acid.

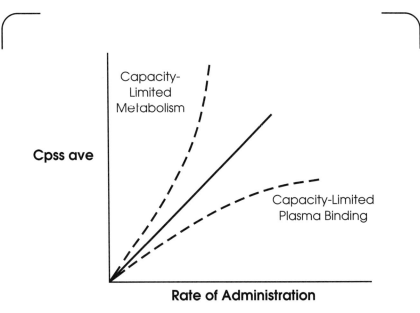

Figure 14.1 Graph Representing the Effects of Capacity-Limited Plasma Protein Binding on the Average Steady-State Plasma Concentration of a Drug. Note that as the rate of drug administration increases, the plasma concentration increases by a less-than-proportional amount, as denoted by the dashed line labeled ''capacity-limited plasma binding.'' An increase in the average steady-state plasma concentration which is less than proportional to the change in dosing rate would result in a decrease in the calculated clearance value. Likewise, the dashed line labeled ''capacity-limited metabolism'' represents the expected disproportionate rise in the average steady-state plasma concentrations with an increase in dose and a corresponding decrease in the calculated clearance. For salicylates, it appears that these two factors are such that the average clearance value within the therapeutic range is approximately linear (solid line). From reference 7.

Time to Sample

Plasma samples of salicylates that are obtained within one week of a change in the dosing regimen should be viewed with some caution. These values can only be used to evaluate the relationship between the salicylate concentration and the patient's clinical response at the time the plasma sample was obtained. Salicylate concentrations measured more than one week following the initiation of a salicylate regimen probably reflect steady state and can be used as a guide to dose adjustment. Although relatively little fluctuation in plasma concentration is expected within the dosing interval ($\tau \leq t\frac{1}{2}$), the rapid absorption of salicylates as well as the capacity-limited plasma protein binding tend to complicate the relationship between dose and measured salicylate concentrations. It is for this reason that trough levels are probably most reproducible and should be obtained whenever possible.

Question #1. **G.L. is a 40-year-old, 65 kg male taking one 325 mg aspirin tablet Q 6 hr for minor joint pain. Calculate the expected steady-state plasma concentration for salicylate in G.L.**

Using the average clearance value of 0.012 L/kg/hr (or 0.78 L/hr for this 65 kg patient), a salt factor (S) of 0.77 and a bioavailability (F) of 1.0 for acetylsalicylic acid (ASA), or aspirin, Equation 35 can be used to predict an average steady-state salicylate concentration.

$$\text{Cpss ave} = \frac{(S)(F)(\text{Dose}/\tau)}{Cl}$$

$$= \frac{(0.77)(1)(325 \text{ mg}/6 \text{ hr})}{0.78 \text{ L/hr}}$$

$$= 53 \text{ mg/L}$$

This predicted salicylate level of 53 mg/L is lower than the usual range of therapeutic concentrations. At concentrations below 100 mg/L, the salicylate clearance is generally much greater than the average literature value (0.012 L/kg/hr). For this reason, the measured serum concentration of salicylate is likely to be considerably less than the predicted value of 53 mg/L. There also is a nonlinear decrease in salicylate clearance as concentrations approach 100 mg/L; pharmacokinetic extrapolations based upon concentrations below the therapeutic range should be avoided.

Question #2. **L.P., a 52-year-old, 50 kg female, is taking three 325 mg aspirin tablets Q 6 hr for her arthritis. What would be the expected steady-state trough salicylate concentration for L.P.?**

Using an average volume of distribution of ≈0.2 L/kg and an average clearance value of 0.012 L/kg/hr, L.P. should have a volume of distribution, clearance, and elimination rate constant of approximately 10 L, 0.6 L/hr, and 0.06 hr^{-1}, respectively, according to the calculations below.

$$\text{Salicylate Vd} = (0.2 \text{ L/kg})(50 \text{ kg})$$
$$= 10 \text{ L}$$

$$\text{Salicylate Cl} = (0.012 \text{ L/kg/hr})(50 \text{ kg})$$
$$= 0.6 \text{ L/hr}$$

$$\text{Kd} = \frac{\text{Cl}}{\text{Vd}}$$
$$= \frac{0.6 \text{ L/hr}}{10 \text{ L}}$$
$$= 0.06 \text{ hr}^{-1}$$

Using these values, an assumed S of 0.77, and an F of 1.0, an anticipated trough concentration of $\approx$175 mg/L can be calculated by use of Equation 47.

$$\text{Cpss min} = \frac{\dfrac{(S)(F)(\text{Dose})}{\text{Vd}}}{(1 - e^{-Kd\tau})}(e^{-Kd\tau})$$

$$= \frac{\dfrac{(0.77)(1)(975 \text{ mg})}{10 \text{ L}}}{(1 - e^{-(0.06 \text{ hr}^{-1})(6 \text{ hr})})}(e^{-(0.06 \text{ hr}^{-1})(6 \text{ hr})})$$

$$= \left[\frac{75 \text{ mg/L}}{0.3}\right][0.7]$$

$$= 175 \text{ mg/L}$$

An alternative method for calculating the trough concentration would be to first estimate the average steady-state level by using Equation 35.

$$\text{Cpss ave} = \frac{(S)(F)(\text{Dose}/\tau)}{Cl}$$

$$= \frac{(0.77)(1)(975 \text{ mg}/6 \text{ hr})}{0.6 \text{ L}/\text{hr}}$$

$$= 208 \text{ mg}/L$$

This average plasma salicylate concentration could then be used to estimate the trough concentration by the following equation:

$$\text{Cpss min} = [\text{Cpss ave}] - \left[(0.5) \frac{(S)(F)(\text{Dose})}{Vd} \right]$$

Eq. 14.1

This equation assumes that the average concentration lies approximately halfway between the peak and the trough and will be reasonably accurate as long as the dosing interval is one half-life or less. For example, in this case the expected trough concentration using Equation 14.1 is ≈ 170 mg/L as compared to the value of 175 mg/L calculated from Equation 47 above.

$$\text{Cpss min} = [208 \text{ mg}/L] - \left[(0.5) \frac{(0.77)(1)(975 \text{ mg})}{10 \text{ L}} \right]$$

$$= 208 \text{ mg} - 37.5 \text{ mg}$$

$$= 170.5 \text{ mg}/L$$

Question #3. **L.P. has experienced some gastrointestinal side effects. What would be the anticipated consequence of adding therapeutic doses of an antacid to her salicylate regimen?**

Antacids markedly decrease serum salicylate levels when taken in therapeutic amounts. Since this decrease can range from 30%

to 70%, L.P.'s serum salicylate concentration should decrease to about one-half of the expected value when antacids are added to her therapy. The decrease in salicylate level is only an approximation, however, and should antacids be utilized, additional salicylate monitoring would be appropriate. In addition, L.P. should be cautioned against altering her antacid regimen since toxicity or a decreased anti-inflammatory response may result. The mechanism for the decrease in salicylate levels is an increase in renal clearance due to the increase in urinary pH associated with antacid therapy.

Question #4. **It was decided that instead of adding an antacid to L.P.'s therapy, she would be changed from acetylsalicylic acid to choline salicylate. Calculate a dose of choline salicylate that would be equivalent to 975 mg ASA every six hours.**

Using Equation 3, one can estimate that the amount of salicylate absorbed from 975 mg aspirin tablets is $\approx$750 mg.

$$\begin{array}{l} \text{Amount of Drug} \\ \text{Absorbed or Amount Reaching} \\ \text{Systemic Circulation} \end{array} = (S)(F)(Dose)$$

$$= (0.77)(1)(975 \text{ mg})$$

$$= 750 \text{ mg}$$

This amount of salicylic acid can then be converted to the equivalent amount of choline salicylate using Equation 4 and the information in Table 14.1.

$$\frac{\text{Dose of New}}{\text{Dosage Form}} = \frac{\begin{array}{c}\text{Amount of Drug Absorbed}\\\text{From Current Dosage Form}\end{array}}{(S)(F) \text{ of New Dosage Form}}$$

$$= \frac{750 \text{ mg}}{(0.57)(1)}$$

$$= 1316 \text{ mg}$$

This new dose of 1316 mg is equivalent to approximately 1.5 teaspoonsful of choline salicylate liquid (870 mg/5 mL). For convenience, the choline salicylate could be administered at a dosing rate of two teaspoonsful or 1740 mg every eight hours. As can be seen from these calculations, the choline salicylate dosage form has been designed so that one teaspoonful is approximately equal to two aspirin tablets. Choline salicylate has an unpleasant flavor and is a relatively expensive form of salicylate.

References

1. Mongan E et al. Tinnitis as an indication of therapeutic serum salicylate levels. JAMA 1973;226:142.

2. Koch-Weser J. Serum concentrations as therapeutic guides. N Engl J Med. 1972;287:227.

3. Rowland M et al. Absorption kinetics of aspirin in man following oral administration of an aqueous solution. J Pharm Sci. 1972;61:379.

4. Graham GG et al. Patterns of plasma concentration and urinary excretion of salicylate in rheumatoid arthritis. Clin Pharmacol Ther. 1977;22:410.

5. Levy G, Yaffe SJ. Relationship between dose and apparent volume of distribution of salicylate in children. Pediatrics. 1974;54:713.

6. Rubin G et al. Concentration dependence of salicylate distribution. J Pharm Pharmacol. 1982;35:115.

7. Furst DE et al. Salicylate clearance, the resultant of protein binding and metabolism. Clin Pharmacol Ther. 1979;26:380.

8. Levy G. Pharmacokinetics of salicylate in man. Drug Metab Rev. 1979;9:3.

9. Levy G, Tsuchiya T. Salicylate accumulation kinetics in man. N Engl J Med. 1972;9:430.

10. Levy G et al. Capacity-limited salicylate formation during prolonged administration of aspirin to healthy human subjects. J Pharm Sci. 1969;58:503.

Theophylline   15

Theophylline is a bronchial smooth muscle relaxant and is widely used to treat bronchial asthma and other respiratory diseases. Theophylline is poorly soluble in water (about 1%) and is usually administered intravenously as the more soluble ethylenediamine salt of theophylline, aminophylline. Dilute solutions of theophylline ($\approx$1 mg/L) also can be administered intravenously. There are numerous oral preparations of theophylline, aminophylline, and other theophylline salts. In addition, aminophylline and other theophylline salts are sometimes administered rectally as suppositories or rectal solutions. The rectal solutions are absorbed slowly and erratically, but tend to have better absorption characteristics than do the suppositories.

Doses vary widely and should be based upon pharmacokinetic considerations and plasma theophylline concentrations. Aminophylline is the most widely used salt of theophylline. An aminophylline loading dose of 250 to 500 mg for an average 70 kg patient (5 to 6 mg/kg) usually is administered by slow intravenous (IV) injection. Typically, the loading dose is followed by intravenous aminophylline infused at a rate of about 30 to 50 mg/hr (0.5 mg/kg/hr). The usual oral maintenance dose of aminophylline tablets is 200 to 300 mg three to four times a day.

Therapeutic and Toxic Plasma Concentrations

The usual therapeutic plasma concentration for theophylline is 10 to 20 mg/L;[1-3] however, improvement in respiratory function can be observed with plasma concentrations as low as 5 mg/L.[1]

Nausea and vomiting are the most common side effects of theophylline. Although these effects can occur at concentrations as low as 13 to 15 mg/L, they are observed more frequently at plasma concentrations exceeding 20 mg/L.[3,4] Cardiac symptoms such as tachycardia are usually minor within the therapeutic range;[5] premature atrial and ventricular contractions are less predictable, but are usually associated with theophylline levels exceeding 40 mg/L.[6] Insomnia and nervousness are side effects that occur over a wide range of concentrations. More severe central nervous system (CNS) manifestations such as seizures usually occur at plasma concentrations exceeding 50 mg/L,[6,7] but have been observed in patients at theophylline concentrations <30 mg/L.[7,8]

Side effects such as nausea and vomiting that usually occur at lower plasma concentrations cannot be used as reliable indicators of excessive

Key Parameters

Therapeutic Plasma Concentration	5–20 mg/L
F	100%
S[a]	See Table 15.1
Vd[b]	0.5 L/kg
Cl[c]	0.04 L/kg/hr
t½	8.3 hr

[a] See Table 15.1
[b] The use of total body versus ideal body weight in obese patients is uncertain. See Theophylline Volume of Distribution (Vd) and Half-Life (t½) sections.
[c] See Tables 15.2 and 15.3 and Theophylline Clearance (Cl) section.

theophylline concentrations. These less severe toxic effects are not always observed, even at high plasma concentrations. In a series of eight patients who suffered from theophylline-induced seizures, only one patient had premonitory signs such as nausea, vomiting, tachycardia, or nervousness which were recognized as signs of toxicity.[7]

The bronchodilating effects of theophylline are proportional to the log of the theophylline concentration. This means that as the theophylline concentration increases, there will be a less than proportional increase in bronchodilation.[6] For this reason, many patients with theophylline concentrations >20 mg/L will experience about the same therapeutic benefit as that associated with concentrations of <20 mg/L; these patients, however, will be at much higher risk for theophylline toxicity. Patients should always be maintained at the lowest possible theophylline plasma concentration that produces a satisfactory therapeutic endpoint. Given the limited bronchodilating effects of theophylline and its potential for toxicity, most clinicians choose an initial target concentration of ≈10 mg/L. Many patients, however, are well controlled on theophylline concentrations in the range of 5 to 10 mg/L and do not require dose adjustments of their theophylline therapy. To optimize the bronchodilating effects of theophylline, it is almost always used in conjunctioin with inhaled beta-antagonists which generally produce more rapid and significant bronchodilating effects than theophylline.

Bioavailability (F)

Nonsustained-Release Dosage Forms. The absorption of theophylline and theophylline derivatives, when administered as either liquid or non-sustained-release oral dosage forms, appears to be rapid and complete. Plasma theophylline concentrations peak about one to two hours after oral administration.[9] Selection of these oral theophylline dosage forms that do not have sustained-release characteristics should be based primarily on cost and convenience if the quality of product can be assured. Theophylline products are available in a large number of salt forms, examples of which are listed in Table 15.1. When changing from one theophylline salt to another, care should be taken to administer an equivalent theophylline dose.

Sustained-Release (SR) Dosage Forms. A large number of sustained-release dosage forms of theophylline have been marketed. These products are designed to release theophylline slowly so that patients who metabolize the drug rapidly (e.g., children and smokers) can maintain theophylline plasma concentrations within the therapeutic range when usual dosing intervals of 6 to 12 hours are used. Most of these drug products are completely absorbed;[9,10] however, there are major differences between these products with regard to duration of absorption. Some of these dosage forms are absorbed over three to four hours, while others appear to be absorbed over a time interval that ranges between 8 and 12 hours.[9,10] For those products that have longer durations of absorption, administration every 8 to 12 hours is usually acceptable. Nevertheless, as the duration of absorption increases, the possibility of incomplete bioavailability increases because the duration of absorption begins to exceed the gastrointestinal transit time.[9]

Dosage forms that can be administered once daily are available; however, the need for these has been questioned.[11,12] The primary concern with the once daily dosing products is the rate and extent of absorption. For example, there is evidence that concurrent administration of Theo-24 with a high-fat meal can accelerate its absorption thereby producing a "dose-dumping" effect.[13] While no "dose dumping" was observed following the ingestion of Uniphyl with a high-fat meal, a change in the rate of absorption was apparent.[14]

In addition to the problems associated with the once daily dosage forms, the variability in absorption among products designed to be administered every 6 to 12 hours may be greater than originally suspected.[15] For these reasons, it is probably wise to avoid the once daily dosage forms until the absorption problems are resolved.

Table 15.1	Selected Theophylline Dosage Forms and Their Salt Factors	
Dosage Form		*S*
Uncoated Tablets and Liquid		
Aminophylline (generic)		0.8 to 0.84
Elixophylline (generic)		1.0
Theophylline (generic)		1.0
Somophyllin		1.0
Slo-Phyllin		1.0
Coated and Sustained Release		
Choledyl		0.64
Aminodur		0.84
Aerolate		1.0
Constant-T		1.0
Respbid		1.0
Slo-bid Gyrocap		1.0
Slo-Phyllin Gyrocap		1.0
Somophyllin-CRT		1.0
Theo-24		1.0
Theobid Duracap		1.0
Theo-Dur		1.0
Theolair-SR		1.0
Theophyl-SR		1.0
Uniphyl		1.0

S = Fraction of labeled dose which is theophylline.

Volume of Distribution (Vd)

The volume of distribution for theophylline is ≈0.5 L/kg,[6,16,17] and distribution follows a two-compartment model. [See Part I: Volume of Distribution (Vd) on page 22.] The bronchioles behave as though they are located in the second or tissue compartment; however, toxic effects are associated with high concentrations in the initial volume of distribution. Therefore, theophylline toxicity may be experienced when theophylline is administered too rapidly or when theophylline accumulates in that first compartment.

The volume of distribution in premature newborns is ≈ 0.7 L/kg.[18] After one year of age, however, the volume of distribution is ≈ 0.5 L/kg.[19,20] The volume of distribution for theophylline is also increased in patients with cystic fibrosis to ≈ 0.6 L/kg.[21,22]

The volume of distribution for theophylline in obese subjects is somewhat controversial. The Food and Drug Administration (FDA) recommends that the ideal or non-obese weight be used to calculate the loading dose or volume of distribution,[23] while others have suggested that use of total body weight may be more appropriate.[24,25] Since the disposition of theophylline in obese subjects is uncertain, a weight that is somewhat less than the actual body weight (but greater than the ideal body weight) should be used when calculating theophylline loading doses. This will result in a smaller volume of distribution and a conservative loading dose. This approach may not be appropriate when calculating theophylline half-lives. [See Theophylline Half-Life (t½) on page 411.]

Clearance (Cl)

The average theophylline clearance is 0.04 L/hr/kg, based on lean or ideal body weight.[16,23,25,26] A number of clinical factors will influence theophylline clearance. (See Table 15.2.)

Table 15.2	Disease States Which Affect Theophylline Clearance	
Disease	*Factor[a]*	*References*
Smoking history	1.6	16, 29
Congestive heart failure	0.4	16, 30, 31
Cystic fibrosis	1.5	21, 22, 51
Acute pulmonary edema	0.5	32
Acute viral illness	0.5	52
Hepatic cirrhosis	0.5	33
Severe obstructive pulmonary disease	0.8	16
Obesity	IBW[b]	24

[a] Indicates the estimate for clearance adjustments. The product of all the factors which are present (also see Table 15.3) should be multiplied by the average clearance value (0.04 L/hr/kg). Multiple factors increase the uncertainty in clearance prediction.

[b] IBW = Ideal body weight should be used.

Obesity. Obese subjects have a theophylline clearance which is most accurately estimated by using non-obese weight.[23,24,25,27] As a general guideline, ideal body weight is estimated using Equations 65 and 66. [See Part I: Creatinine Clearance (Cl_{Cr}) on page 96.]

Smoking. Cigarette smokers have a theophylline clearance about 1.5 to 2 times that of non-smokers.[16,28,29] The effects of smoking (one pack of cigarettes per day) appear to last several months after the cigarettes have been discontinued.[29] Therefore, patients admitted to the hospital with a recent history of smoking should be considered smokers throughout their hospitalization even if they refrain from smoking during hospitalization.

Diseases. Congestive heart failure (CHF), in contrast to cigarette smoking, reduces theophylline clearance to about 40% of normal.[16,26,30,31] Pulmonary edema has also been reported to reduce theophylline clearance,[32] although this effect may be secondary to the associated congestive heart failure. Severe pulmonary disease reduces theophylline clearance to about 85% of the average value.[16] Hepatic cirrhosis also can significantly reduce theophylline clearance.[16,33] Premature newborns have a theophylline clearance that is very low even when adjusted for weight or body surface area.[34]

Diet also influences the metabolism of theophylline. Patients ingesting high-protein, low-carbohydrate diets generally metabolize theophylline more rapidly, presumably because the diet induces hepatic enzymes.[35] Dietary intake of other methylxanthines such as caffeine can decrease the rate of theophylline metabolism to a limited extent.[36] While the effects of diet have been well documented, they usually produce relatively minor changes in theophylline therapy if the patient's diet remains reasonably consistent.

Drug Interactions. Many drug interactions with theophylline have been documented,[26,37] but only the most common of these will be presented. Macrolide antibiotics such as triacetyloleandomycin and erythromycin reduce theophylline clearance by as much as 25% to 50%;[37–39] the interaction with erythromycin has been disputed.[39] Phenobarbital increases theophylline metabolism in some individuals by as much as 30%,[40] but this induction of theophylline metabolism has not been observed by all investigators.[41] Phenytoin (Dilantin) increases theophylline clearance by a factor of ≈ 1.5.[37]

Cimetidine (Tagamet), a drug commonly used in patients receiving theophylline, appears to reduce theophylline metabolism by about 40%. In these patients, the theophylline clearance should be multiplied by 0.6.[37] Similar effects on theophylline clearance were not observed when ranitidine (Zantac) was administered at doses ten times greater than those generally prescribed.[42] Rifampin can increase theophylline metabolism; however, the increase in clearance is only about 20% to 25%.[37] Intravenous isoproterenol (Isuprel) has also been shown to increase the clearance of theophylline by about 20%.[43] Unfortunately, the predictability of clearance changes secondary to the addition of these drugs is poor, indicating that while some change may be expected, each patient will need to be evaluated individually. This concept applies to disease states as well (See Table 15.3).

When multiple factors which influence theophylline clearance are present, the prediction of theophylline drug levels is difficult; therefore, theophylline plasma levels should be monitored.

Half-Life (t½)

The usual theophylline half-life in adult patients is approximately eight hours; however, it is quite variable. For example, the theophylline half-life can be as short as three to four hours in patients who smoke or in those receiving drugs known to induce theophylline metabolism. In contrast, the theophylline half-life can be as long as 18 to 24 hours in patients with severe congestive heart failure or in those receiving drugs which inhibit theophylline metabolism.

The theophylline half-life in obese subjects is frequently longer than eight hours. When attempting to estimate whether steady state has been

Table 15.3	Selected Drugs Which Affect Theophylline Clearance	
Drug		**Factor[a]**
Cimetidine		0.6
Ciprofloxacin		0.7
Erythromycin		0.75
Influenza vaccine		0.5
Phenobarbital		1.3
Phenytoin		1.6
Propranolol		0.6
Rifampin		1.3

[a] Adapted from references 27,53, and 54. Indicates the estimate for clearance adjustments. The product of all of the factors present (see Table 15.2) should be multiplied by the average clearance value (0.04 L/kg/hr). Multiple factors increase the uncertainty value in clearance prediction.

achieved in obese subjects, it may be wise to utilize a total body weight instead of an ideal body weight in calculating the volume of distribution. This will ensure that the longest possible half-life is being used.

Time to Sample

Since the average theophylline half-life is approximately eight hours, routine monitoring of theophylline plasma concentrations can usually begin approximately 24 hours after the initiation of therapy or a change in the maintenance regimen. Plasma samples obtained earlier, especially those obtained within the first 18 hours of therapy, should be interpreted cautiously because steady state may not have been achieved. Patients admitted to acute care centers frequently have been taking sustained-release theophylline products as outpatients. For these individuals, plasma samples obtained within the first 12 to 24 hours after admission may represent an unknown rate of theophylline absorption from doses taken before admission.

In patients receiving nonsustained-release or liquid dosage forms of theophylline, routine monitoring of theophylline plasma concentrations is probably most reliable when trough levels are obtained. Some patients may have relatively short theophylline half-lives; peak theophylline plasma concentrations should be estimated by adding the increase in theophylline concentration expected from a single dose to the trough concentration, as in Equation 15.1:

$$\text{Cpss max} = [\text{Cpss min}] + \left[\frac{(S)(F)(\text{Dose})}{Vd}\right]$$

Eq. 15.1

This equation is only applicable to rapidly-absorbed dosage forms, since the change in concentration following the administration of a sustained-release theophylline product is much less than the value calculated by Equation 15.1. In patients receiving sustained-release theophylline products, the time of sampling is less critical. While trough concentrations are recommended, samples obtained at the midpoint of the dosing interval may also be acceptable.

Question 1. K.M., who is receiving an aminophylline infusion, has a plasma theophylline concentration of 30 mg/L.

If the aminophylline infusion rate is decreased by one-half, so that the new plasma theophylline concentration is 15 mg/L, will the pharmacologic (bronchodilating) effect also be reduced by one-half?

No. The bronchodilating effect of theophylline is proportional to the log of the theophylline concentration.[1] A 50% reduction in the plasma theophylline concentration in K.M. may be well tolerated, since the bronchodilating effect will be decreased by much less than 50%. However, before any alteration in the theophylline plasma concentration is considered, the clinical status of the patient must be assessed. In some cases, a change in dosage may have serious consequences: toxicity may appear if an increase in plasma concentration is attempted or increased bronchospasm may occur if the concentration is reduced.

Question #2. **R.J., an 80 kg, 50-year-old male, is seen in the emergency room with asthma that is unresponsive to epinephrine. Estimate a loading dose of aminophylline that will produce a plasma theophylline concentration of 15 mg/L.**

Assuming R.J. has received no recent aminophylline doses, Equation 11 can be used to determine the loading dose:

$$\text{Loading Dose} = \frac{(Vd)(Cp)}{(S)(F)}$$

The salt form (S) of aminophylline is either 0.80 or 0.84 depending upon whether the hydrous (0.80) or anhydrous (0.84) form was used to compound the drug product. The usual volume of distribution for theophylline is approximately 0.4 to 0.5 L/kg.[3,16,17] If 0.5 L/kg is used,[16] R.J.'s volume of distribution is 40 L.

$$\text{Theophylline Vd} = (0.5 \text{ L/kg})(\text{Weight})$$
$$= (0.5 \text{ L/kg})(80 \text{ kg})$$
$$= 40 \text{ L}$$

The calculated loading dose of aminophylline would be 750 mg.

$$\text{Loading Dose} = \frac{(Vd)(Cp)}{(S)(F)}$$

$$= \frac{(40 \text{ L})(15 \text{ mg/L})}{(0.8)(1.0)}$$

$$= \frac{600 \text{ mg}}{0.8}$$

$$= 750 \text{ mg}$$

This aminophylline dose is somewhat larger than the usual 300 to 500 mg loading dose for two reasons. First, the target level of 15 mg/L is higher than the usual target of 10 mg/L[1] that can be achieved with the standard loading dose of 5 to 6 mg/kg of aminophylline. Second, R.J. is larger than average and, therefore, should require a larger loading dose.

Question #3. What would be a reasonable loading dose for R.J. if he is obese and has an estimated ideal body weight of 60 kg?

The Food and Drug Administration (FDA) recommends that ideal body weight be used to calculate the loading dose.[23] Others have argued that the volume of distribution (which is the major determinant of loading dose) correlates best with total body weight rather than lean or ideal body weight.[24,25] Because there is uncertainty with regard to the relationship between ideal or total body weight and the apparent volume of distribution for theophylline, some care should be taken when calculating loading doses for obese patients. In general, it is sufficient to calculate a theophylline loading dose that will produce a theophylline concentration below the usual target level of 10 mg/L. This should not be a problem as long as a theophylline concentration of at least 5 mg/L is achieved. If a target level >10 mg/L is desired, one should ensure that the upper end of the therapeutic range (20 mg/L) is not exceeded.

For obese patients whose ideal body weight is less than one-half their total body weight, the calculated loading dose of theophylline will be substantially different when the calculation is based upon ideal body weight. In these individuals, it may be more appropriate to use a value somewhere between the ideal and total body weights to calculate the volume of distribution. In any case, theophylline plasma concentrations should be monitored and the loading dose is usually limited to no more than 500 mg. A theophylline level taken approximately one to two hours after the initial loading dose will help establish the approximate volume of distribution for obese subjects.

Question #4. What factors will influence the theophylline loading dose?

A major factor (other than obesity) which is known to influence the loading dose of theophylline is the presence of theophylline in the plasma. The pre-existing theophylline concentration can be accounted for in the calculation of a theophylline loading dose by use of Equation 12:

$$\text{Incremental Loading Dose} = \frac{(Vd)(Cp \text{ desired} - Cp \text{ initial})}{(S)(F)}$$

Since "stat" theophylline levels are not widely available, it is common clinical practice to obtain a plasma sample and administer an empiric loading dose of 3 mg/kg of aminophylline if the patient has taken theophylline within the past 12 to 24 hours, but is not believed to have taken this drug on a regular basis. This reduced loading dose increases the plasma theophylline concentration by about 5 mg/L, which will produce some bronchodilation if the initial plasma theophylline concentration is zero. Hopefully, this increment will not cause toxicity if the patient's initial theophylline concentration is >10 to 20 mg/L.

If the patient is believed to have been compliant with the outpatient theophylline dosing regimen, the loading dose should be omitted and the patient should be started on a maintenance regimen. Care should be taken, however, to obtain an accurate outpatient medication history because many patients receiving sustained-release theophylline products will continue to absorb drug for 8 to 24 hours after admission. This will depend upon the time of the last outpatient dose and the type of product prescribed.

Question #5. **How rapidly should the aminophylline loading dose be administered if it is given intravenously?**

Theophylline displays two-compartment pharmacokinetics in which the therapeutic or bronchodilating effects correlate more closely with concentrations in the second or tissue compartment.[44] Since the toxic effects of theophylline correlate with high concentrations in the initial volume of distribution, the loading dose is usually infused over 30 minutes to minimize accumulation within the first compartment and to avoid toxicity.[1,17,44]

Question #6. **R.J., the patient described in Question 2, received the 750 mg loading dose of aminophylline and a theophylline plasma concentration of 15 mg/L was achieved. What aminophylline infusion rate will maintain an average steady-state level of 15 mg/L?**

Since this problem involves a constant infusion which will be given to maintain a steady-state plasma concentration, Equation 16 can be used:

$$\text{Maintenance Dose} = \frac{(Cl)(Cpss\ ave)(\tau)}{(S)(F)}$$

Using an average theophylline clearance of 0.04 L/kg/hr (3.2 L/hr for R.J. who weighs 80 kg),[16] a salt factor (S) of 0.8, and a bioavailability (F) of 100% (F = 1.0), the maintenance infusion dose would be 60 mg/hr of aminophylline based on the following calculation:

$$
\begin{aligned}
\text{Maintenance Dose} &= \frac{(Cl)(Cpss\ ave)(\tau)}{(S)(F)} \\
&= \frac{(3.2\ \text{L/hr})(15\ \text{mg/L})(1\ \text{hr})}{(0.8)(1.0)} \\
&= \frac{48\ \text{mg}}{0.8} \\
&= 60\ \text{mg aminophylline}
\end{aligned}
$$

Question #7. Calculate a maintenance dose for R.J. if he had been an obese individual with a total body weight of 80 kg and an ideal body weight of 60 kg.

Unlike volume of distribution, which may correlate better with total body weight, the clearance of theophylline appears to correlate better with ideal body weight.[23-25] If R.J.'s ideal body weight is 60 kg, the assumed clearance would be 2.4 L/hr (0.04 L/kg/hr × 60 kg) and the maintenance dose would be 45 mg/hr of aminophylline according to the calculations below.

$$\text{Maintenance Dose} = \frac{(Cl)(Cpss\ ave)(\tau)}{(S)(F)}$$
$$= \frac{(2.4\ L/hr)(15\ mg/L)(1\ hr)}{(0.8)(1.0)}$$
$$= \frac{36\ mg}{0.8}$$
$$= 45\ mg\ aminophylline$$

Question #8. Assume that R.J. (80 kg non-obese weight) has severe obstructive pulmonary disease, CHF, and smokes more than 1 pack/day. Calculate a maintenance dose of aminophylline that will maintain the average steady-state theophylline plasma concentration at 15 mg/L.

If none of the factors known to alter theophylline clearance were present, R.J.'s expected theophylline clearance would be 3.2 L/hr (0.04 L/kg/hr × 80 kg). However, smoking, severe obstructive pulmonary disease, and congestive heart failure alter theophylline clearance by a factor of 1.6, 0.8, and 0.4, respectively (see Table 15.2). The product of these factors is 0.512.

$$(1.6)(0.4)(0.8) = 0.512$$

The average theophylline clearance value should be multiplied by this factor of 0.512 to estimate the theophylline clearance.

$$(3.2\ L/hr)(0.512) = 1.64\ L/hr$$

This clearance could then be used in Equation 16 (see below) to calculate a maintenance dose of ≈30 mg/hr of aminophylline.

$$\text{Maintenance Dose} = \frac{(Cl)(Cpss\ ave)(\tau)}{(S)(F)}$$

$$= \frac{(1.64\ L/hr)(15\ mg/L)(1\ hr)}{(0.80)(1.0)}$$

$$= \frac{24.6\ mg}{0.8}$$

$$= 30.75\ mg \quad or \quad \approx 30\ mg$$

When multiple factors are known to alter theophylline clearance in a patient, the ability to accurately predict theophylline clearance diminishes. In these situations, initial doses may be adjusted based upon literature estimates; however, theophylline plasma concentrations should be monitored to ensure that the patient does not develop excessive or subtherapeutic theophylline plasma concentrations. Even though R.J. will probably discontinue smoking during the acute exacerbation of his respiratory disease, the smoking factor should still be used when estimating theophylline clearance. Most clinicians assume the induction of theophylline metabolism continues for at least three months and perhaps for as long as a year after a patient has stopped smoking.

Question #9. **Approximate R.J.'s theophylline half-life, assuming the clearance is 1.64 L/hr (as calculated in Question 8) and the volume of distribution is 40 L (as calculated in Question 2).**

The half-life is a function of clearance and volume of distribution and can be calculated using Equation 32 as shown below.

$$t^{1/2} = \frac{(0.693)(Vd)}{Cl}$$

$$= \frac{(0.693)(40\ L)}{1.64\ L/hr}$$

$$= \frac{27.7\ L}{1.64\ L/hr}$$

$$= 16.9\ hr$$

This half-life is considerably longer than the average value of six to ten hours because R.J. has multiple factors that are known to alter theophylline clearance.

Question #10. **How long should the aminophylline infusion be continued before a plasma sample is obtained to monitor the plasma theophylline concentration for R.J.?**

The earliest time to sample plasma for a theophylline concentration is 14 to 20 hours after starting the maintenance infusion (approximately two times the usual half-life). Although the expected theophylline half-life for R.J. is 16 hours, obtaining a sample early minimizes the time during which plasma concentrations are low (if the clearance is greater than expected) and prevents excessive accumulation (if the clearance is less than expected). Plasma theophylline concentrations obtained within two half-lives, however, cannot be reliably used to calculate R.J.'s clearance or to predict the steady-state concentration, since both clearance and steady-state concentration are very sensitive to small errors in the assay or in volume of distribution estimates.

If the theophylline concentration at 14 to 20 hours is significantly higher than expected (clearance is less than expected), the infusion rate should be reduced at that time. A second plasma concentration should then be obtained the following day to reevaluate R.J.'s clearance and predicted steady-state concentration.

If the theophylline concentration is much lower than expected, then an incremental loading dose might be calculated to increase the concentration from the observed level to a desired concentration by use of Equation 12.

$$\frac{\text{Incremental}}{\text{Loading Dose}} = \frac{(Vd)(Cp\ \text{desired} - Cp\ \text{initial})}{(S)(F)}$$

Increasing the infusion rate at this time should be undertaken with extreme caution, however, because the low theophylline concentrations may be due in part to a larger than expected volume of distribution rather than a higher than expected clearance.

Question #11. M.K., a 58-year-old, 60 kg female, was admitted to the hospital in status asthmaticus. She received an IV aminophylline loading dose of 375 mg at 9 p.m., followed by a constant aminophylline infusion of 60 mg/hr. The next morning at 7 a.m. (ten hours after the bolus and initiation of the infusion) a plasma sample was obtained and the reported theophylline concentration was 18 mg/L. Calculate the apparent clearance and half-life of theophylline in M.K.

The reported plasma concentration of 18 mg/L probably does not represent a steady-state concentration because the sample was obtained only ten hours after the infusion was begun. The plasma concentration-versus-time curve (which describes a bolus followed by a constant infusion) and the plasma concentration which is produced by this mode of administration are depicted in Part I: Figure 25 on page 64.

As illustrated in that figure, the reported plasma concentration of 18 mg/L is actually the sum of the plasma concentration produced by the loading dose (Equation 50) and that produced by the infusion (Equation 37):

$$Cp_1 = \begin{bmatrix} \text{Loading Dose and} \\ \text{Decay Equation} \end{bmatrix} + \begin{bmatrix} \text{Nonsteady-State} \\ \text{Infusion Equation} \end{bmatrix}$$

$$18 \text{ mg/L} = \left[\frac{(S)(F)(\text{Loading Dose})}{Vd} (e^{-Kdt_1}) \right] + \left[\frac{(S)(F)(\text{Dose}/\tau)}{Cl} (1 - e^{-Kdt_1}) \right]$$

If the following are assumed: S and F are 0.8 and 1.0, respectively; t_1 is ten hours, the loading dose is 375 mg; the maintenance dose is 60 mg/hr; Kd = Cl/Vd (see Equation 27); and Vd is 0.5 L/kg (30 L for this 60 kg patient), the above equation can be reduced to the following:

$$18 \text{ mg/L} = \left[\frac{(0.8)(1.0)(375 \text{ mg})}{Vd} \left(e^{-\left(\frac{Cl}{Vd}\right)(10 \text{ hr})} \right) \right]$$

$$+ \left[\frac{(0.8)(1.0)(60 \text{ mg/hr})}{Cl} \left(1 - e^{-\left(\frac{Cl}{Vd}\right)(10 \text{ hr})} \right) \right]$$

$$= \left[\left(10 \text{ mg/I} \right) \left(e^{-\left(\frac{Cl}{30 \text{ L}}\right)(10 \text{ hr})} \right) \right]$$

$$+ \left[\left(\frac{48 \text{ mg/hr}}{Cl} \right) \left(1 - e^{-\left(\frac{Cl}{30 \text{ L}}\right)(10 \text{ hr})} \right) \right]$$

Unfortunately, clearance cannot be solved for directly, but must be determined through trial and error by finding a value which will result in a theophylline concentration of 18 mg/L. If one has a good clinical history, the factors known to alter clearance should aid in making the initial estimate for clearance. In this case, no history is provided, so a clearance of 0.04 L/kg/hr could be tried in the above equation. Substitution of this clearance value in Equation 35 would result in a final steady-state theophylline concentration of only 20 mg/L as shown below.

$$\begin{aligned} \text{Theophylline Clearance} &= (0.04 \text{ L/kg/hr})(\text{Weight}) \\ &= (0.04 \text{ L/kg/hr})(60 \text{ kg}) \\ &= 2.4 \text{ L/hr} \end{aligned}$$

$$\begin{aligned} \text{Cpss ave} &= \frac{(S)(F)(\text{Dose}/\tau)}{Cl} \\ &= \frac{(0.8)(1.0)(60 \text{ mg/1 hr})}{2.4 \text{ L/hr}} \\ &= 20 \text{ mg/L} \end{aligned}$$

It is unlikely that a theophylline concentration which has increased from 10 mg/L to 18 mg/L in ten hours will plateau at 20 mg/L. Therefore, M.K.'s clearance must be <2.4 L/hr. Furthermore, if a clearance of 2.4 L/hr is inserted into the previous equation, the predicted theophylline concentration at the ten hours would only be 15 mg/L. If a new clearance estimate of 2.0 L/hr is used, the calculated theophylline concentration at ten hours is 17 mg/L.

$$
\begin{aligned}
\text{Cp}_{10 \text{ hr}} &= [(10 \text{ mg/L})(e^{-(2.0/30)(10)})] + \left[\left(\frac{(0.8)(60 \text{ mg/hr})}{2.0 \text{ L/hr}} \right)(1 - e^{-(2.0/30)(10)}) \right] \\
&= [(10 \text{ mg/L})(e^{-(0.066)(10)})] + [(24 \text{ mg/L})(1 - e^{-(0.066)(10)})] \\
&= [(10 \text{ mg/L})(0.51)] + [(24 \text{ mg/L})(1 - 0.51)] \\
&= 5.1 \text{ mg/L} + 11.8 \text{ mg/L} \\
&= 16.9 \text{ mg/L } \textit{ or } \approx 17 \text{ mg/L}
\end{aligned}
$$

Since this predicted plasma theophylline concentration is also less than that which was observed, the clearance must be <2.0 L/hr. Further trials would demonstrate that a clearance value of 1.65 L/hr results in a predicted theophylline level of 18 mg/L.

Because the plasma theophylline sample was taken after only one half-life (approximately), there may be considerable error in the clearance estimate of 1.65 L/hr. However, if it is assumed that this clearance estimate is correct, the calculated theophylline half-life would be 12.6 hours (Equation 32).

$$
\begin{aligned}
t_{1/2} &= \frac{(0.693)(Vd)}{Cl} \\
&= \frac{(0.693)(30 \text{ L})}{1.65 \text{ L/hr}} \\
&= 12.6 \text{ hr}
\end{aligned}
$$

Because the time interval between the initial plasma concentration of 10 mg/L and the observed 18 mg/L was less than one half-life, the accuracy of this revised clearance is questionable. It does suggest, however, that M.K.'s clearance is substantially less than the average literature value of 2.5 L/hr and that some adjustment in dose at this point is appropriate.

Question #12. **Assuming that the desired steady-state plasma theophylline concentration for M.K. is <20 mg/L, determine whether the maintenance dose needs to be adjusted.**

Since clearance is the primary determinant of the steady-state plasma concentration, this adjusted value (1.65 L/hr) can be used to estimate the plasma theophylline concentration which will be produced by an aminophylline infusion of 60 mg/hr (Equation 35).

$$
\begin{aligned}
\text{Cpss ave} &= \frac{(S)(F)(Dose/\tau)}{Cl} \\
&= \frac{(0.8)(1.0)(60 \text{ mg}/1 \text{ hr})}{1.65 \text{ L/hr}} \\
&= \frac{48 \text{ mg/hr}}{1.65 \text{ L/hr}} \\
&= 29 \text{ mg/L}
\end{aligned}
$$

Since the predicted steady-state plasma theophylline concentration of 29 mg/L exceeds 20 mg/L, the infusion rate should be adjusted. The new infusion rate can be calculated from Equation 16 by inserting the desired steady-state plasma concentration and using the clearance estimate of 1.65 L/hr. If a steady-state plasma concentration of 15 mg/L is desired, the new maintenance infusion will be 30.9 mg/hr of aminophylline.

$$
\begin{aligned}
\text{Maintenance Dose} &= \frac{(Cl)(Cpss \text{ ave})(\tau)}{(S)(F)} \\
&= \frac{(1.65 \text{ L/hr})(15 \text{ mg/L})(1 \text{ hr})}{(0.8)(1.0)} \\
&= \frac{24.75 \text{ mg}}{0.8} \\
&= 30.9 \text{ mg } or \approx 30 \text{ mg}
\end{aligned}
$$

Another plasma theophylline concentration should be measured the following morning after the infusion rate has been reduced to ensure that the clearance estimate used (1.65 L/hr) is reasonably close to M.K.'s actual value.

Question #13. O.P., a 72 kg male, became nauseated after receiving IV aminophylline 85 mg/hr for several days. A plasma sample for theophylline was obtained and the infusion was discontinued. Twelve hours later a second plasma sample was obtained. The reported plasma theophylline concentrations were 32 mg/L and 16 mg/L, respectively. Estimate the hourly dose of aminophylline required to maintain the plasma theophylline concentration at 15 mg/L.

In this case, there are two ways to calculate a new maintenance dose. One method entails using Equation 28 to estimate the elimination rate constant based on the established theophylline decay pattern in O.P. The estimated Kd is used with an assumed volume of distribution to calculate clearance. Once clearance is known, the new maintenance dose can be calculated.

$$Kd = \frac{\ln\left(\dfrac{Cp_1}{Cp_2}\right)}{t}$$

Where Cp_1 is 32 mg/L, Cp_2 is 16 mg/L, and t is the 12 hours between the two plasma concentrations. Therefore,

$$Kd = \frac{\ln\left(\dfrac{32}{16}\right)}{12 \text{ hr}}$$
$$= \frac{\ln(2)}{12 \text{ hr}}$$
$$= \frac{0.693}{12 \text{ hr}}$$
$$= 0.058 \text{ hr}^{-1}$$

If the volume of distribution is assumed to be 0.5 L/kg or 36 L (0.5 L/kg × 72 kg), the clearance can be estimated from Equation 33 as shown below.

$$Cl = (Kd)(Vd)$$
$$= (0.058 \text{ hr}^{-1})(36 \text{ L})$$
$$= 2.1 \text{ L/hr}$$

Now, using Equation 16, the maintenance dose can be calculated. Assuming S, F, and τ are 0.8, 1.0, and 1 hr, respectively:

$$\text{Maintenance Dose} = \frac{(Cl)(Cpss \text{ ave})(\tau)}{(S)(F)}$$
$$= \frac{(2.1 \text{ L/hr})(15 \text{ mg/L})(1 \text{ hr})}{(0.8)(1.0)}$$
$$= \frac{31.5 \text{ mg}}{0.8}$$
$$= 39.3 \text{ mg}$$

Thus, an aminophylline infusion of 40 mg/hr should result in a steady-state plasma theophylline concentration of ≈15 mg/L.

A second method to calculate the new maintenance dose assumes that the plasma concentration of 32 mg/L represents a steady-state level. Then, the apparent theophylline clearance can be calculated directly by Equation 15 as follows:

$$Cl = \frac{(S)(F)(\text{Dose}/\tau)}{Cpss \text{ ave}}$$
$$= \frac{(0.8)(1.0)(85 \text{ mg}/1 \text{ hr})}{32 \text{ mg/L}}$$
$$= \frac{68 \text{ mg/hr}}{32 \text{ mg/L}}$$
$$= 2.1 \text{ L/hr}$$

In this particular case, both methods of calculation resulted in identical estimates of theophylline clearance for O.P. The first method should be used if steady state has not been achieved or if the dosing history is unreliable. This method, however, requires a reasonable time interval (one half-life or more) between plasma samples Cp_1 and Cp_2 and a reliable estimate of the volume of distribution. The second method is preferred when the volume of distribution estimate is questionable or when the elimination rate constant cannot be estimated accurately. However, it does require an accurate dosing history and steady-state conditions.

***Question #14.* E.C., a 56-year-old, 50 kg female receiving 25 mg/hr of aminophylline, has a steady-state theophylline level of 12 mg/L. She is to be started on cimetidine. How should her theophylline infusion be adjusted?**

Cimetidine reduces theophylline clearance[9,26,42] by about 40%, although this percentage is highly variable. E.C.'s theophylline clearance, therefore, should be about 60% of her current clearance after cimetidine is initiated. One approach to adjusting the theophylline infusion rate is to calculate E.C.'s theophylline clearance before cimetidine therapy using Equation 15 and to multiply this clearance value by a factor of 0.6.

$$Cl = \frac{(S)(F)(Dose/\tau)}{Cpss\ ave}$$
$$= \frac{(0.8)(1)(25\ mg/hr)}{12\ mg/L}$$
$$= 1.67\ L/hr$$

$$\begin{array}{c} Clearance \\ (After\ Cimetidine) \end{array} = (Clearance\ Before\ Cimetidine)(0.6)$$
$$= [1.67\ L/hr][0.6]$$
$$= 1\ L/hr$$

Cimetidine inhibition of theophylline metabolism should be observed as soon as reasonable cimetidine plasma concentrations are achieved. Therefore, the aminophylline (theophylline) infusion rate should be reduced at the time, or shortly after, cimetidine therapy is initiated. Using the clearance value of 1 L/hr in Equation 16, the new infusion rate would be 15 mg/hr, assuming the target concentration is still 12 mg/L.

$$\text{Maintenance Dose} = \frac{(Cl)(Cpss\ ave)(\tau)}{(S)(F)}$$

$$= \frac{(1\ L/hr)(12\ mg/L)(1\ hr)}{(0.8)(1.0)}$$

$$= 15\ mg$$

Not all patients receiving concomitant cimetidine therapy experience a reduction in theophylline clearance, or a reduction to the degree that was assumed in this example.[45,46] Therefore, one may elect not to change the infusion rate at the time cimetidine is initiated. Instead, one could monitor theophylline plasma concentrations to ensure that they do not rise to excessive levels. This second approach is most appropriate for patients who are poorly controlled on theophylline and in whom a reduced plasma concentration of theophylline may seriously compromise the respiratory status. This latter approach also may be more reasonable when the initial theophylline concentrations are in the low therapeutic range (i.e., ≥ 12 mg/L). When plasma theophylline concentrations are <12 mg/L, a cimetidine-induced reduction in the theophylline clearance by 40% is unlikely to result in a new steady-state theophylline concentration above 20 mg/L.

Question #15. S.R., a 70 kg, 40-year-old male, has been receiving an IV aminophylline infusion at a rate of 35 mg/hr. His steady-state plasma theophylline concentration is 15 mg/L. Calculate an appropriate oral dosing regimen and estimate the peak and trough levels that would be produced by this regimen.

One method used to convert an intravenous dose to an equivalent oral dose is to multiply the hourly intravenous dose by the dosing interval to be used for oral therapy. For example, if theophylline is to be dosed at six-hour intervals for S.R., the equivalent oral dose would be 210 mg every six hours (35 mg/hr ×

6 hr = 210 mg). It is assumed here that the same salt form (aminophylline) will be used and the bioavailability of the oral form is 100% (F = 1.0). (See Key Parameters and Table 15.1). The usual aminophylline dosage form of 200 mg is reasonably close to the calculated dose of 210 mg and would probably be prescribed.

The peak and trough plasma concentrations produced by intermittent dosing will be higher and lower, respectively, than the average concentration achieved during the infusion. There are two methods that can be used to estimate Cpss max and Cpss min.

Method I. A quick way to estimate the peak and trough plasma concentrations when the *same average dose* is given on an intermittent schedule is to first calculate the expected difference between the peak and trough concentrations by dividing the dose by the volume of distribution. Then, by adding one-half of this value to the average plasma concentration, the peak concentration can be estimated. Similarly, by subtracting this value from the average plasma concentration, the trough concentration can be estimated.

The plasma concentration after a dose is administered is the sum of the existing plasma concentration before the dose (trough concentration) and the change in plasma concentration (Δ Cp) produced by that dose. If absorption is assumed to be rapid, the maximum difference between peak and trough plasma concentrations (Δ Cp) can be estimated by use of Equation 15.2.

$$\Delta Cp = \frac{(S)(F)(Dose)}{Vd}$$

Eq. 15.2

Assuming S is 0.8, F is 1.0, and Vd is 0.5 L/kg, each 200 mg dose of aminophylline should produce a 4.6 mg/L increment in the plasma theophylline concentration.

$$\Delta Cp = \frac{(S)(F)(Dose)}{Vd}$$

$$= \frac{(0.8)(1.0)(200 \text{ mg})}{(0.5 \text{ L/kg})(70 \text{ kg})}$$

$$= \frac{160 \text{ mg}}{35 \text{ L}}$$

$$= 4.6 \text{ mg/L}$$

One-half of this change in plasma concentration is 2.3 mg/L. Therefore, the peak and trough concentrations produced by the prescribed regimen should be approximately 17.3 mg/L and 12.7 mg/L, respectively, as shown below using Equations 15.3 and 14.1:

$$Cpss \text{ max} = [Cpss \text{ ave}] + \left[(0.5)\frac{(S)(F)(Dose)}{Vd} \right]$$

Eq. 15.3

$$= 15 \text{ mg/L} + 2.3 \text{ mg/L}$$
$$= 17.3 \text{ mg/L}$$

$$Cpss \text{ min} = [Cpss \text{ ave}] - \left[(0.5)\frac{(S)(F)(Dose)}{Vd} \right]$$
$$= 15 \text{ mg/L} - 2.3 \text{ mg/L}$$
$$= 12.7 \text{ mg/L}$$

This approach (i.e., Method I) assumes that 1) the oral dose will produce the same average plasma concentration as the intravenous infusion; 2) the oral dosage form will be absorbed rapidly and completely; and 3) the dosing interval is equal to or shorter than the theophylline half-life. If the dosing interval is greater than one half-life, the exponential decay results in a Cpss ave which is below the arithmetic average of the peak and trough concentrations.

Method II. A second method to calculate the peak and trough plasma concentrations is to estimate the clearance, volume of distribution, and elimination rate constant in S.R. and then to use Equations 43 and 46 to estimate the maximum and minimum plasma concentrations:

$$\text{Cpss max} = \frac{\dfrac{(S)(F)(Dose)}{Vd}}{(1 - e^{-Kd\tau})}$$

$$\text{Cpss min} = (\text{Cpss max})(e^{-Kd\tau})$$

To use these equations, the elimination rate constant (Kd) must first be estimated. The theophylline Kd for S.R. is a function of his theophylline clearance and volume of distribution. The clearance can be calculated from the observed steady-state plasma theophylline concentration using Equation 15.

$$
\begin{aligned}
Cl &= \frac{(S)(F)(Dose/\tau)}{\text{Cpss ave}} \\
&= \frac{(0.8)(1.0)(35 \text{ mg}/1 \text{ hr})}{15 \text{ mg/L}} \\
&= \frac{28 \text{ mg/hr}}{15 \text{ mg/L}} \\
&= 1.87 \text{ L/hr}
\end{aligned}
$$

If the volume of distribution is assumed to be 35 L (0.5 L/kg $\times$ 70 kg), the elimination rate constant can be calculated from Equation 27.

$$
\begin{aligned}
Kd &= \frac{Cl}{Vd} \\
&= \frac{1.87 \text{ L/hr}}{35 \text{ L}} \\
&= 0.053 \text{ hr}^{-1}
\end{aligned}
$$

Based upon this Kd of 0.053 hr^{-1}, a Vd of 35 L, and a τ of six hours, the calculated maximum plasma theophylline concentration after each 200 mg aminophylline dose is 16.9 mg/L.

$$
\begin{aligned}
\text{Cpss max} &= \frac{\dfrac{(S)(F)(Dose)}{Vd}}{(1 - e^{-Kd\tau})} \\[2em]
&= \frac{\dfrac{(0.8)(1.0)(200 \text{ mg})}{35 \text{ L}}}{(1 - e^{-(0.053 \text{ hr}^{-1})(6 \text{ hr})})} \\[2em]
&= \frac{\dfrac{160 \text{ mg}}{35 \text{ L}}}{1 - e^{-0.32}} \\[2em]
&= \frac{4.57 \text{ mg/L}}{0.27} \\[1em]
&= 16.9 \text{ mg/L}
\end{aligned}
$$

And the minimum plasma concentration before each dose would be 12.3 mg/L.

$$
\begin{aligned}
\text{Cpss min} &= (\text{Cpss max})(e^{-Kd\tau}) \\
&= (16.9 \text{ mg/L})(e^{-(0.053 \text{ hr}^{-1})(6 \text{ hr})}) \\
&= (16.9 \text{ mg/L})(e^{-0.32}) \\
&= 12.3 \text{ mg/L}
\end{aligned}
$$

These estimates are reasonably close to those calculated by Method I, and differ primarily because the average steady-state theophylline concentration from the oral regimen will be slightly lower than the assumed level of 15 mg/L. This is in part because the oral dose is 200 mg rather than the actual dose of 210 mg (35 mg/hr $\times$ 6 hr) given by intravenous infusion. Also, the true "average" concentration is a little closer to the trough than the peak concentration due to the exponential decay.

Question #16. What types of patients are likely to experience wide fluctuations in their plasma theophylline concentrations when taking oral doses Q 6 hr?

Patients with a short theophylline half-life (i.e., less than six hours) will tend to have higher peak plasma concentrations and lower trough concentrations when the dosing interval is six hours or more. Since the volume of distribution of theophylline is reasonably constant, patients who have a large theophylline clearance will have a short theophylline half-life (Equation 32).

$$t\frac{1}{2} = \frac{(0.693)(Vd)}{Cl}$$

In general, pediatric patients tend to have higher theophylline clearances and shorter theophylline half-lives than the average adult.[47–49] Adults who smoke but do not have other disease states (i.e., congestive heart failure) also tend to have theophylline half-lives shorter than six hours.[28,29] Wide fluctuations in the plasma theophylline concentration can be minimized in these cases by shortening the dosing interval or by prescribing a sustained-release preparation.

Question #17. When should plasma samples for theophylline concentrations be obtained for a patient who is on an oral regimen with a constant dosing interval?

Plasma samples should be obtained immediately before a scheduled dose because trough concentrations are more predictable than peak concentrations. Peak plasma concentrations can be delayed by slow absorption, resulting in substantial error. (See Part I: Figure 29 on page 74.)

Since the theophylline half-life is short in many patients, the difference between the trough and peak concentrations can be substantial. Theophylline toxicity frequently occurs when the dose is increased to bring trough concentrations into the usually accepted therapeutic range of 10 to 20 mg/L. Such toxicity may be prevented by estimating the peak plasma concentration. Adding the increment in plasma concentration that will be produced by each dose to the observed trough concentration usually will give a reasonable approximation of the peak plasma concentration. This principle is illustrated in the following question.

Question #18. **M.G., who weighs 31 kg, has been receiving 200 mg of aminophylline Q 6 hr for several days. A plasma theophylline sample drawn immediately before a scheduled dose was 5.0 mg/L. Estimate the peak plasma concentration after each dose and the expected t½ based upon the observed trough concentration of 5 mg/L.**

The reported plasma theophylline concentration of 5.0 mg/L is a trough concentration. The peak plasma concentration will be the sum of this plasma concentration and the expected change in theophylline concentration resulting from each dose. The change in theophylline concentration can be calculated by use of Equation 15.2. (See Question 15.)

$$\Delta Cp = \frac{(S)(F)(Dose)}{Vd}$$

If the average Vd of 0.5 L/kg is assumed, M.G.'s Vd would be 15.5 L (0.5 L/kg × 31 kg). Therefore,

$$\Delta Cp = \frac{(0.8)(1.0)(200 \text{ mg})}{15.5 \text{ L}}$$
$$= 10.3 \text{ mg/L}$$

Thus, each 200 mg dose of aminophylline will increase the trough theophylline concentration by ≈10 mg/L, so the peak plasma concentration will be 15 mg/L (Equation 15.1).

$$Cpss \text{ max} = [Cpss \text{ min}] + \left[\frac{(S)(F)(Dose)}{Vd} \right]$$
$$= 5 \text{ mg/L} + 10.3 \text{ mg/L}$$
$$= 15.3 \text{ mg/L}$$

Actually, the peak concentration will be somewhat lower because oral absorption is not instantaneous.

To calculate the expected half-life, use Equation 28 to estimate the elimination rate constant and then Equation 31 to estimate the half-life. Note that in Equation 28 the peak concentration would be 15.3 mg/L and t would be the entire dosing interval of six hours. This is because the peak concentration is assumed to occur directly over the trough in the bolus dose model, resulting in a decay time equal to the dosing interval. (See Part I: Choosing a Model to Revise or Estimate a Patient's Clearance at Steady State on page 82.)

$$Kd = \frac{\ln\left(\frac{Cp_1}{Cp_2}\right)}{t} \qquad \text{(Eq. 28)}$$

$$= \frac{\ln\left(\frac{15.3 \text{ mg/L}}{5 \text{ mg/L}}\right)}{6 \text{ hr}}$$

$$= \frac{\ln (3.06)}{6 \text{ hr}}$$

$$= \frac{1.12}{6 \text{ hr}}$$

$$= 0.187 \text{ hr}^{-1}$$

$$t\tfrac{1}{2} = \frac{0.693}{Kd} \qquad \text{(Eq. 31)}$$

$$= \frac{0.693}{0.187 \text{ hr}^{-1}}$$

$$= 3.7 \text{ hr}$$

If the maintenance dose for M.G. were to be doubled for a steady-state trough concentration of 10 mg/L, the peak concentration would also be doubled to ≈30 mg/L. Clearly, peak concentrations of 30 mg/L are above the usual accepted therapeutic range. Given the patient's estimated theophylline half-life of ≈3.7 hours, one may have to be satisfied with relatively low trough concentrations which may be appropriate. If higher theophylline concentrations are desired, a sustained-release drug product should be used since intervals shorter than six hours would make it very difficult for a patient to maintain compliance.

Question #19. E.L. is a 48 kg male receiving an aminophylline infusion of 50 mg/hr; his steady-state plasma theophylline concentration is 15 mg/L. Parenteral aminophylline is discontinued and oral aminophylline is prescribed (300 mg at 9 a.m., 1 p.m., 5 p.m., and 9 p.m.). What problems would you anticipate with this dosing regimen?

Since the average daily administration rate is the same (1200 mg/day) for both regimens, the *average* steady-state level will be the same. However, because the interval between doses is irregular (every four hours between 9 a.m. and 9 p.m. followed by an interval of 12 hours between 9 p.m. and 9 a.m.), the plasma theophylline concentration will be increasing above the Cpss ave during the day and declining below the Cpss ave during the night and early morning hours (see Figure 15.1).

The two plasma levels of most interest are the peak concentration just after the 9 p.m. dose and the trough concentration just before the 9 a.m. dose. These plasma levels should represent the highest and lowest levels produced by this dosing regimen.

Since the dosing interval is irregular, the usual steady-state Cpss max and Cpss min equations cannot be used. Instead, the plasma level at any given time must be thought of as the sum of that produced by four separate doses, each of which is given every 24 hours (i.e., each 9 a.m. dose is given every 24 hours, each 1 p.m. dose is given every 24 hours). As illustrated by Equation 48, the plasma level produced by any *one* of the four regimens is the Cpss max for that dose multiplied by the fraction of drug remaining at that point in time.

$$Cp_1 = (Cpss\ max)(Fraction\ Remaining)$$

$$Cpss_1 = \frac{\frac{(S)(F)(Dose)}{Vd}}{(1 - e^{-Kd\tau})} (e^{-Kdt_1})$$

Figure 15.1 Plasma Level Time Curve For a Dosing Regimen of 300 mg Aminophylline at 9 a.m., 1 p.m., 5 p.m., and 9 p.m. Note that plasma concentrations are lowest just before the 9 a.m. dose and highest just after the 9 p.m. dose. Even though the interval between doses is irregular, each dose is given every 24 hours, at 9 a.m., 1 p.m., 5 p.m., and 9 p.m., respectively. (See Equation 15.4.)

The actual plasma level at any given time will be the sum of the levels produced by each of the four regimens. Since each regimen is given every 24 hours, τ is 24 hours.

$$Cp = \left[\frac{\frac{(S)(F)(Dose)}{Vd}}{[1 - e^{-(Kd)(24\ hr)}]} (e^{-Kdt_1}) \right] + \left[\frac{\frac{(S)(F)(Dose)}{Vd}}{[1 - e^{-(Kd)(24\ hr)}]} (e^{-Kdt_2}) \right] + \ldots$$

Or, more simply stated:

$$Cp = \frac{\frac{(S)(F)(Dose)}{Vd}}{[1 - e^{-(Kd)(24\ hr)}]} (e^{-Kdt_1} + e^{-Kdt_2} + e^{-Kdt_3} + e^{-Kdt_4})$$

$$\text{Eq. } 15.4$$

where t_1, t_2, t_3, and t_4 represent the time intervals between the time of administration for each dose and the time at which one wishes to predict the plasma theophylline level.

To solve the above equation for Cp, first calculate Kd which can be derived from the clearance and volume of distribution. Since a steady-state level (15 mg/L) and dose (50 mg/hr) are known, clearance can be calculated through the use of Equation 15.

$$Cl = \frac{(S)(F)(Dose/\tau)}{Cpss \ ave}$$
$$= \frac{(0.8)(1.0)(50 \ mg/1 \ hr)}{15 \ mg/L}$$
$$= 2.67 \ L/hr$$

If the volume of distribution is assumed to be 24 L (0.5 L/kg × 48 kg), the elimination rate constant can be calculated using Equation 27.

$$Kd = \frac{Cl}{Vd}$$
$$= \frac{2.67 \ L/hr}{24 \ L}$$
$$= 0.11 \ hr^{-1}$$

The plasma level after the 9 p.m. dose can now be determined by considering t_1 through t_4 as the number of hours since the last 9 a.m., 1 p.m., 5 p.m., and 9 p.m. doses were administered. Therefore, t_1 through t_4 would be 12, 8, 4, and 0 hours, respectively. This assumes that the 9 p.m. dose was administered and rapidly absorbed.

$$\text{Cp at 9 p.m.} = \frac{\frac{(0.8)(1.0)(300 \text{ mg})}{24 \text{ L}}}{[1 - e^{-(0.11)(24 \text{ hr})}]} [e^{-(0.11)(12 \text{ hr})}$$

$$+ e^{-(0.11)(8 \text{ hr})} + e^{-(0.11)(4 \text{ hr})} + e^{-(0.11)(0 \text{ hr})}]$$

$$= \frac{10 \text{ mg/L}}{[1 - e^{-2.64}]} (e^{-1.32} + e^{-0.88} + e^{-0.44} + e^{-0})$$

$$= \left[\frac{10 \text{ mg/L}}{1 - 0.071}\right][0.27 + 0.41 + 0.64 + 1]$$

$$= \left[\frac{10 \text{ mg/L}}{0.929}\right][2.32]$$

$$= 25 \text{ mg/L}$$

The plasma concentration just before the 9 a.m. dose could be calculated using the same equation and the appropriate time intervals. In this case, the time intervals since the last 9 a.m., 1 p.m., 5 p.m., and 9 p.m. dose would be 24 hours, 20 hours, 16 hours, and 12 hours, respectively.

Another method which could be used to determine the level just before the morning dose would be to multiply the peak concentration of 25 mg/L by the fraction remaining after 12 hours (Equation 26).

$$Cp = (Cp^{\circ})(e^{-Kdt})$$
$$= (25 \text{ mg/L})(e^{-(0.11 \text{ hr}^{-1})(12 \text{ hr})})$$
$$= (25 \text{ mg/L})(0.27)$$
$$= 6.7 \text{ mg/L (Immediately Prior to 9 a.m. Dose)}$$

In summary, while it is possible that E.L. could be well controlled clinically on this irregular dosing schedule, a regular dosing interval of six hours would result in lower peaks and higher trough concentrations (20.8 mg/L and 10.8 mg/L, respectively). Thus, toxicity would be minimized and the therapeutic response maximized (Equations 43 and 46).

$$Cpss\ max = \cfrac{\cfrac{(S)(F)(Dose)}{Vd}}{(1 - e^{-Kd\tau})}$$

$$= \cfrac{\cfrac{(0.8)(1.0)(300\ mg)}{24\ L}}{1 - e^{-(0.11\ hr^{-1})(6\ hr)}}$$

$$= \cfrac{10\ mg/L}{1 - e^{-0.66}}$$

$$= \cfrac{10\ mg/L}{1 - 0.52}$$

$$= \cfrac{10\ mg/L}{0.48}$$

$$= 20.8\ mg/L$$

$$
\begin{aligned}
Cpss\ min &= (Cpss\ max)(e^{-Kd\tau}) \\
&= (20.8\ mg/L)(e^{-(0.11\ hr^{-1})(6\ hr)}) \\
&= (20.8\ mg/L)(e^{-0.66}) \\
&= (20.8\ mg/L)(0.52) \\
&= 10.8\ mg/L
\end{aligned}
$$

An alternative to the six-hour dosing interval is the use of a sustained-release product which can be administered less frequently. Such a product would minimize the fluctuation in the theophylline plasma concentrations between dosing intervals and would thus decrease the possibility of toxic peak levels and subtherapeutic trough levels in a patient who requires a high Cpss ave for clinical control.

Question #20. **If E.L. were placed on a sustained-release dosage form, such as Theo-Dur 600 mg Q 12 hr, how would one calculate the expected theophylline concentrations?**

Assuming Theo-Dur has slow-release characteristics, the plasma concentrations of theophylline should not change very much even if the dosing interval is 12 hours. The administration of this oral form could thus be treated as an infusion described by Equation 35.

$$\text{Cpss ave} = \frac{(S)(F)(\text{Dose}/\tau)}{Cl}$$

In this case, S is 1.0 (since Theo-Dur is theophylline) and F appears to be ≈ 1.0.[50]

$$\begin{aligned}
\text{Cpss ave} &= \frac{(1.0)(1.0)(600 \text{ mg}/12 \text{ hr})}{2.67 \text{ L/hr}} \\
&= \frac{50 \text{ mg/hr}}{2.67 \text{ L/hr}} \\
&= 18.7 \text{ mg/L}
\end{aligned}$$

Calculation of peak and trough levels using Equations 43 and 46 would be inappropriate since the levels should fluctuate relatively little within the dosing interval.

As an alternative, an intermittent infusion model could be used to calculate the "peak" theophylline concentration which should occur at the end of the absorption time. The subsequent trough concentration will occur t_2 hours after the end of the absorption process and just before the next dose (Equation 57). (Also see Part I: Selecting the Appropriate Equation: Sustained-Release Dosage forms on page 69.)

$$\text{Cpss}_2 = \frac{\dfrac{(S)(F)(\text{Dose}/t_{in})}{Cl}(1 - e^{-Kdt_{in}})}{(1 - e^{-Kd\tau})}(e^{-Kdt_2})$$

For Theo-Dur, the t_{in} or duration of absorption is estimated to be between 8 and 12 hours. If a t_{in} of 12 hours is selected, it can be seen that E.L.'s theophylline concentration would be essentially a continuous infusion, as calculated previously. If the shorter duration of eight hours is selected, then the peak concentration would be expected to occur approximately eight hours after the administration of the dose, and the trough concentration would occur approximately four hours after that, or just before the next dose. Using an eight-hour duration of absorption, the expected peak concentration would be 22 mg/L.

$$\text{Cpss } t_2 = \left[\frac{\dfrac{(1)(1)(600 \text{ mg}/8 \text{ hr})}{2.67 \text{ L/hr}} (1 - e^{-(0.11 \text{ hr}^{-1})(8 \text{ hr})})}{(1 - e^{-(0.11 \text{ hr}^{-1})(12 \text{ hr})})} \right] [(e^{-(0.11 \text{ hr}^{-1})(0 \text{ hr})})]$$

$$= \frac{(28 \text{ mg/L})(0.58)}{(0.73)} (1)$$

$$= 22 \text{ mg/L}$$

The corresponding trough concentration four hours later would be 14 mg/L (Equation 26).

$$Cp = (Cp^{\circ})(e^{-Kdt})$$
$$= [22 \text{ mg/L}][e^{-(0.11 \text{ hr}^{-1})(4 \text{ hr})}]$$
$$= 14 \text{ mg/L}$$

Because of the potentially elevated peak concentrations and the uncertainty regarding the actual rate of the absorption from sustained-release drug products, a reduction in dose might be warranted. In addition, because the half-life for E.L. is relatively short, a dosing interval of eight hours might be more appropriate. The shorter dosing interval would diminish the possibility of excessive peak and lower trough concentrations to some extent. If the intermittent infusion model is used and if shorter dosing intervals are selected, the duration of absorption (t_{in}) in Equation 57 should always be equal to or less than the dosing interval (τ). If the expected duration of absorption is longer than the dosing interval, one normally would use a continuous infusion model (Equation 35 for Cpss ave) because the overlapping infusions would tend to minimize the fluctuation in plasma concentrations.

$$\text{Cpss ave} = \frac{(S)(F)(Dose/\tau)}{Cl}$$

When patients are converted from intravenous to oral theophylline therapy, it should be considered a change in the dosing regimen even if they are receiving approximately the same amount of theophylline per day. This is because theophylline concentrations obtained soon after changing the route of administration may be very sensitive to the specific model selected for predicting the drug concentration (i.e., bolus versus infusion; short versus long t_{in}) rather than the patient's pharmacokinetic parameters (i.e., clearance and volume of distribution). For this reason, theophylline levels should normally be obtained no sooner than one day (approximately three to four half-lives) after the route of administration has been changed.

References

1. Mitenko PA, Ogilvie RI. Rational intravenous doses of theophylline. N Engl J Med. 1973;289:600.

2. Bierman CW et al. Acute and chronic therapy in exercise induced bronchospasm. Pediatrics. 1977;60:845.

3. Jenne JW. Pharmacokinetics of theophylline: application to adjustment of the clinical dose of aminophylline. Clin Pharmacol Ther. 1972;13:349.

4. Jacobs MH et al. Clinical experience with theophylline: relationships between dosage, serum concentration and toxicity. JAMA. 1976; 235:1983.

5. Ogilvie R et al. Cardiovascular response to increasing theophylline concentrations. Eur Clin Pharmacol. 1977;12:409.

6. Piafsky KM, Ogilvie RI. Dosage of theophylline in bronchial asthma. N Engl J Med. 1975;292:1218.

7. Zillich CW et al. Theophylline-induced seizures in adults. Ann Intern Med. 1975;82:784.

8. Yarnell PR, Chu NS. Focal seizures and aminophylline. Neurology. 1975;25:819.

9. Hendeles L et al. A clinical and pharmacokinetic basis for the selection and use of slow-release theophylline products. Clin Pharmacokinet. 1984;9:95.

10. Upton RA et al. Evaluation of the absorption from some commercial sustained-release theophylline products. J Pharmacokinet Biopharm. 1980;8:131.

11. Barr WH. The once-daily theophylline controversy. Pharmacotherapy. 1984;4:167. Editorial.

12. Weinberger MM. Theophylline: QID, TID, BID, and now QD? Pharmacotherapy. 1984;4:181.

13. Hendeles L et al. Food-induced dose-dumping from a "once-a-day" theophylline product as a cause of theophylline toxicity. Chest. 1984; 87:758.

14. Karim A et al. Food-induced changes in theophylline absorption from controlled-release formulations. Part I: substantial increased and decreased absorption with Uniphyl tablets and Theo-Dur sprinkle. Clin Pharmacol Ther. 1985;38:77.

15. Dietrich R et al. Intra-subject variation and sustained-release theophylline absorption. J Allergy Clin Immunol. 1981;67:465.

16. Powell JR et al. Theophylline disposition in acutely ill hospitalized patients. Am Rev Respir Dis. 1978;118:229.

17. Mitenko PA, Ogilvie RI. Pharmacokinetics of intravenous theophylline. Clin Pharmacol Ther. 1972;14:509.

18. Aranda J et al. Pharmacokinetic aspects of theophylline in premature infants. N Engl J Med. 1976;295:413.

19. Loughnan PM et al. Pharmacokinetic analysis of the disposition of intravenous theophylline in young children. J Pediatr. 1976;88:874.

20. Rosen JP et al. Theophylline pharmacokinetics in the young infant. Pediatrics. 1979;64:248.

21. Isles A et al. Theophylline disposition in cystic fibrosis. Am Rev Respir Dis. 1983;127:417.

22. Larsen GI et al. Intravenous aminophylline in patients with cystic fibrosis. Am J Dis Child. 1980;134:1143.

23. FDA Drug Bulletin. IV guidelines for theophylline products. 1980 (Feb.); Vol. 10.

24. Gal P et al. Theophylline disposition in obesity. Clin Pharmacol Ther. 1978;24:438.

25. Koup JR, Vawter TK. Theophylline pharmacokinetics in an extremely obese patient. Clin Pharm. 1983;2:181.

26. Hendeles L, Weinberger M. Theophylline: a "state of the art" review. Pharmacotherapy. 1983;3:2.

27. Edwards DJ et al. Theophylline. In: Evans WE et al, eds. Applied Pharmacokinetics: Principles of Therapeutic Drug Monitoring. 3rd ed. Vancouver: Applied Therapeutics Inc;1992:13:1–38.

28. Powell JR et al. The influence of cigarette smoking and sex on theophylline disposition. Am Rev Respir Dis. 1977;116:17.

29. Hunt SN et al. Effects of smoking on theophylline disposition. Clin Pharmacol Ther. 1976;19:546.

30. Jenne JW et al. Apparent theophylline half-life fluctuations during treatment of acute left ventricular failure. Am J Hosp Pharm. 1977; 34:408.

31. Jusko WJ et al. Intravenous theophylline therapy: nomogram guideline. Ann Intern Med. 1977;86:400.

32. Piafsky KM et al. Theophylline kinetics in acute pulmonary edema. Clin Pharmacol Ther. 1977;21:310.

33. Piafsky KM et al. Theophylline disposition in patients with hepatic cirrhosis. N Engl J Med. 1977;296:1495.

34. Aranda JV et al. Pharmacokinetic aspects of theophylline in premature newborns. N Engl J Med. 1976;295:413.

35. Kappas A et al. Influence of dietary protein and carbohydrate on antipyrine and theophylline metabolism in man. Clin Pharmacol Ther. 1976;20:643.

36. Monks T et al. The effect of increased caffeine intake on the metabolism and pharmacokinetics of theophylline in man. Biopharm Drug Dispos. 1981;2:31.

37. Jonkman JHG, Upton RA. Pharmacokinetic drug interactions with theophylline. Clin Pharmacokinet. 1984;9:309.

38. Weinberger M et al. Inhibition of theophylline clearance by triacetyloleandomycin. J Allergy Clin Immunol. 1977;59:228.

39. Pfeifer HJ et al. Effects of three antibiotics on theophylline kinetics. Clin Pharmacol Ther. 1979;26:36.

40. Landay RA. Effect of phenobarbital on theophylline disposition. J Allergy Clin Immunol. 1978;62:27.

41. Piafsky KM et al. Effect of phenobarbital on the disposition of intravenous theophylline. Clin Pharmacol Ther. 1977;22:336.

42. Kelly HW et al. Ranitidine at very large doses does not inhibit theophylline elimination. Clin Pharmacol Ther. 1986;39:577.

43. Hemstreet MP et al. Effect of intravenous isoproterenol on theophylline kinetics. J Allergy Clin Immunol. 1982;69:360.

44. Mitenko PA, Ogilvie RI. Rapidly achieved plasma concentrations plateaus, with observation on theophylline kinetics. Clin Pharmacol Ther. 1972;13:329.

45. Ambrose PJ, Harralson AF. Lack of effect of cimetidine on theophylline clearance. Drug Intell Clin Pharm. 1981;15:389.

46. Bauman JH, Kimmelblatt BJ. Cimetidine as an inhibitor of drug metabolism: therapeutic implications and drug review of the literature. Drug Intell Clin Pharm. 1982;16:380.

47. Levy G et al. Pharmacokinetic analysis of the effect of theophylline on pulmonary function in asthmatic children. J Pediatr. 1978;86:789.

48. Maselli R et al. Pharmacologic effect of intravenously administered aminophylline in asthmatic children. J Pediatr. 1970;76:777.

49. Wyatt R et al. Oral theophylline dosage for the management of chronic asthma. J Pediatr. 1978;92:125.

50. Weinberger M et al. The relation of product formulation to absorption of oral theophylline. N Engl J Med. 1978;299:852.

51. Knoppert DC et al. Cystic fibrosis: enhanced theophylline metabolism may be linked to the disease. Clin Pharmacol Ther. 1988;44:254–64.

52. Chang K et al. Altered theophylline pharmacokinetics during acute respiratory viral illness. Lancet. 1978;1:1132.

53. Upton RA. Pharmacokinetic interactions between theophylline and other medications (Part I). Clin Pharmacokinet. 1991;20:66–80.

54. Upton RA. Pharmacokinetic interactions between theophylline and other medications (Part II). Clin Pharmacokinet. 1991;20:135–50.

Tricyclic Antidepressants: 16
Amitriptyline, Desipramine, Imipramine, Nortriptyline

Tricyclic antidepressants (TCAs) have been used clinically for approximately 40 years; however, it is only recently that assay procedures for clinical monitoring have become widely available. While the number of agents used as antidepressants is increasing, this chapter will focus on amyitriptyline, desipramine, imipramine, and nortriptyline because assay procedures for these agents are widely available and therapeutic ranges have been established. For many other antidepressants, the reported "therapeutic ranges" primarily represent the usual plasma concentrations produced by standard doses. Most clinicians adjust tricyclic antidepressant doses by monitoring the drug's efficacy and side effects; plasma levels are monitored only in specific situations (See Tricyclic Antidepressants: Time to Sample on page 451). When tricyclic antidepressants are used for clinical indications other than depression [e.g., enuresis, attention deficit disorder (ADD), and other mood disorders], dose adjustments are based primarily on clinical observations. Because very little data are available on target plasma concentrations for these alternate therapeutic uses, most clinicians tend to use the therapeutic range established for depression.

A number of factors make plasma level monitoring of tricyclic antidepressants difficult. One major problem lies in the inability to establish a clearly defined therapeutic end-point. Also, active metabolites and altered plasma protein-binding can complicate the ability to relate measured plasma concentrations to a therapeutic response. The wide variability in the dose to plasma concentration ratio stimulated investigators to establish a therapeutic range.[1] To a great extent, the variability in plasma concentrations can be attributed to a high first-pass hepatic clearance of the tricyclic antidepressants which results in a relative low and variable bioavailability. While some of these agents are available in parenteral dosage forms, they are not commonly administered by this route. In addition, the maximum therapeutic effect is usually not apparent for several weeks following the initiation of tricyclic antidepressants even though steady-state plasma concentrations usually are achieved within one week.[2,3,4]

Therapeutic and Toxic Plasma Concentrations

The therapeutic range for the tricyclic antidepressants is not as well established as it is for many of the other drugs described in this text.

Table 16.1	Tricyclic Antidepressants
Drug	*Dosage Forms Available[a]*
Amitriptyline	10, 25, 50, 75, 100, and 150 mg tablets 10 mg/mL 10 mL injectable (multidose vial)
Desipramine	10, 25, 50, 75, 100, and 150 mg tablets 25, 50 mg capsules
Imipramine	10, 25, and 50 mg tablets 75, 100, 125, and 150 mg capsules (Tofranil-PM) 12.5 mg/mL 2 mL injectable ampule
Nortriptyline	10, 25, 50, 75 mg capsules 10 mg/5mL oral solution

[a] The usual maximum recommended adult daily dose orally is approximately 300 mg.

Plasma protein binding to various blood elements accounts for some of the difficulty in interpreting the plasma concentrations of these basic compounds. Tricyclic antidepressants bind to α_1-acid glycoprotein (AAG) with a relatively high affinity but somewhat low capacity. They also bind to serum albumin.[5] Lipoprotein concentrations may be important[6] since the degree of binding for amitriptyline and nortriptyline has been associated with cholesterol and triglyceride concentrations. Elevated concentrations of AAGs in response to certain inflammatory processes alter the plasma binding and potential therapeutic range for the TCAs.[7] It is also difficult to determine whether or not the alterations in plasma protein-binding for the tricyclic antidepressants are due to patient variations or to the collection techniques and the assay methodologies used to determine the unbound drug concentrations. While the plasma protein-binding of the various tricyclic antidepressants is not identical, they all have a free fraction of less than 10%; for most, about 5% of the drug in plasma is unbound or free.[5,7,26] While higher free fractions have been reported,[8,9] it is unclear whether these studies represent actual variations in plasma protein-binding or artifacts in the assay methodology.

The therapeutic range for *nortriptyline* of 50 to 150 µg/L (ng/mL) is more clearly established than that for other tricyclic agents.[2,3,10] Desipramine has an accepted therapeutic range of approximately 100 to 250 µg/L.[10,11] One study indicated that plasma concentrations above 115 µg/L strongly correlated with positive therapeutic outcomes, while others have suggested that plasma concentrations as low as 75 µg/L were potentially therapeutic.[12,13]

Imipramine is metabolized to desipramine. To date, no one has been able to distinguish a therapeutic difference between these two com-

Key Parameters

Therapeutic Range

    Amitriptyline   120–250 µg/L[a]

    Desipramine   100–250 µg/L

    Imipramine   180–350 µg/L[b]

    Nortriptyline   50–150 µg/L

Free fraction (α)[c]

    Amitriptyline, Desipramine,   <0.1
    Imipramine, Nortriptyline

F

    Amitriptyline, Desipramine,   0.4
    Imipramine

    Nortriptyline   0.5

Vd[d]

    Amitriptyline   15 L/kg

    Desipramine, Imipramine,   20 L/kg
    Nortriptyline

Cl[d]

    Amitriptyline   0.7 L/kg/hr

    Desipramine   0.6 L/kg/hr

    Imipramine   0.9 L/kg/hr

    Nortriptyline   0.4 L/kg/hr

$t_{1/2}$[d]

    Amitriptyline, Desipramine,   20 hr
    Imipramine

    Nortriptyline   30 hr

[a] Therapeutic range includes sum of amitriptyline + nortriptyline.
[b] Therapeutic range is the sum of imipramine + desipramine.
[c] Free fraction is variable with significant plasma protein binding to serum proteins other than albumin.
[d] These values represent average estimates from the literature and, therefore, use of any two to extract a third parameter may not result in the reported average value.

pounds; therefore, plasma concentration ranges usually are described as the sum of the imipramine and desipramine concentrations. Most studies suggest that the combined concentration range should be at least 150 µg/L and perhaps as high as 240 µg/L.[10,14] While the therapeutic range of imipramine is somewhat variable depending upon the source, many clinicians use a relatively wide range of 180 to 350 µg/L.[10,15]

Amitriptyline is metabolized to an active metabolite, nortriptyline; therefore, its therapeutic range represents the sum of these two compounds. While the therapeutic range is not clearly established, most clinicians accept a range of 120 to 250 µg/L.[10,16] It is generally felt that concentrations above this range, and especially concentrations >450 µg/L, are not likely to result in a therapeutic response for patients who have failed to respond at lower concentrations. They can, however, develop significant anticholinergic side effects including dry mouth, blurred vision, confusion, and delirium.[17]

While most clinicians simply monitor the patient's clinical response to tricyclic antidepressants, plasma concentration monitoring is useful occasionally. (See Tricyclic Antidepressants: Time to Sample on page 451.)

Bioavailability (F)

Although gastrointestinal absorption of orally administered tricyclic antidepressants is almost complete, the significant first-pass metabolism that occurs as the drugs pass through the liver reduces their bioavailability to less than 50% in most patients. As with most drugs exhibiting significant first-pass metabolism, the bioavailability range is broad and difficult to estimate in any individual patient. Amitriptyline is generally considered to have a bioavailability of approximately 30% to 60%,[18,26,35] desipramine 30% to 50%,[19,26,35] imipramine 20% to 70%,[20,36] and nortriptyline is 45% to 70%.[21,35] The rate of absorption is also variable with peak concentrations occurring two to eight hours following a single dose.[20] In general, the various dosage forms of the tricyclic antidepressants are considered to be bioequivalent and there is little information suggesting that their absorption is altered by drug interactions or food. There may be some differences, however, between oral and parenteral dosage forms. The high liver extraction and metabolic conversion of orally-administered tricyclic compound does not occur following parenteral administration. Thus, the parent compound to metabolite ratio may differ when the same drug is given orally and parenterally. This factor could be important if the metabolites and parent compound have different therapeutic effects.[22]

Volume of Distribution (Vd)

Tricyclic antidepressants are widely distributed throughout the body, and considering their extensive binding to plasma proteins, their tissue binding is impressive. While estimates for the volume of distribution of the tricyclic antidepressants vary, most values are in the range of 15 to 20 L/kg.[18,19,21,35] Volume of distribution is a pharmacokinetic parameter that is not used clinically, since loading doses of tricyclic antidepressants are not administered. The large volume of distribution and high plasma protein-binding do indicate that hemodialysis is not likely to remove a significant amount of drug from the body.

Clearance (Cl)

Tricyclic antidepressants are cleared almost exclusively by the liver; less than 5% of these compounds are eliminated by the kidney.[20,23] As previously mentioned, metabolites of some tricyclic antidepressants are active and need to be considered when monitoring the plasma concentrations. Clearances estimated for the tricyclic antidepressants reported in the literature vary by up to three to five times. Average values are usually in the range of 10 mL/kg/min (0.6 L/kg/hr). Some of this variance is due to intra- and interindividual variation in hepatic metabolism and drug interactions. For example, cimetidine decreases the hepatic metabolism of imipramine; this not only reduces its clearance but also increases its bioavailability by decreasing the first-pass effect.[24]

Many compounds and liver disease appear to increase the plasma concentrations of the tricyclic antidepressants. Those which decrease hepatic metabolism, such as chloramphenicol, disulfiram, and alcoholic liver disease, are easy to predict. Others, such as haloperidol, fluoxetine, and oral contraceptives, may not come to mind readily as inhibitors of hepatic metabolism, but have reportedly increased the plasma concentrations of tricyclic antidepressants.[25,35] Most of the drugs that have been reported to increase the metabolism of the tricyclic antidepressants are easy to predict and include carbamazepine, phenytoin, barbiturates, smoking, and chloral hydrate.[35] It is difficult to estimate the clinical significance of any of these drug interactions since some patients appear to exhibit substantial changes in metabolism while others exhibit relatively little change in TCA concentrations when these agents are added to or deleted from a therapeutic regimen. Because the intrinsic metabolism of TCAs varies widely among patients, and because the magnitude of drug interactions is difficult to predict, all patients should be carefully monitored any time concurrent drug therapy is changed. While plasma concentration monitoring may help to sort out some of these problems, careful observation of the patient's clinical symptoms is also warranted.

Half-Life (t½)

As mentioned previously, the tricyclic antidepressants have an exceptionally large volume of distribution and a high clearance which results in an average half-life of ≈20 hours.[26,35] As with the volume of distribution and clearance, half-life also has an extremely wide reported range: 9 to >50 hours. It is difficult to know whether or not this wide range reflects true alterations in pharmacokinetic parameters or the limitations that exist when attempting to estimate a drug's half-life within a dosing interval that is approximately equal to the drug's half-life. In any case, it is unclear whether the half-life of the drug would be used clinically to establish a dosing interval for the TCAs. The significant lag between the onset of clinical response relative to the time plasma concentrations plateau suggests that the therapeutic response is associated with a more slowly equilibrating deep tissue compartment or some other biochemical change associated with TCA therapy. Therefore, daily changes in drug levels may not be important with regard to therapeutic control of the depression but could be an issue with regard to side effects of the TCAs.

Time to Sample

Several factors should be considered in selecting the appropriate time to sample tricyclic antidepressants. First, unless there are overt signs of clinical toxicity, plasma samples obtained before steady state has been achieved are not recommended because they can be misleading. For this reason, most clinicians wait at least one week before obtaining a plasma concentration. Using steady-state concentrations, adjustments in the dosing regimens can be made in proportion to the desired change in plasma concentration. The appropriate time to obtain the sample within a dosing interval, however, is a bit more complex. Peak concentrations obtained a few hours after the dose is administered are unpredictable because the rate of absorption is so variable; trough concentrations are often inconvenient because these agents are normally dosed at bedtime. Therefore, most clinicians attempt to standardize the sampling time at about 12 hours after an oral dose, which is usually in the morning if the TCA is administered at bedtime. Mid-interval plasma concentrations should approximate the average steady-state concentration; thus, any revision of pharmacokinetic parameters will focus on estimates of clearance and bioavailability (Equation 35).

$$Cpss\ ave\ =\ \frac{(S)(F)(Dose/\tau)}{Cl}$$

A large number of techniques have been employed to help clinicians select an initial dosing regimen that will achieve a target concentration.[27] One method utilizes the principle of mean residence time (See Part I: Figure 32 on page 89) and recommends measuring a plasma concentration at a specified point in time (usually 24 to 36 hours after an initial dose).[28–30] As previously discussed, these techniques are most effective when the sampling time occurs at ≈1.5 half-lives.

The first question that one should consider is whether or not plasma concentrations ought to be monitored in the patient under treatment. Although wide variations in both bioavailability and clearance might make tricyclic antidepressants ideal candidates for therapeutic drug monitoring, most clinicians do not routinely monitor tricyclic antidepressant concentrations. Instead, they rely on clinical observations and limit drug level monitoring to specific circumstances. Some have suggested TCA monitoring early in therapy to allow adjustment of the dosing regimen one or two weeks after initiating therapy. This method should result in a more rapid dose adjustment since clinicians must wait three or more weeks to adjust the dose based upon the antidepressant clinical response. While this technique is not routinely employed, early drug level monitoring for agents that have a delayed therapeutic benefit makes sense. Drug concentrations also are used to differentiate noncompliant patients from those who are unresponsive. However, differentiation between noncompliant patients and those who exhibit unusual metabolism or low bioavailability is difficult; this assessment is made most easily when the tricyclic antidepressant concentrations are exceedingly low (<30 μg/L). These low levels are unlikely to be due to unusual pharmacokinetic disposition, assuming a dose that would be expected to achieve therapeutic concentrations has been prescribed. Occasionally, tricyclic antidepressant levels are used to document suspected drug toxicity; concentrations >500 μg/L are often associated with side effects, and concentrations >1000 μg/L are usually considered inappropriate and warrant withholding the tricyclic antidepressant.[17] Many clinicians believe that plasma concentrations should only be measured to support clinically observed side effects such as changes in visual accommodation, dry mouth, and mental changes which include confusion and, potentially, seizures. Cardiovascular side effects also should be considered. Orthostatic hypotension and electrocardiogram (ECG) changes such as widening QRS intervals or obvious arrhythmias require adjustment in the tricyclic antidepressant dose. Because these agents can exacerbate cardiovascular diseases, some clinicians start patients with pre-existing heart disease on minimal doses and slowly adjust their doses upward with careful clinical and drug level monitoring. Other patients who are likely to be susceptible to cardiovascular side effects include the elderly and patients whose concurrent drug therapy is known to influence the pharmacokinetics of tricyclic antidepressants.

Question #1. A.R., a 39-year-old, 65 kg female, is to be given desipramine for depression. She has no other significant medical history and takes acetaminophen or ibuprofen rarely for headaches. Describe a reasonable starting dose and schedule for increasing her maintenance regimen.

Because the bioavailability and intrinsic hepatic clearance of TCAs varies over a wide range, most clinicians start therapy with conservative doses in a divided daily schedule. Doses are increased only after the initial dose has achieved steady state and side effects can be evaluated. Because A.R. has no other concurrent illnesses or medications that would be expected to alter her TCA metabolism, a starting desipramine dose of 25 mg twice daily is reasonable. Given the expected half-life of ≈20 hours, steady state should be achieved in approximately four days, although most clinicians would probably wait five to seven days before considering an increase in her maintenance schedule. Although the plasma concentrations of desipramine can be expected to plateau relatively quickly, full therapeutic effects will not be evident for several weeks. If at the end of the first week of therapy A.R. is experiencing no significant side effects, the dose would probably be increased to a total daily dose of 75 to 100 mg even though the full therapeutic benefit from the initial dose is unlikely to be evident. Maintenance doses are increased before the full therapeutic effect is achieved because an excessively long titration period would accrue if the interval between dose escalation were a month or more. If A.R. begins to experience significant side effects from her desipramine [e.g., central nervous system (CNS) depression or anticholinergic side effects], future dose increases would probably be withheld. With time, these side effects may diminish somewhat, once again permitting an increase in the daily dose if required.

Question #2. After three weeks of titration, A.R. has been stabilized on 150 mg/day of desipramine for one week. She has relatively few side effects but her depression has im-

proved minimally. Would plasma levels of desipramine be useful? What would one expect the average steady-state desipramine concentration to be?

One would not expect to see full therapeutic effects of the tricyclic antidepressants within three weeks of initiating therapy. Some clinicians believe that early plasma concentration monitoring may help to identify those patients with low plasma concentrations and therefore at higher risk for therapeutic failure. Depending upon the severity of A.R.'s depression, one approach would be to continue her current regimen for another few weeks. If a satisfactory response is not obtained, the dose could be increased to ≈200 mg/day in an attempt to achieve adequate control of her depression. It would not be irrational, however, to obtain a plasma concentration from A.R. now to determine if it is anywhere near the therapeutic range (100 to 250 µg/L.) If her plasma concentration is low and compliance could be assured, it would be logical to escalate her dose at this time. This saves waiting the additional three weeks to evaluate the full therapeutic response and diminishes the total time required to achieve optimal dose titration.

The expected average steady-state desipramine concentrations can be calculated using Equation 35:

$$\text{Cpss ave} = \frac{(S)(F)(\text{Dose}/\tau)}{Cl}$$

Substituting 1.0 and 0.4 for S and F, respectively; 39 L/hr for Cl (0.6 L/kg/hr × 65 kg); and 150,000 µg/24 hr for dose/τ, a value of 64 µg/L (ng/mL) is estimated.

$$\text{Cpss ave} = \frac{(S)(F)(\text{Dose}/\tau)}{Cl}$$

$$= \frac{(1)(0.4)(150{,}000\ \mu g/24\ hr)}{39\ L/hr}$$

$$= 64.1\ \mu g/L$$

Question #3. S.U., a 68-year-old, 65 kg male, is in good health following a mild myocardial infarction (MI) two years ago. He has been treated intermittently for the past 20 years for endogenous depression and is now to be started on nortriptyline. His most frequent complaints have been a general lack of interest in his usual activities. What would be a reasonable starting dose? Would plasma concentration monitoring be useful?

S.U.'s age and history of cardiac disease place him at higher risk for tricyclic toxicity than other patients.[33,34] Therefore, he should be started on the lowest available dose (10 to 25 mg/day). Even though these low doses are unlikely to result in a therapeutic response, concern for both the cardiovascular and other side effects in the elderly is sufficient to warrant caution. Most clinicians would carefully evaluate S.U. weekly and, if no side effects are observed (e.g., changes in visual acuity, dry mouth, orthostatic hypotension, cardiac arrhythmias), increase the dose by approximately 10 to 25 mg until he is stabilized on a dose of 50 to 75 mg/day. If S.U. has not responded adequately after a sufficient time interval and there are no obvious side effects, it will be necessary to decide whether or not a further increase in dose is appropriate. Many clinicians feel that the elderly and patients with pre-existing cardiac disease are candidates for therapeutic drug level monitoring. Thus, it might be appropriate to obtain a plasma nortriptyline level at this point. If the plasma concentrations are low and an adequate therapeutic response has been attained, the dose should not be increased. If, however, low concentrations are associated with a poor therapeutic response, a further escalation of the dose is probably warranted. If nortriptyline concentrations are within the usual therapeutic range (50 to 150 µg/L) and there is an inadequate therapeutic response, a decision to increase the dose would be difficult. As an alternative a drug with a lower toxicity profile could be considered.

Question #4. O.N., a 38-year-old, 60 kg female, is being titrated on increasing doses of desipramine and, for the past month, has been receiving 150 mg HS. In the past she has complained of dry mouth; lately she does not feel this is a problem and has no other symptoms which might be considered side effects of desipramine. She takes no other concurrent medication except for acetaminophen occasionally and smokes one pack of cigarettes per day. Estimate her desipramine concentration.

In order to calculate O.N.'s steady-state desipramine concentration, it will first be necessary to select a pharmacokinetic model. The average steady-state desipramine concentration can be calculated by using Equation 35.

$$\text{Cpss ave} = \frac{(S)(F)(\text{Dose}/\tau)}{Cl}$$

When the appropriate values are inserted, S = 1.0, F = 0.4, dose/τ = 150,000 µg/24 hr, and Cl = 0.6 L/kg/hr × 60 kg, an average expected steady-state concentration of ≈70 µg/L (ng/mL) is calculated.

$$\text{Cpss ave} = \frac{(1)(0.4)(150{,}000\ \mu g/24\ hr)}{(0.6\ L/kg/hr)(60\ kg)}$$
$$= \frac{2.500\ \mu g/hr}{36\ L/hr}$$
$$= 69.44\ \mu g/L$$

Since the expected half-life of desipramine is ≈20 hours and the dosing interval is 24 hours, the continuous infusion model is not appropriate. The intermittent steady-state bolus dose model is appropriate when a nonsustained-release product is used and absorption occurs over a short time period relative to the drug half-life. Equation 48:

$$\text{Cpss}_1 = \frac{\dfrac{(S)(F)(\text{Dose})}{Vd}}{(1 - e^{-Kd\tau})}(e^{-Kdt_1})$$

By inserting the appropriate parameters as listed above, as well as the usual Vd of 1200 L (20 L/kg × 60 kg), Kd of 0.0347 hr^{-1} (Kd = 0.693/20 hr), and t_1 of 24 hr, the predicted steady-state trough concentration would be ≈40 µg/L.

$$\text{Cpss}_1 = \frac{\dfrac{(1)(0.4)(150{,}000\ \mu g)}{1{,}200\ L}}{(1\ -\ e^{-(0.0347\ hr^{-1})(24\ hr)})}\ (e^{-(0.0347\ hr^{-1})(24\ hr)})$$

$$= \frac{50\ \mu g/L}{(1\ -\ 0.435)}\ (0.435)$$

$$= 38.4\ \mu g/L$$

Note that while there are differences between the calculated average steady-state and trough concentrations, they are somewhat similar. If the measured concentrations differ from the predicted levels, it will be difficult to explain. For example, if a measured trough concentration is reported to be 60 $\mu g/L$, one could revise the bioavailability, clearance, or volume of distribution since all of these parameters can vary significantly. However, while Vd is a variable, it would require an *exceedingly large* Vd to increase the trough concentration to 60 $\mu g/L$ when the average concentration is expected to be 69.4 $\mu g/L$. Therefore, the most common approach would be to adjust the clearance value since this parameter is thought to be more variable than either bioavailability or volume of distribution for most of the TCAs. However, hepatic clearance and the first-pass effect are the predominant reasons for the low bioavailability; thus, if a patient has a lower-than-average clearance, one should anticipate an increase in her bioavailability.

Question #5. O.N. did not respond well to her therapy, and a trough desipramine level was obtained. The laboratory reported a value of 68 ng/mL ($\mu g/L$). Because she is not responding, the physician plans to increase O.N.'s desipramine concentration to 100 to 150 ng/mL. What dose adjustment is likely to achieve this goal?

One approach is to calculate a new set of pharmacokinetic parameters as described in Part I: Interpretation of Plasma Drug Concentrations: Choosing a Model for Revision of Clearance at Steady State on page 82. As described, the peak concentration would first be estimated by adding the observed trough concentration to the expected change associated with the dose (Equation 15.1).

$$\text{Cpss max} = \left[\text{Cpss min} \right] + \left[\frac{(S)(F)(\text{Dose})}{\text{Vd}} \right]$$

Again, by substituting the appropriate values, a maximum concentration of approximately 118 µg/L can be calculated.

$$\text{Cpss max} = 68 \text{ µg/L} + \frac{(1)(0.4)(150{,}000 \text{ µg})}{1{,}200 \text{ L}}$$

$$= 68 \text{ µg/L} + 50 \text{ µg/L}$$

$$= 118 \text{ µg/L}$$

Using the equation below, a derivitive of Equation 28 (see page 41), the revised elimination rate constant (Kd) can be calculated and is 0.023 hr^{-1}; this corresponds to a half-life of about 30 hours.

$$\text{Kd} = \frac{\ln\left(\dfrac{\text{Cp max}}{\text{Cp min}}\right)}{\Delta t}$$

$$= \frac{\ln\left(\dfrac{118 \text{ µg/L}}{68 \text{ µg/L}}\right)}{24 \text{ hr}}$$

$$= 0.023 \text{ hr}^{-1}$$

$$t^{1/2} = \frac{0.693}{\text{Kd}} \qquad \text{(Eq. 31)}$$

$$= \frac{0.693}{0.023 \text{ hr}^{-1}}$$

$$= 30 \text{ hr}$$

This data can then be used along with Equation 1.9, a rearrangement of Equation 48, and the assumed values of S, F, and Vd to calculate a dose. Assuming the Cpss$_1$ is a trough value, t$_1$ would be 24 hours and the calculated dose would be ≈300 mg.

$$Cpss_1 = \frac{\dfrac{(S)(F)(Dose)}{Vd}}{(1 - e^{-Kd\tau})}(e^{-Kdt_1})$$

$$
\begin{aligned}
Dose &= \frac{(Cpss_1)(Vd)(1 - e^{-Kd\tau})}{(S)(F)(e^{-Kdt_1})} \\[2mm]
&= \frac{(150\ \mu g/L)(1{,}200\ L)(1 - e^{-(0.023\ hr^{-1})(24\ hr)})}{(1)(0.4)(e^{-(0.023\ hr^{-1})(24\ hr)})} \\[2mm]
&= \frac{(180{,}000\ \mu g)(1 - 0.576)}{(1)(0.4)(0.576)} \\[2mm]
&= 331{,}250\ \mu g \quad or \quad \approx 300\ mg
\end{aligned}
$$

It is unlikely that the maintenance dose would be increased by this amount because it is a large percentage increase in dose (though consistent with the desired increase in plasma concentration) and because the new dose is approaching or exceeding the maximum recommended dose. While it may be necessary to increase O.N.'s dose to the range of 300 mg/day to achieve a plasma concentration of 150 µg/L, most clinicians would probably increase O.N.'s maintenance dose by approximately 25 to 50 mg/day and observe her for clinical improvement and side effects as described previously. This step-wise approach is more rational because some patients respond at lower plasma concentrations and the chances of side effects are substantial with larger doses.

Question #6. **N.H., a 27-year-old male, has been stabilized on imipramine 100 mg/day (50 mg BID) with good response to his depression. Two weeks ago his physician prescribed 100 mg capsules (Tofranil PM) at bedtime to simplify the regimen. Unfortunately, N.H. continued to take two doses a day (200 mg) at bedtime and now presents with confusion, dry mouth, and blurred vision. Would a drug plasma level be useful to establish a course of action for N.H. and an apparent imipramine toxicity?**

Many clinicians believe that cases of suspected tricyclic toxicity are indications for obtaining plasma concentrations. Plasma levels help the clinician distinguish tricyclic-induced dementia from other potential causes.[31,32] However, the relationship between tricyclic antidepressant concentrations and side effects is variable and cannot be relied upon as an absolute indicator. Many clinicians believe that any plasma concentration >500 µg/L is reason to withhold or reduce the maintenance dose and that concentrations >1000 µg/L warrant withholding the drug and monitoring the patient for cardiovascular side effects.[35] In N.H.'s case, the diagnosis is not in question; therefore, the use of a plasma concentration for this purpose is not warranted. If an imipramine plasma concentration could be rapidly obtained, it might provide the clinician with enough information to determine if N.H.'s side effects could be treated in an outpatient setting. This would also depend upon the severity of the side effects. Some clinicians obtain a plasma concentration for medical legal reasons, even if it will not alter the immediate care of the patient.

References

1. Hammer W, Sjoqvist F. Plasma levels of monomethylated tricyclic antidepressants during treatment with imipramine-like compounds. Life Sci. 1967;6:1895–903.

2. Kragh-Sorensen P et al. Self-inhibiting action of nortriptyline's antidepressant effect at high plasma levels. Psychopharmacology. 1976; 45:305–14.

3. Perry PJ et al. Two prospective dosing methods for nortriptyline. Clin Pharmacokinet. 1984;9:555–63.

4. Gram LF et al. Drug level monitoring in psychopharmacology: usefulness and clinical problems, with special reference to tricyclic antidepressants. Ther Drug Monit. 1982;4:17–25.

5. Piafsky KM, Borga O. Plasma binding of basic drugs II: Importance of α_1-acid glycoprotein for interindividual variation. Clin Pharmacol Ther. 1977;22:545–9.

6. Pike E, Skuterud B. Plasma binding variations of amitriptyline and nortriptyline. Clin Pharmacol Ther. 1982;32:228–34.

7. Freilich DI, Giardina E-GV. Imipramine binding to α_1-acid glycoprotein in normal subjects and cardiac patients. Clin Pharmacol Ther. 1984;35:670–4.

8. Potter WZ et al. Binding of imipramine to plasma protein and to brain tissue: relationship to CSF tricyclic levels in man. Psychopharmacology. 1979;63:187–92.

9. Weder HJ, Bickel MH. Interactions of drugs with proteins. I. Binding of tricyclic thymoleptics to human and bovine plasma proteins. J Pharm Sci. 1970;59:1505–7.

10. Pollock BG, Perel JM. Tricyclic antidepressants: contemporary issues for therapeutic practice. Can J Psychiatry. 1989;34:609–71.

11. Jarvis MR. Clinical pharmacokinetics of tricyclic antidepressant overdose. Psychopharmacol Bull. 1991;27:541–50.

12. Nelson JC et al. Desipramine plasma concentration and antidepressant response. Arch Gen Psychiatry. 1982;39:1419–22.

13. Friedel RO et al. Desipramine plasma levels and clinical response in depressed outpatients. Commun Psychopharmacol. 1979;2:81–7.

14. Costa D et al. Edogenous depression and imipramine levels in the blood. Psychopharmacology. 1980;70:291–4.

15. Glassman AH et al. Tricyclic antidepressant blood level measurements and clinical outcome. Am J Psychiatry. 1985;142:155–63.

16. Breyer-Pfaff U et al. Validation of a therapeutic plasma level range in amitriptyline treatment of depression. J Clin Psycholpharmacol. 1989; 9:116–21.

17. Preskorn SH, Irwin HA. Toxicity of tricyclic antidepressants—kinetics, mechanism, intervention: a review. J Clin Psychiatry. 1982;43:151–6.

18. Jorgensen A, Hanson V. Pharmacokinetics of amitriptyline infused intravenously in man. Eur J Clin Pharmacol. 1976;10:337–41.

19. DeVane CL et al. Desipramine and 2-hydroxy-desipramine pharmacokinetics in normal volunteers. Eur J. Clin Pharmacol. 1981;19:61–4.

20. Sutfin TA et al. The analysis and disposition of imipramine and its active metabolites in man. Psychopharmacology. 1984;82:310–17.

21. Alexanderson B. Pharmacokinetics of desmethylimipramine and nortriptyline in man after single and multiple oral doses—a cross-over study. Eur J Clin Pharmacol. 1972;5:1–10.

22. Randup A, Braestrup C. Uptake inhibition of biogenic amines by newer antidepressant drugs: relevance to the dopamine hypothesis of depression. Psychopharmacology. 1977;53:309–14.

23. Potter WZ, Calil HM. Metabolites in tricyclic antidepressants. Biological activity and clinical implications. In: Usdin E et al, eds. *Clinical Pharmacology in Psychiatry.* New York: Elsevier; 1981:311–24.

24. Abernethy DR et al. Imipramine-cimetidine interaction: impairment of clearance and enhanced absolute bioavailability. J Pharmacol Exp Ther. 1984;229:702–5.

25. Ciraulo DA, Shader RI. Fluoxetine drug-drug interactions. J Clin Psychopharmacol. 1990;10:48–50, 213–7.

26. Benet LZ, Williams RL. Appendix II: Design and optimization of dosage regimen: Pharmacokinetic data. In: Gilman AG et al, eds. *Goodman and Gilman's The Pharmacologic Basis of Therapeutics.* 8th edition. New York: Pergamon Press; 1990:1650–1735.

27. Nelson JC, Jatlow PI. Nonlinear desipramine kinetics: prevalence and importance. Clin Pharmacol Ther. 1987;41:666–70.

28. Dawling S et al. Nortriptyline therapy in elderly patients: dosage prediction after single dose pharmacokinetic study. Eur J Pharmacol. 1980;18:147–50.

29. Potter WZ et al. Single-dose kinetics predict steady-state concentrations of imipramine and desipramine. Arch Gen Psychiatry. 1980; 37:314–20.

30. Cooper TB et al. Prediction of steady-state plasma and saliva levels of desmethylimipramine using a single dose, single time point procedure. Psychopharmacology. 1981;74:115–21.

31. Crome P, Braithwaite RA. Relationship between clinical features of tricyclic antidepressant poisoning and plasma concentrations in children. Arch Dis Child. 1978;53:902–5.

32. Pederson OL et al. Overdosage of antidepressants: clinical and pharmacokinetic aspects. Eur J Clin Pharmacol. 1982;23:513–21.

33. Nelson JC et al. Major adverse reactions during desipramine treatment. Arch Gen Psychiatry. 1982;39:1055–61.

34. Glassman AH, Bigger JT. Cardiovascular effects of therapeutic doses of tricyclic antidepressants. Arch Gen Psychiatry. 1981;38:815–20.

35. DeVane CL, Jarecke CR. Cyclic Antidepressants. In: Evans WE et al., eds. Applied Pharmacokinetics: Principles of Therapeutic Drug Monitoring, 3rd ed. Vancouver: Applied Therapeutics; 1992:1.

Valproic Acid   17

Valproic acid is currently used to treat various seizure disorders. The mechanism of action for valproic acid is uncertain; it purportedly increases the brain concentrations of gamma aminobutyric acid (GABA), an inhibitory neurotransmitter in the central nervous system. The usual initial dose of valproic acid is ≈15 mg/kg/day. Many patients receive doses of ≈30 mg/kg/day and in a few cases, daily doses as high as 60 mg/kg/day have been used.[1-3] Valproic acid is interesting from a pharmacokinetic point of view for several reasons. First, valproic acid is known to influence the pharmacokinetics of a number of other drugs. The metabolism of phenobarbital and the major metabolite of carbamazepine appear to be inhibited by valproic acid.[4,5] The metabolism of phenytoin also appears to be inhibited; however, this interaction is difficult to evaluate accurately because valproic acid also displaces phenytoin from its binding sites on serum albumin.[6,7] In addition, valproic acid is highly bound to serum albumin, and at therapeutic plasma concentrations, saturates plasma protein binding sites.[1,8]

Therapeutic and Toxic Plasma Concentrations

The therapeutic range for valproic acid is 50 to 100 mg/L;[1,2,9] however, valproic acid concentrations in excess of 100 mg/mL are often required in patients with partial seizures. There is some evidence that the therapeutic effect of valproic acid lags behind the attainment of steady-state plasma concentrations. This observation is consistent with the fact that some patients continue to experience persistent side effects for several days after the drug has been discontinued.[10] In most cases, the dose-limiting side effects are gastrointestinal in nature (e.g., nausea, vomiting, diarrhea, and abdominal cramps). Sedation and drowsiness do occur but may, in part, be due to the interaction between valproic acid and other concomitant anticonvulsant therapy. Other infrequent side effects include alopecia, a benign essential tremor, thrombocytopenia, and hepatotoxicity. Although not clearly established, elevated levels of valproic acid have been associated with hepatotoxicity.[1,11,12] While the hepatotoxicity associated with valproic acid is rare, it is a serious complication of therapy and should be considered in any patient with elevated liver enzymes.

Bioavailability (F)

Both sodium valproate and valproic acid appear to be rapidly and completely absorbed. Plasma valproate concentrations usually peak one

Key Parameters

Therapeutic Plasma Concentration	50–100 mg/L
F	100%
S	1.0
Vd[a]	0.14 (0.1–0.5) L/kg
Cl[a,b]	
Children	13 mL/kg/hr
Adults	8 mL/kg/hr
t½	
Children	6–8 hr
Adults	10–12 hr

[a] Vd and Cl may be increased in patients with end-stage renal disease; hypo-albuminemia; or valproic acid levels >50 mg/L because of altered plasma protein binding.
[b] Cl may be increased in patients receiving other anticonvulsant drug therapy.

to three hours after oral administration when fasting.[13] Meals, however, appear to slow the rate of absorption of valproic acid; serum concentrations peak as late as six to eight hours after oral administration when taken with food.[14] The amount of sodium valproate in the oral solution formulation and the amount of valproic acid in the capsule preparation are labeled in mg of valproic acid. Consequently, both the bioavailability (F) and the salt form (S) are 1.0 for the oral solution and capsules.

Enteric-coated valproic acid tablets are not sustained in their release characteristics, but absorption is delayed and is markedly influenced by the timing of meals.[15] The bead-filled capsule (Depakote Sprinkles) does appear to have a more sustained plasma profile and more closely approximates a continuous infusion model. Valproic acid oral solution has also been diluted with equal parts water and administered rectally with apparently good absorption.[16]

Volume of Distribution (Vd)

The apparent volume of distribution for valproic acid is variable and ranges from 0.1 to 0.5 L/kg.[1,17,18] Alterations in plasma protein binding (e.g., in patients with low serum albumin or end-stage renal disease) as well as the capacity-limited binding to plasma protein by this drug account for the variable volume of distribution of valproic acid. Valproic acid's binding to serum albumin appears to become saturated when valproic acid concentrations exceed 50 mg/L.[19] For most patients with valproic acid concentrations in the range of 25 to 50 mg/L, an average volume of distribution of 0.14 L/kg is a reasonable value to use for pharmacokinetic calculations, assuming the patient has normal serum albumin concentrations and normal renal function.

Clearance (Cl)

Valproic acid is almost entirely eliminated from the body through hepatic metabolism; less than 5% of the drug is eliminated by the renal route.[1,8,17] The usual clearance values for valproic acid are 6 to 10 mL/kg/hr with an average value of 8 mL/kg/hr. In pediatric patients and in patients receiving additional anti-epileptic drugs, the clearance values may be substantially higher (10 to 13 mL/kg/hr).[20] In addition, capacity-limited plasma protein binding may result in nonlinear changes in the plasma concentration of valproic acid, especially when concentrations exceed 50 mg/L. As long as the trough concentrations are ≤50 mg/L, the changes in trough concentrations should be reasonably proportional to the dose. Therefore, a one-compartment linear model can be used to describe the valproic trough concentrations for most patients in the clinical setting.

Half-Life (t½)

The half-life for valproic acid ranges from 4 to 17 hours, with an average value of six to eight hours. In children and patients receiving other anti-epileptic drugs, the half-life of valproate is reduced. Since the usual half-life is relatively short, valproic acid plasma concentrations appear to plateau within 24 hours after therapy is initiated. Loading doses are not given. The short half-life, coupled with the dosing interval of 8 to 12 hours, results in wide fluctuations in plasma concentrations within a dosing interval.[1,8,18,20]

Time to Sample

Due to wide fluctuations in plasma valproate concentrations within a dosing interval, monitoring both the peak and trough concentrations of this drug would seem to be desirable. Nevertheless, only trough concentrations are routinely monitored because of the uncertainty about the time at which peak plasma concentrations will occur and the difficulty evaluating markedly elevated valproic acid concentrations given its capacity-limited plasma protein binding. In general, valproic acid concentrations in plasma are monitored within two to four days following: 1) initiation of therapy; 2) change in a dosing regimen; or 3) addition of other anti-epileptic drugs to the patient's regimen. Valproic acid concentrations are also measured whenever the patient's clinical course has changed (e.g., a decrease in seizure control or laboratory or physical findings consistent with valproic acid toxicity). As stated previously, there is some evidence that even though valproic acid concentrations may have plateaued relatively rapidly, increased therapeutic effects may continue to be observed for some time following the achievement of steady-state valproic acid concentrations.

> *Question #1.* A.H., an eight-year-old, 25 kg male, is receiving 250 mg of valproic acid Q 12 hr for absence seizures. While the seizure frequency has declined with this therapy, he is still experiencing one to two absence seizures per day. A.H. has experienced no obvious side effects from the valproic acid therapy and has normal renal and hepatic function. What is the expected trough concentration for A.H. on his current regimen?

First, the clearance for A.H. can be calculated by using an average valproic acid clearance for children of 13 mL/kg/hr. Then, A.H.'s volume of distribution can be calculated by using the average volume of distribution value of 0.14 L/kg (see Valproic Acid Key Parameters on page 464). According to the calculations shown below, A.H. would have a valproic acid clearance of 0.325 L/hr and a volume of distribution of 3.5 L.

$$Cl = (13 \text{ mL/kg/hr})(25 \text{ kg})$$
$$= 325 \text{ mL/hr } or \text{ } 0.325 \text{ L/hr}$$

$$Vd = (0.14 \text{ L/kg})(25 \text{ kg})$$
$$= 3.5 \text{ L}$$

Using these values for clearance and volume of distribution, Equations 27 and 31 can be used as follows to calculate A.H.'s elimination rate constant of 0.093 hr^{-1} and the corresponding half-life of 7.5 hours.

$$Kd = \frac{Cl}{Vd}$$

$$= \frac{0.325 \text{ L/hr}}{3.5 \text{ L}}$$

$$= 0.093 \text{ hr}^{-1}$$

$$t\frac{1}{2} = \frac{0.693}{Kd}$$

$$= \frac{0.693}{0.093 \text{ hr}^{-1}}$$

$$= 7.5 \text{ hr}$$

Assuming steady state has been achieved and the salt form and bioavailability are 1.0, Equation 47 can be used to calculate the expected steady-state trough concentration of ≈35 mg/L as follows:

$$Cpss\ min = \frac{\frac{(S)(F)(Dose)}{Vd}}{(1 - e^{-Kd\tau})} (e^{-Kd\tau})$$

$$= \frac{\frac{(1)(1)(250 \text{ mg})}{3.5 \text{ L}}}{(1 - e^{-(0.093\ \text{hr}^{-1})(12\ \text{hr})})} (e^{-(0.093\ \text{hr}^{-1})(12\ \text{hr})})$$

$$= 34.8 \text{ mg/L } or \approx 35 \text{ mg/L}$$

Question #2. A.H. had a measured trough concentration of 25 mg/L. Because of the inadequate seizure control and the lack of apparent side effects, it is decided to increase the trough concentration to 50 mg/L. What dose will be required to achieve the target trough concentration of 50 mg/L if the dosing interval is decreased from Q 12 hr to Q 8 hr?

If the dosing interval had remained unchanged (12 hours), the trough concentration would have changed in proportion to the maintenance dose. The trough concentration will not be directly proportional to the dose, however, because the dosing interval is to be decreased. Therefore, it will be necessary to estimate A.H.'s apparent pharmacokinetic parameters. If the serum concentration of valproic acid of 25 mg/L represents a steady-state trough value, Equation 15.1 can be used to estimate a peak concentration of ≈96 mg/L as shown below (also see 15: Theophylline on page 405).

$$\text{Cpss max} = [\text{Cpss min}] + \left[\frac{(S)(F)(Dose)}{Vd}\right]$$

$$= [25 \text{ mg/L}] + \frac{(1)(1)(250 \text{ mg})}{3.5 \text{ L}}$$

$$= 96.4 \text{ mg/L}$$

By substituting the peak concentration of 96 mg/L for Cp_1, the measured trough concentration of 25 mg/L for Cp_2, and the dosing interval of 12 hours for t, Equation 28 (below) can be used to estimate an elimination rate constant (Kd) of 0.112 hr^{-1}. This Kd value can be used in Equation 31 to estimate a half-life of 6.2 hours as follows:

$$Kd = \frac{\ln\left(\frac{Cp_1}{Cp_2}\right)}{t}$$

$$= \frac{\ln\left(\frac{96}{25}\right)}{12 \text{ hr}}$$

$$= 0.112 \text{ hr}^{-1}$$

$$t\tfrac{1}{2} = \frac{0.693}{Kd}$$

$$= \frac{0.693}{0.112 \text{ hr}^{-1}}$$

$$= 6.2 \text{ hr}$$

The assumed volume of distribution of 3.5 L and the calculated elimination rate constant of 0.112 hr^{-1} then can be used in Equation 33 to calculate a clearance of 0.39 L/hr (15.6 mL/kg/hr).

$$Cl = (Kd)(Vd)$$
$$= (0.112 \text{ hr}^{-1})(3.5 \text{ L})$$
$$= 0.392 \text{ L/hr}$$

Equation 47 for Cpss min can be rearranged so that the dose required to achieve a desired trough concentration can be calculated:

$$Cpss \text{ min} = \frac{\dfrac{(S)(F)(Dose)}{Vd}}{(1 - e^{-Kd\tau})} (e^{-Kd\tau})$$

$$Dose = \frac{(Cpss \text{ min})(Vd)(1 - e^{-Kd\tau})}{(S)(F)(e^{-Kd\tau})}$$ **Eq. 18.3**

By making the appropriate substitutions for the steady-state drug level, elimination rate constant, dosing interval, and volume of distribution, the dose required to achieve a trough concentration of 50 mg/L would be ≈250 mg given every eight hours.

$$Dose = \frac{(50 \text{ mg/L})(3.5 \text{ L})(1 - e^{-(0.112 \text{ hr}^{-1})(8 \text{ hr})})}{(1)(1)(e^{-(0.112 \text{ hr}^{-1})(8 \text{ hr})})}$$
$$= 253 \ or \approx 250 \text{ mg}$$

The actual measured trough concentration, however, may not coincide with the calculations for a number of reasons. First, the volume of distribution of 3.5 L (0.14 L/kg) is an assumed value and may not correspond to A.H.'s actual volume of distribution. Second, the target concentration of 50 mg/L is approaching the range where capacity-limited plasma protein binding may be observed. If the plasma protein binding sites become saturated, the measured or total drug concentration may be lower than calculated. Sampling at the trough concentration helps to avoid this capacity-limited binding problem because the measured drug levels are at their lowest concentration and are least likely to be at a concentration range where protein-binding can become saturated.

Question #3. S.N., a 23-year-old, 70 kg female, is receiving phenobarbital 60 mg BID and phenytoin 300 mg QD. The steady-state plasma drug concentrations are 18 mg/L for phenobarbital and 10 mg/L for phenytoin. Because of poor seizure control, valproic acid 500 mg Q 8 hr was added to this drug treatment regimen. Two months later, S.N. complained of increased drowsiness. At that time, plasma drug concentrations were measured and reported as follows: phenobarbital 30 mg/L; phenytoin 6 mg/L; and valproic acid 75 mg/L. How can the increased phenobarbital concentration and decreased phenytoin concentration be explained?

Valproic acid decreases the clearance of phenobarbital by about 40%.[21,22] The increase in plasma phenobarbital concentration from 18 mg/L to 30 mg/L 60 days after valproic acid was added is consistent with a 40% decrease in the phenobarbital clearance. If the original steady-state phenobarbital concentration of 18 mg/L is desired, the daily phenobarbital dose should be decreased by about 40%.

The decline in the plasma phenytoin concentration from 10 mg/L to 6 mg/L is probably the result of competition for plasma protein binding between valproic acid and phenytoin. In patients with normal serum albumin concentrations and normal renal function, valproic acid (at a concentration of ≈70 mg/L) produces a 30% to 40% decline in phenytoin plasma concentrations.[19,23,24] This acute decline in the plasma concentration of phenytoin is due to a decrease in the bound concentration. The unbound or therapeutically active plasma phenytoin concentration appears to remain unchanged because any bound phenytoin which is displaced re-equilibrates with the large tissue compartment. Since the tissue space is large, the increased tissue concentrations will be negligible. There is less well-documented evidence that chronic valproic acid therapy increases the unbound phenytoin concentration; this may be caused by inhibition of phenytoin metabolism. To minimize the impact of competitive plasma protein binding on the assessment of drug concentrations, both phenytoin and valproic acid samples should be obtained when valproic acid concentrations are at their lowest (that is, at trough, or just before the next dose).

Question #4. **C.B., a 10-year-old, 32 kg female, is receiving valproic acid sprinkles 250 mg (2 × 125 mg) PO Q 8 hr for her seizure disorder. Calculate her valproic acid level at steady state.**

Because C.B. is receiving valproic acid as the sprinkle product, one would not expect a great deal of fluctuation within the dosing interval. For this reason, Equation 35 is a reasonable model to use to predict her valproic acid concentration.

$$\text{Cpss ave} = \frac{(S)(F)(\text{Dose}/\tau)}{\text{Cl}}$$

Assume C.B.'s clearance of valproic acid is 0.416 L/hr:

$$\text{Cl} = (13 \text{ mL/kg/hr})(32 \text{ kg})$$
$$= 416 \text{ mL/hr } or \text{ } 0.416 \text{ L/hr}$$

If S and F are assumed to be 1.0, C.B.'s valproic acid concentration should be $\approx$75 mg/L.

$$\text{Cpss ave} = \frac{(S)(F)(\text{Dose}/\tau)}{\text{Cl}} \qquad \text{(Eq. 35)}$$
$$= \frac{(1)(1)(250 \text{ mg}/8 \text{ hr})}{0.416 \text{ L/hr}}$$
$$= 75.1 \text{ mg/L}$$

This predicted valproic acid concentration is within the usually accepted therapeutic range of 50 to 100 mg/L. However, plasma concentration monitoring would be useful to confirm this prediction if satisfactory therapeutic effects are not achieved or toxicities occur.

References

1. Pinder RM et al. Sodium valproate: a review of its pharmacological properties in therapeutic efficacy in epilepsy. Drugs. 1977;13:81.

2. Sherard ES et al. Treatment of childhood epilepsy with valproic acid: result of the first 100 patients in a 6-month trial. Neurology. 1980;30:31.

3. Bowdle TA et al. Valproic acid dosage and plasma protein binding and clearance. Clin Pharmacol Ther. 1980;28:486–92.

4. Levy RH et al. Carbamazepine-valproic acid interaction in man and rhesus monkey. Epilepsia. 1984;25:338–45.

5. Patel IH et al. Phenobarbital-valproic acid interaction. Clin Pharmacol Ther. 1980:27:515–21.

6. Cramer JA, Matson RH. Valproic acid: *In vitro* plasma protein binding and interaction with phenytoin. Ther Drug Monit. 1979;1:105–16.

7. Haidukewych D et al. Derivation and evaluation of an equation for prediction of free phenytoin concentration in patients comedicated with valproic acid. Ther Drug Monit. 1989;11:134–9.

8. Gugler R et al. Disposition of valproic acid in man. Eur J Clin Pharm. 1977;12:125.

9. Graham L et al. Sodium valproate, serum level, and critical effect in epilepsy: a controlled study. Epilepsia. 1979;20:303.

10. Lockard JS, Levy RH. Valproic acid: Reversibly acting drug? Epilepsia. 1976;17:477–9.

11. Suchy FJ et al. Acute hepatic failure associated with the use of sodium valproate. N Engl J Med. 1979;300:962.

12. Donat JT et al. Valproic acid and fatal hepatitis. Neurology. 1979; 29:273.

13. Klotz U, Antonin KH. Pharmacokinetics and bioavailability of sodium valproate. Clin Pharm Ther. 1977; 21:736.

14. Chun AHC et al. Bioavailability of valproic acid under fasting-non-fasting regimens. J Crit Pharm. 1980;20:30.

15. Cloyd JC et al. Bioavailability of coated particle versus enteric-coated Divalproex sodium tablets in patients on monotherapy. Neurology. 1989;39(Suppl 1):119.

16. Cloyd JC, Brundage RC. Valproic acid. In: Taylor WJ et al. A Text for the Clinical Drug Monitoring. Irving: Abbott Laboratories Diagnostic Division; 1986:269–80.

17. Gugler R, Unruh GE. Clinical pharmacokinetics of valproic acid. Clin Pharmacokinet. 1980;5:67.

18. Mihaly GW et al. Single and chronic dose pharmacokinetic studies of sodium valproate in epileptic patients. Eur J Clin Pharmacol. 1979; 16:23.

19. Monks A, Richens A. Effect of a single dose of sodium valproate on serum phenytoin levels and protein binding in epileptic patients. Clin Pharm Ther. 1980;27:89.

20. Kriel RL et al. The pharmacokinetics of valproic acid in children. Ann Neurol. 1979;6:179.

21. Bruni J et al. Valproic acid and plasma levels of phenobarbital. Neurology. 1980;30:94.

22. Patel IH et al. Phenobarbital-valproic acid interaction. Clin Pharm Ther. 1980;27:515.

23. Friel PM et al. Valproic acid-phenytoin interaction. Ther Drug Monit. 1979;1:243.

24. Perucca E et al. Interaction between phenytoin and valproic acid; plasma protein binding and metabolic effects. Clin Pharm Ther. 1980;28:779.

Vancomycin 18

Vancomycin is a bactericidal antibiotic with a gram-positive spectrum of activity that is effective in the treatment of nafcillin-resistant *Staphylococcus aureus* (NRSA). It is also an alternative to penicillin in patients who have a history of serious penicillin allergy.[1–4] There has been a resurgence in the use of vancomycin because of the increased incidence of nafcillin-resistant staphylococcus.

Vancomycin is poorly absorbed orally and has been used to treat gastrointestinal overgrowths of gram-positive bacteria. When used to treat systemic infections, vancomycin must be given by the intravenous route or intraperitoneally for those patients on continuous ambulatory peritoneal dialysis (CAPD). The usual dose is 1 gm (10 to 15 mg/kg) administered over 60 minutes every 12 hours.[4] Although 2 gm/day (20 to 30 mg/kg/day) of vancomycin has been recommended historically, this dose can be excessive, particularly in the elderly and in patients with diminished renal function. In these individuals, doses should be adjusted. Vancomycin is not administered intramuscularly because it is painful and causes local irritation and a histamine reaction.

Therapeutic and Toxic Plasma Concentrations

The ideal vancomycin dosing regimen is one that results in peak vancomycin plasma concentrations that are less than 30 to 50 mg/L and trough concentrations that are in the range of 5 to 15 mg/L.[1,2,5–7] Peak concentrations above 50 mg/L have been associated with ototoxicity; however, vancomycin-induced ototoxicity has been primarily reported in patients with vancomycin concentrations >80 mg/L.[1,3,8]

Although the above concentrations are widely accepted, there is some controversy over their validity and the necessity for routinely monitoring plasma vancomycin concentrations.[9,10] This problem in part arises from the fact that peak concentrations are often obtained at different times relative to the end of the infusion. Furthermore, the minimum inhibitory concentration (MIC) for most bacteria is <5 mg/L, making it difficult to establish exactly when and how long over the dosing interval plasma concentrations should exceed 5 mg/L. It is the author's opinion that patients most likely to require vancomycin plasma concentration monitoring are those at highest risk for therapeutic failure or potential drug toxicity. These include pediatric patients because they have high clearances and short half-lives. Consequently, trough concentrations frequently are well

Key Parameters

Therapeutic Plasma Concentration[a]	
Peak	<40–50 mg/L
Trough	≈10 ± 5 mg/L
F	<5%
Vd[b]	0.7 (0.5–1) L/kg
Cl[c]	[0.65][Cl_{Cr} mL/kg/min] [TBW]
t½	7 hr

[a] A peak concentration in the range of 30 mg/L is probably a reasonable target; however, to ensure efficacy, trough concentrations should be maintained at or above 5 mg/L.

[b] TBW = Total body weight, including any excess adipose and third space fluid weight, when calculating vancomycin volume of distribution.

[c] TBW = Total body weight for obese and non-obese subjects but should not include excess third space fluid weight when calculating vancomycin clearance.

below 5 mg/L. Patients with poor renal function in whom the initial vancomycin dosing regimen has not been adjusted also deserve to be monitored for vancomycin concentrations that greatly exceed those required for efficacy.

Other major side effects associated with vancomycin therapy include phlebitis and a histamine reaction which presents as flushing, tachycardia, and hypotension. To minimize the histamine response, vancomycin should be infused slowly over 60 minutes. Even at this rate of infusion, some patients will experience the flushing and tachycardia.[11,12] Although renal toxicity was originally associated with vancomycin, this was probably due to an impurity present in the original formulation; there have been no recent reports of vancomycin-induced renal toxicity when administered as a single agent.[1,12] While vancomycin by itself has relatively little nephrotoxicity, there is evidence that when it is combined with aminoglycoside antibiotics, the incidence may be as high as 30%.[8] It is difficult to know whether this high incidence of nephrotoxicity is a result of the patient population selected (i.e., critically ill patients) or a synergistic nephrotoxicity caused by the concurrent use of vancomycin and aminoglycosides.

The minimum inhibitory concentration for most strains of staphylococcus is below 5 mg/L; therefore, trough concentrations should be maintained in the range of 5 to 15 mg/L. Many clinicians recommend maintaining trough concentrations above 10 mg/L since there is evidence of increased efficacy in patients with endocarditis and there is no known increased risk of toxicity at these concentrations.[5,7,13]

Bioavailability (F)

Vancomycin is poorly absorbed following oral administration (i.e., <5%); as a result, parenteral or intraperitoneal administration is necessary for the treatment of systemic infections. Vancomycin's limited oral bioavailability has been used advantageously to treat enterocolitis.[1,4,7] Oral vancomycin and metronidazole are commonly used to treat *Clostridium difficile*-produced pseudomembranous colitis, a clinical condition that can be precipitated by the use of broad spectrum antibiotics. Metronidazole is currently the drug of choice because it is less expensive than vancomycin.

Volume of Distribution (Vd)

The volume of distribution for vancomycin ranges between 0.5 and 1 L/kg.[14] In clinical practice, an average value of 0.7 L/kg usually is used. A two- or three-compartment model best describes its distribution and the complexity of this model can cause problems when peak plasma samples are obtained during the distribution phase.

Clearance (Cl)

Vancomycin is eliminated primarily by the renal route; approximately 5% of the dose is metabolized. The clearance of vancomycin approximates 65% of creatinine clearance.[14,15] However, because vancomycin clearance appears to correlate better with total body weight in obese subjects, creatinine clearance is often expressed as mL/kg/min and this value is multiplied by the patient's total body weight in kg even if the patient is obese.[6]

$$\text{Vancomycin Cl} = (0.65)(\text{Cl}_{Cr} \text{ in mL/kg/min}) \left(\frac{\text{Total Body}}{\text{Weight in kg}} \right)$$

Eq. 18.1

Creatinine clearance in mL/kg/min can be calculated by dividing the creatinine clearance by the patient's weight initially used to calculate the creatinine clearance. The total body weight in kg should exclude excessive third space fluid since this weight would not be expected to be associated with an increase in vancomycin renal clearance. Two additional issues should be considered when calculating vancomycin clearance. The first is whether or not $SrCr_{ss}$ should be normalized to 1.0 mg/dL. (See Part I: Creatinine Clearance on page 94.) The second is whether the factor by which Cl_{Cr} in Equation 18.1 should be >0.65. Many clinicians currently use a value of ≈1.0 because in their clinical experience more accurate and less biased estimates can be made by assuming a vancomycin clearance in Cl_{Cr}.[26]

Very little vancomycin is cleared by standard hemo- or peritoneal dialysis.[7,16,17] In patients undergoing continuous ambulatory peritoneal dialysis (CAPD), the small but continuous drug loss due to peritoneal dialysis exchanges is significant. As discussed in Part I, the usual approach is to replace vancomycin with intermittent intravenous injections on a somewhat more frequent basis than is usually done for patients with end-stage renal disease (in some cases as often as every three to five days) or to instill vancomycin directly into the peritoneal space to treat peritonitis and achieve systemic concentrations of vancomycin.[18,19] Some caution should be used in evaluating plasma concentrations in patients receiving CAPD. Many assays overestimate actual vancomycin concentrations due to an accumulation of metabolites.[20] In patients undergoing high-flux or high-efficiency hemodialysis, a significant amount of vancomycin can be removed. Early studies estimated that as much as 30% of vancomycin was removed during high-flux hemodialysis; recent reports indicate only 17% of vancomycin is removed during these procedures. Early investigators did not recognize that a redistribution of vancomycin occurs after the completion of dialysis.[21,22]

Half-Life (t½)

The usual serum half-life of vancomycin is six to ten hours; in patients with end-stage renal disease the half-life may approach seven days.[7,14,15] This wide range in the serum half-life of vancomycin partially explains the variability in the dose and dosing intervals used for vancomycin. Patients with normal renal function may receive the drug every 12 hours, while those with end-stage renal disease may receive a dose every one to two weeks.[7,16]

Nomograms

Dosing nomograms for vancomycin are available.[7] However, an understanding of the desired therapeutic range and the pharmacokinetic parameters of vancomycin enables the clinician to select doses and dosing intervals which meet the specific needs of the patient.

Time to Sample

Wide swings in vancomycin serum concentrations within a normal dosing interval suggest that both peak and trough concentrations should be monitored. In general, however, steady-state trough concentrations are probably adequate. As a general rule, vancomycin is dosed with an interval of approximately one half-life. Assuming an average volume of distribution of ≈0.7 L/kg, coupled with the dose administered and a measured trough, it is the author's opinion that peak concentrations can be estimated with reasonable accuracy. While the bulk of the literature suggests that both peak and trough concentrations are appropriate, the concept of using only trough concentrations is supported by both the pharmacokinetic and clinical characteristics of the drug.[10,23]

If the highest expected peak concentration for a dose that produces a trough concentration of 5 to 15 mg/L is below 40 to 50 mg/L, the dose is acceptable. If the trough concentration is known, the peak concentration (Cpss max) can be calculated using Equation 15.1.

$$\text{Cpss max} = \left[\text{Cpss min} \right] + \left[\frac{(S)(F)(\text{Dose})}{V_d} \right] \qquad \text{(Eq. 15.1)}$$

The $\frac{(S)(F)(\text{Dose})}{V_d}$ represents the change in concentration (ΔCp) following a dose.

As described in Part I, the use of the above equation requires that several conditions be met. They are:

1) Steady-state has been achieved.

2) The measured plasma concentration is a trough concentration.

3) The bolus dose is an acceptable model.

In the clinical setting, trough concentrations often are obtained slightly before the true trough. Because vancomycin has a relatively long half-life, most plasma concentrations obtained within one hour of the true trough can be assumed to have met condition 2 above.

Since vancomycin follows a multicompartmental model, it is difficult to avoid the distribution phase when obtaining peak plasma concentrations.[24] If peak levels are to be measured, samples should be obtained at least one or possibly two hours after the end of the infusion period. It is difficult to evaluate the appropriateness of a dosing regimen that is based upon plasma samples obtained before steady state. Additional plasma concentrations are required to more accurately estimate a patient's apparent clearance and half-life, and to ensure that any dosing adjustments based on a non-steady-state trough concentration actually achieve the targeted steady-state concentrations.

Question #1. B.C., a 65-year-old, 45 kg male with a serum creatinine of 2.2 mg/dL, is being treated for a presumed hospital-acquired, nafcillin-resistant *S. aureus* infection. Design a dosing regimen that will produce peak concentrations less than 40 to 50 mg/L and trough concentrations of 5 to 15 mg/L.

Calculate Parameters. The first step in calculating an appropriate dosing regimen for B.C. is to estimate his pharmacokinetic parameters (i.e., volume of distribution, clearance, and elimination rate constant or half-life).

The volume of distribution for B.C. can be calculated by using the average volume of distribution for vancomycin of 0.7 L/kg (see Vancomycin Key Parameters on page 475). According to the calculations shown below, B.C.'s expected volume of distribution would be 31.5 L.

$$[0.7 \text{ L/kg}][45 \text{ kg}] = 31.5 \text{ L}$$

Using Equation 63, B.C.'s creatinine clearance is estimated to be approximately 21.3 mL/min or 0.473 mL/kg/min as shown:

$$\begin{aligned} \frac{\text{Cl}_{Cr} \text{ for Males}}{\text{(mL/min)}} &= \frac{(140 - \text{Age})(\text{Weight})}{(72)(\text{SrCr}_{ss})} \\ &= \frac{(140 - 65)(45)}{(72)(2.2)} \\ &= 21.3 \text{ mL/min} \quad or \quad 0.473 \text{ mL/kg/min} \end{aligned}$$

The corresponding vancomycin clearance for B.C. is 0.83 L/hr.

$$\begin{aligned} \text{Vancomycin Cl} &= (0.65)(\text{Cl}_{Cr} \text{ in mL/kg/min})(\text{Total Body Weight in kg}) \\ &= (0.65)(0.473 \text{ mL/kg/min})(45 \text{ kg}) \\ &= 13.84 \text{ mL/min} \end{aligned}$$

or

$$= 13.84 \text{ mL/min} \times \frac{60 \text{ min/hr}}{1000 \text{ mL/L}}$$

$$= 0.83 \text{ L/hr}$$

Note that because B.C. was not considered to be obese, the process of calculating clearance in mL/kg/min and then multiplying by the same weight was not a necessary step; however, it serves as a reminder to consider the body weight in obese patients.

The calculated clearance of 0.83 L/hr and the calculated volume of distribution of 31.5 L then can be used to estimate the elimination rate constant (Equation 27) and corresponding half-life (Equation 32) for vancomycin in B.C.

$$\begin{aligned} \text{Kd} &= \frac{\text{Cl}}{\text{Vd}} \\ &= \frac{0.83 \text{ L/hr}}{31.5 \text{ L}} \\ &= 0.026 \text{ hr}^{-1} \end{aligned}$$

$$\begin{aligned} t\text{½} &= \frac{(0.693)(\text{Vd})}{\text{Cl}} \\ &= \frac{(0.693)(31.5 \text{ L})}{0.83 \text{ L/hr}} \\ &= 26 \text{ hr} \end{aligned}$$

Loading Dose. In clinical practice, loading doses of vancomycin are seldom administered. This is probably because most clinicians prescribe about 15 mg/kg as their maintenance dose. Using Equation 49 and substituting the usual maintenance dose as mg/kg and volume of distribution as L/kg, it can be seen that the initial plasma concentration should be $\approx$20 mg/L.

$$Cp^{\circ} = \frac{(S)(F)(\text{Loading Dose})}{Vd}$$

$$= \frac{(1)(1)(15 \text{ mg/kg})}{0.7 \text{ L/kg}}$$

$$= 21 \text{ mg/L}$$

Although this value is below the usual target level of 30 mg/L, it is well above that needed for efficacy (5–15 mg/L). If one wanted to calculate an initial dose, Equation 11 and the assumed volume of distribution of 31.5 L could be used. The salt form and bioavailability are assumed to be 1.0. Using an initial target of 30 mg/L, the loading dose would be $\approx$1000 mg.

$$\text{Loading Dose} = \frac{(Vd)(Cp)}{(S)(F)}$$

$$= \frac{(31.5 \text{ L})(30 \text{ mg/L})}{(1)(1)}$$

$$= 945 \text{ mg } or \approx 1000 \text{ mg}$$

There are no known renal or ototoxicities associated with elevated vancomycin levels that occur during the distribution phase. However, to minimize the cardiovascular effects associated with rapid administration, the initial and subsequent doses should be administered over $\approx$60 minutes. In addition, if peak concentrations are measured, samples should be drawn at least one to two hours after completion of the infusion period to avoid the distribution phase.

Maintenance Dose. The maintenance dose can be calculated by a number of methods. One approach might be to first approximate the hourly infusion rate required to maintain the desired average concentration. Then, the hourly infusion rate can be multiplied by an appropriate dosing interval to calculate a reasonable dose to be given on an intermittent basis. For example, if an average concentration of 20 mg/L is selected (approximately halfway between the desired peak concentration of 30 mg/L and trough concentration of $\approx$10 mg/L), the hourly administration rate would be 17 mg/hr (Equation 16).

$$\text{Maintenance Dose} = \frac{(Cl)(Cpss\ ave)(\tau)}{(S)(F)}$$
$$= \frac{(0.83\ L/hr)(20\ mg/L)(1\ hr)}{(1)(1)}$$
$$= 17\ mg$$

Although a number of dosing intervals could be selected, 24 hours is reasonable because it is a convenient interval and approximates B.C.'s half-life for vancomycin of 26 hours. A dosing interval of less than one half-life should result in peak concentrations that are below 40 to 50 mg/L and trough concentrations that are above the 5 to 15 mg/L range. If an interval of 24 hours is selected, the dose would be $\approx$400 mg.

$$\text{Maintenance Dose} = \frac{(0.83\ L/hr)(20\ mg/L)(24\ hr)}{(1)(1)}$$
$$= 398\ mg\ \ or\ \approx 400\ mg$$

A second approach that can be used to calculate the maintenance dose is to select a desired peak and trough concentration that is consistent with the therapeutic range and B.C.'s vancomycin half-life. For example, if steady-state peak concentrations of 30 mg/L are desired, it would take approximately two half-lives for that peak level to fall to 7.5 mg/L (a level of 30 mg/L declines to 15 mg/L in one half-life and to 7.5 mg/L in the second half-life). Since the vancomycin half-life in B.C. is approximately one day, the dosing interval would be 48 hours. The dose to be administered every 48 hours can be calculated using Equation 18.2.

$$\text{Dose} = \frac{(Vd)(Cpss\ max - Cpss\ min)}{(S)(F)}$$

Eq. 18.2

$$= \frac{(31.5\ L)(30\ mg/L - 7.5\ mg/L)}{(1)(1)}$$

$$= 709\ mg\ \ or\ \ \approx 700\ mg$$

The peak and trough concentrations which can be expected using this dosing regimen can be calculated by using Equations 43 and 47, respectively:

$$Cpss\ max = \frac{\dfrac{(S)(F)(Dose)}{Vd}}{(1 - e^{-Kd\tau})}$$

(Eq. 43)

$$= \frac{\dfrac{(1)(1)(700\ mg)}{31.5\ L}}{(1 - e^{-(0.026\ hr^{-1})(48\ hr)})}$$

$$= 31\ mg/L$$

Note that although 31 mg/L is an acceptable peak, the actual clinical peak would normally be obtained approximately two hours after this calculated concentration and would be ≈29 mg/L as calculated by Equation 26.

$$Cp = Cp^{o}(e^{-Kdt})$$

(Eq. 26)

$$= 31\ mg/L\ (e^{-(0.026)(2\ hr)})$$

$$= 31\ mg/L\ (0.95)$$

$$= 29.4\ mg/L$$

The calculated trough concentration would be ≈ 9 mg/L (Equation 47).

$$\text{Cpss min} = \frac{\dfrac{(S)(F)(Dose)}{Vd}}{(1 - e^{-Kd\tau})}(e^{-Kd\tau}) \qquad \text{(Eq. 47)}$$

$$= [31 \text{ mg/L}][e^{-(0.026 \text{ hr}^{-1})(48 \text{ hr})}]$$

$$= (31 \text{ mg/L})(0.29)$$

$$= 8.99 \text{ mg/L}$$

This process of checking the expected peak and trough concentrations is most appropriate when the dosing interval or the dose has been changed from a theoretical or calculated value to a practical value.

A third alternative is to rearrange Equation 47 such that the dose can be calculated (Equation 17.1).

$$\text{Cpss min} = \frac{\dfrac{(S)(F)(Dose)}{Vd}}{(1 - e^{-Kd\tau})}(e^{-Kd\tau})$$

$$\text{Dose} = \frac{(\text{Cpss min})(Vd)(1 - e^{-Kd\tau})}{(S)(F)(e^{-Kd\tau})}$$

Note that it is the Cpss min or trough concentration that is used to solve for dose. This is because it is the trough concentration which has been associated with efficacy and therefore is the primary target for dosing. Making the appropriate substitutions for the parameters indicated in Equation 17.1 and choosing a target trough concentration of 10 mg/L and a dosing interval of 48 hours, a dose of ≈ 750 mg is calculated.

$$\text{Dose} = \frac{(10 \text{ mg/L})(31.5 \text{ L})(1 - e^{-(0.026)(48 \text{ hr})})}{(1)(1)(e^{-(0.026)(48 \text{ hr})})}$$

$$= \frac{(10 \text{ mg/L})(31.5 \text{ L})(1 - 0.29)}{(1)(1)(0.29)}$$

$$= 771.2 \text{ mg} \ \text{ or } \ \approx 750 \text{ mg}$$

The discrepancy between the 750 mg calculated by Method 3 and the 700 mg calculated from Method 2 can be attributed to the fact that Method 2 assumes that the average concentration is half way between the peak and trough. As mentioned in Part I, this is approximately correct as long as the dosing interval is less than or equal to the drug's half-life. When dosing intervals greatly exceed the half-life, the true average concentration is much lower than halfway between the peak and trough levels.

Question #2. E.K., a 60-year old, 50 kg female with a serum creatinine of 1.0 mg/dL, has been empirically started on 500 mg of vancomycin Q 8 hr for treatment of a hospital-acquired staphylococcal infection. What would be the expected peak and trough vancomycin concentrations for E.K.?

Determine Patient's Parameters. To calculate the peak and trough concentrations, E.K.'s volume of distribution, clearance, and elimination rate constant or half-life have to be estimated. Assuming E.K. has an average volume of distribution of 0.7 L/kg, the expected volume of distribution would be 35 L.

$$[0.7 \text{ L/kg}][50 \text{ kg}] = 35 \text{ L}$$

E.K.'s vancomycin clearance can be calculated using Equation 64 to calculate creatinine clearance, and then a vancomycin clearance of 1.8 L/hr can be calculated as shown below.

$$\frac{\text{Cl}_{Cr} \text{ for Females}}{\text{(mL/min)}} = (0.85) \frac{(140 - \text{Age})(\text{Weight})}{(72)(\text{SrCr}_{ss})}$$

$$= (0.85) \frac{(140 - 60)(50 \text{ kg})}{(72)(1.0 \text{ mg/dL})}$$

$$= 47.2 \text{ mL/min} \ or \ 0.944 \text{ mL/kg/min}$$

Using Equation 18.1 to calculate vancomycin clearance:

$$\text{Vancomycin Cl} = (0.65)(\text{Cl}_{\text{Cr}} \text{ in mL/kg/min})(\text{Total Body Weight in kg})$$
$$= (0.65)(0.944 \text{ mL/kg/min})(50 \text{ kg})$$
$$= 30.68 \text{ mL/min}$$

or

$$= \left(30.68 \text{ mL/min}\right)\left(\frac{60 \text{ min/hr}}{1000 \text{ mL/L}}\right)$$
$$= 1.8 \text{ L/hr}$$

Equation 27 can now be used to calculate E.K.'s elimination rate constant and Equation 32 to calculate the corresponding half-life.

$$\text{Kd} = \frac{\text{Cl}}{\text{Vd}}$$
$$= \frac{1.8 \text{ L/hr}}{35 \text{ L}}$$
$$= 0.051 \text{ hr}^{-1}$$

$$t\tfrac{1}{2} = \frac{(0.693)(\text{Vd})}{\text{Cl}}$$
$$= \frac{(0.693)(35 \text{ L})}{1.8 \text{ L/hr}}$$
$$= 13.5 \text{ hr}$$

And Equations 43 and 46 can be used to calculate the expected peak and trough concentrations for E.K.

$$\text{Cpss max} = \frac{\dfrac{(S)(F)(\text{Dose})}{\text{Vd}}}{(1 - e^{-\text{Kd}\tau})} \qquad \text{(Eq. 43)}$$
$$= \frac{\dfrac{(1)(1)(500 \text{ mg})}{35 \text{ L}}}{(1 - e^{-(0.051 \text{ hr}^{-1})(8 \text{ hr})})}$$
$$= 42.6 \text{ mg/L}$$

In order to calculate the clinical peak concentration which is usually sampled two hours after the start of a vancomycin infusion (one hour after the end of a one-hour infusion), the Cpss max could be decayed for two hours using Equation 26.

$$Cp = Cp^o \ (e^{-Kdt}) \qquad\qquad \text{(Eq. 26)}$$
$$= 42.6 \ mg/L \ (e^{-(0.051)(2 \ hr)})$$
$$= 42.6 \ mg/L \ (0.90)$$
$$= 38.34 \ mg/L \ \text{two hr after starting infusion}$$

$$Cpss \ min = (Cpss \ max)(e^{-Kd\tau}) \qquad\qquad \text{(Eq. 46)}$$
$$= (42.6 \ mg/L)(e^{-(0.051 \ hr^{-1})(8 \ hr)})$$
$$= 28.3 \ mg/L$$

Although the expected peak concentration of ≈ 40 mg/L is not above the usually accepted peak concentration range, the trough concentration of ≈ 30 mg/L is well above that required for efficacy. This suggests that decreasing the dose and/or increasing the dosing interval, as well as monitoring plasma concentrations of vancomycin, would be appropriate.

Question #3. A steady-state trough concentration was obtained for E.K. and was reported as 35 mg/L. Design a dosing regimen that will produce lower therapeutic vancomycin concentrations for E.K.

Revise Patient's Parameters. To design such a regimen, E.K.'s pharmacokinetic parameters should first be revised so that they are consistent with the observed trough concentration of 35 mg/L. Some assumptions will have to be made. For E.K., the percent fluctuation between peak and trough concentrations should be relatively small at steady state because her dosing interval of eight hours is much shorter than her predicted half-life of 13.5 hours. Therefore, the best approach is to estimate the volume of distribution and then calculate the corresponding elimination rate constant and clearance values.

If E.K.'s volume of distribution is assumed to be 0.7 L/kg (see Vancomycin Key Parameters) and the observed trough concentration of 35 mg/L is used, a peak concentration of 49 mg/L can be calculated using Equation 15.1 as follows.

$$Cpss\ max = [Cpss\ min] + \left[\frac{(S)(F)(Dose)}{Vd} \right]$$

$$= [35\ mg/L] + \frac{(1)(1)(500\ mg)}{(0.7\ L/kg)(50\ kg)}$$

$$= 49\ mg/L$$

Using the observed trough concentration of 35 mg/L and the predicted peak concentration of 49 mg/L, an elimination rate constant (Kd) can be calculated using Equation 28, where Cp_1 is the peak concentration of 49 mg/L, Cp_2 is the trough concentration of 35 mg/L, and the interval between those two concentrations, t, is the dosing interval of eight hours.

$$Kd = \frac{\ln\left(\dfrac{Cp_1}{Cp_2}\right)}{t}$$

$$= \frac{\ln\left(\dfrac{49\ mg/L}{35\ mg/L}\right)}{8\ hr}$$

$$= 0.042\ hr^{-1}$$

This apparent elimination rate constant of 0.042 hr^{-1} corresponds to a half-life of approximately 16.5 hours (Equation 31) as shown below.

$$t\tfrac{1}{2} = \frac{0.693}{Kd}$$

$$= \frac{0.693}{0.042\ hr^{-1}}$$

$$= 16.5\ hr$$

The apparent elimination rate constant of 0.042 hr^{-1} and the assumed volume of distribution of 35 L (0.7 L/kg $\times$ 50 kg) can be used in Equation 33 to calculate E.K.'s vancomycin clearance.

$$
\begin{aligned}
\text{Cl} &= (\text{Kd})(\text{Vd}) \\
&= (0.042 \text{ hr}^{-1})(35 \text{ L}) \\
&= 1.5 \text{ L/hr}
\end{aligned}
$$

Note that because the revised t½ is $\leq \tau$ clearance could have been calculated by assuming Cpss ave is approximately equal to:

$$
\text{Cpss ave} = \text{Cpss min} + (\tfrac{1}{2}) \frac{(\text{S})(\text{F})(\text{Dose})}{\text{Vd}}
$$

and then calculating clearance by using Equation 15.

$$
\text{Cl} = \frac{(\text{S})(\text{F})(\text{Dose}/\tau)}{\text{Cpss ave}}
$$

(See Part I: Choosing a Model to Revise or Estimate a Patient's Clearance at Steady State on page 82.)

Maintenance Dose. The maintenance dose can then be calculated by rearranging Equation 47 to Equation 17.1. Because the apparent half-life is $\approx$16 hours, the most logical dosing interval and Cpss min would be 24 hours and 10 mg/L, respectively.

$$
\text{Cpss min} = \frac{\dfrac{(\text{S})(\text{F})(\text{Dose})}{\text{Vd}}}{(1 - e^{-\text{Kd}\tau})} (e^{-\text{Kd}\tau})
$$

$$
\begin{aligned}
\text{Dose} &= \frac{(\text{Cpss min})(\text{Vd})(1 - e^{-\text{Kd}\tau})}{(\text{S})(\text{F})(e^{-\text{Kd}\tau})} \\
&= \frac{(10 \text{ mg/L})(35 \text{ L})(1 - e^{-(0.042)(24)})}{(1)(1)(e^{-(0.042)(24)})} \\
&= 622 \text{ mg } or \approx 600 \text{ mg}
\end{aligned}
$$

This dosing regimen of 600 mg every 24 hours should result in a peak concentration of approximately 25 mg/L (Equation 48).

$$\text{Cpss}_1 = \frac{\dfrac{(S)(F)(\text{Dose})}{\text{Vd}}}{(1 - e^{-Kd\tau})} (e^{-Kdt_1})$$

$$= \frac{\dfrac{(1)(1)(600 \text{ mg})}{35 \text{ L}}}{(1 - e^{-(0.042)(24)})} (e^{-(0.042)(2)})$$

$$= \frac{17.1 \text{ mg/L}}{(1 - 0.36)} (0.92)$$

$$= 24.6 \text{ mg/L}$$

The target trough concentration of 10 mg/L should be acceptable since the goal is to maintain trough concentrations in the therapeutic range (5 to 15 mg/L).

Question #4. **A.C., a 60 kg female with end-stage renal disease and a serum creatinine of 9 mg/dL, is undergoing intermittent hemodialysis treatments three times a week and currently has an apparent shunt infection which is to be treated with vancomycin. Calculate an appropriate dose for A.C.**

Vancomycin is extensively cleared by the kidneys; consequently, patients with end-stage renal disease have prolonged half-lives that average five to seven days. This extended half-life is consistent with a residual vancomycin clearance of 3 to 4 mL/70 kg/min (0.18 to 0.24 L/70 kg/hr) and a volume of distribution of ≈ 0.7 L/kg. Depending upon A.C.'s residual renal function, the half-life may be shorter or longer than this average range. Note that for dialysis patients it is not appropriate to use the patients SrCr to estimate creatinine clearance with Equation 63 or 64, because the SrCr is not at steady state. The duration and frequency of hemodialysis is not a factor in vancomycin dosing, since the amount of vancomycin cleared during standard hemodialysis is negligible.

The standard approach to the use of vancomycin in patients on intermittent hemodialysis is to administer 1 gm every five days to two weeks. Using average parameters for a patient with end-stage renal disease in Equation 49, one can see that the first 1 gm dose should result in an initial peak concentration of 25 mg/L.

$$Cp^\circ = \frac{(S)(F)(\text{Loading Dose})}{Vd}$$

$$= \frac{(1)(1)(1000 \text{ mg})}{42 \text{ L}}$$

$$= 23.8 \text{ mg/L } or \approx 25 \text{ mg/L}$$

Steady-state peak and trough levels of 42 mg/L and 18 mg/L, respectively, can be calculated using an average vancomycin clearance of 3.5 mL/min (0.21 L/hr), a volume of distribution of 42 L (0.7 L/kg × 60 kg), and a corresponding elimination rate constant of 0.005 hr^{-1} (Equations 43 and 46):

$$\text{Cpss max} = \frac{\dfrac{(S)(F)(\text{Dose})}{Vd}}{(1 - e^{-Kd\tau})} \qquad \text{(Eq. 43)}$$

$$= \frac{\dfrac{(1)(1)(1000 \text{ mg})}{42 \text{ L}}}{(1 - e^{-(0.005 \text{ hr}^{-1})(24 \text{ hr/day})(7 \text{ days})})}$$

$$= 41.9 \text{ mg/L } or \approx 42 \text{ mg/L}$$

$$\text{Cpss min} = (\text{Cpss max})(e^{-Kd\tau}) \qquad \text{(Eq. 46)}$$

$$= (41.9 \text{ mg/L})(e^{-(0.005 \text{ hr}^{-1})(24 \text{ hr/day})(7 \text{ days})})$$

$$= 18 \text{ mg/L}$$

If the 1 gm dose had been administered every two weeks, the expected peak and trough vancomycin concentrations would have been approximately 29 mg/L and 5 mg/L, respectively.

If an extended course of therapy is anticipated, it probably is advisable to obtain vancomycin plasma levels to make certain that A.C.'s actual plasma levels are within an acceptable range. In seriously ill patients it might be appropriate to obtain an initial vancomycin level three to five days after the initiation of therapy. The purpose is to ensure that the patient's actual clearance is not unusually large resulting in vancomycin levels that are below the desired therapeutic range.

If A.C. had been receiving CAPD as her method of dialysis, it is probable that the vancomycin would be administered via her peritoneal dialysis fluid. The usual approach is to place 15 to 30 mg/kg of vancomycin (approximately 1 to 2 gm for A.C.) into an initial dialysate exchange which should result in about one-half that dose being absorbed during the usual four to six hour dwell time. Her maintenance dose would then be administered in one of two ways. An additional 15 to 30 mg/kg dose could be administered in single exchanges every three to five days such that her pre-dose trough vancomycin concentration would be maintained at $\approx$10 mg/L. Alternatively, a concentration of 15 to 20 mg/L could be placed in each dialysis exchange (30 to 40 mg/2 L exchange.) This technique of placing vancomycin in each exchange results in a steady-state plasma concentration approximately equal to the concentration of vancomycin in the dialysate fluid.[18,19]

Question #5. K.G., a 50-year-old, 70 kg male with a serum creatinine of 1.2 mg/dL, is receiving vancomycin 1000 mg IV Q 12 hr at 10:00 a.m. and 10:00 p.m. for a nafcillin-resistant *S. aureus* (NSRA) infection. A steady-state vancomycin level was drawn with morning labs at 6:00 a.m. and was reported to be 18 mg/L. (Note: This level was drawn eight hours after the start of the vancomycin infusion and is four hours before the trough.) Based upon this information, estimate K.G.'s vancomycin Cl and Kd values and the true trough concentration.

Because this level was drawn four hours early, Equation 15.1 should not be used to estimate the peak concentration.

$$\text{Cpss max} = \left[\text{Cpss min}\right] + \left[\frac{(S)(F)(Dose)}{Vd}\right]$$

Instead, an iterative search technique must be used to determine K.G.'s pharmacokinetic parameters. The usual technique is to use Equation 48 where t_1 is eight hours from the start of the infusion and to assume K.G. has an average volume of distribution of $\approx$49 L (0.7 L/kg $\times$ 70 kg). Then, by trial and error, solve for the elimination-rate constant (Kd) that predicts a plasma concentration equal to the observed value of 18 mg/L. For example, if a Kd of 0.058 hr^{-1} is inserted into the equation, a concentration of 25.7 mg/L is calculated. This value is greater than the observed concentration of 18 mg/L and therefore does not satisfy the equation. By trial and error, one can discover that an elimination rate constant of 0.078 hr^{-1} calculates a concentration very close to 18 mg/L.

$$Cpss_1 = \frac{\dfrac{(S)(F)(Dose)}{Vd}}{(1 - e^{-Kd\tau})} (e^{-Kdt_1})$$

$$18 = \frac{\dfrac{(1)(1)(1000 \text{ mg})}{49 \text{ L}}}{(1 - e^{-Kd(12 \text{ hr})})} (e^{-Kd(8 \text{ hr})})$$

$$Cpss_1 = \frac{\dfrac{(1)(1)(1000 \text{ mg})}{49 \text{ L}}}{(1 - e^{-(0.058)(12)})} (e^{-(0.058)(8)})$$

$$= \frac{20.4 \text{ mg/L}}{(1 - 0.5)} (0.63)$$

$$= 25.7 \text{ mg/L}$$

$$= \frac{\dfrac{(1)(1)(1000 \text{ mg})}{49 \text{ L}}}{(1 - e^{-(0.078)(12 \text{ hr})})} (e^{-(0.078)(8)})$$

$$= \frac{20.4 \text{ mg/L}}{(1 - 0.392)} (0.54)$$

$$= 18.11 \text{ mg/L}$$

It can be reasonably assumed, then, that this elimination rate constant of 0.078 hr^{-1} is the value which would be most appropriate for K.G. When this Kd is coupled with Equations 31 and 33, a revised half-life and vancomycin clearance can be calculated for K.G.

$$t^{1/2} = \frac{0.693}{Kd}$$

$$= \frac{0.693}{0.078 \text{ hr}^{-1}}$$

$$= 8.88 \text{ hr}$$

$$Cl = (Kd)(Vd)$$
$$= (0.078 \text{ hr}^{-1})(49 \text{ L})$$
$$= 3.82 \text{ L/hr}$$

In addition, Equation 26 can be used to calculate the expected trough concentration (12 hours after the dose was administered) by decaying the reported value at eight hours an additional four hours.

$$Cp = (Cp^\circ)(e^{-Kdt}) \qquad \text{(Eq. 26)}$$
$$= (18 \text{ mg/L})(e^{-(0.078)(4 \text{ hr})})$$
$$= (18 \text{ mg/L})(0.73)$$
$$= 13.14 \text{ mg/L}$$

This concentration is reasonable considering the usual target trough concentrations are 5 to 15 mg/L. If the estimated trough concentration was not acceptable, then the revised half-life and clearance coupled with the assumed volume of distribution for K.G. could be used to establish a new dosing regimen.

Question #6. C.U. is a 40-year-old, five foot seven inch, 105 kg male with a serum creatinine of 1.2 mg/dL. He has a penicillin allergy history and for that reason, vancomycin is being considered for empiric therapy. Should the dosing regimen of vancomycin be based on C.U.'s total or ideal body weight?

Although renal function appears to correlate best with ideal rather than total body weight in obese subjects, evidence suggests that both the volume of distribution and clearance of vancomycin in obese subjects correlates best with the actual rather than the ideal body weight.[6,25]

To calculate the expected pharmacokinetic parameters for C.U., first estimate his creatinine clearance and ideal body weight using Equations 65 and 63.

$$\frac{\text{Ideal Body Weight}}{\text{for Males in kg}} = 50 + (2.3)(\text{Height in inches} > 60)$$

$$\frac{\text{Cl}_{\text{Cr}} \text{ for Males}}{(\text{mL/min})} = \frac{(140 - \text{Age})(\text{Weight})}{(72)(\text{SrCr}_{ss})}$$

Alternatively, the weight could be eliminated from the numerator in Equation 63 so that creatinine clearance would be calculated as mL/kg/min as shown below.

$$\frac{\text{Cl}_{\text{Cr}} \text{ for Males}}{(\text{mL/kg/min})} = \frac{(140 - \text{Age})}{(72)(\text{SrCr}_{ss})}$$

Using the above equation, C.U.'s creatinine clearance is ≈ 1.16 mL/kg/min and corresponds to a vancomycin clearance of 4.75 L/hr.

$$\frac{\text{Cl}_{\text{Cr}} \text{ for Males}}{(\text{mL/kg/min})} = \frac{(140 - 40 \text{ years})}{(72)(1.2 \text{ mg/dL})}$$
$$= 1.16 \text{ mL/kg/min}$$

$$\text{Vancomycin Cl} = (0.65)(\text{Cl}_{\text{Cr}} \text{ in mL/kg/min})(\text{Total Body Weight in kg})$$
$$= (0.65)(1.16 \text{ mL/kg/min})(105 \text{ kg})$$
$$= 79.17 \text{ mL/min}$$

or

$$= (79.17 \text{ mL/min})\left(\frac{60 \text{ min/hr}}{1000 \text{ mL/L}}\right)$$
$$= 4.75 \text{ L/hr}$$

Again, using C.U.'s total body weight to calculate his volume of distribution of 73.5 L, C.U.'s elimination rate constant (Kd) would be 0.065 hr^{-1} which corresponds to a half-life of approximately ten hours.

$$Vd = (0.7\ L/kg)(105\ kg)$$
$$= 73.5\ L$$

$$Kd = \frac{Cl}{Vd} \qquad \text{(Eq. 27)}$$
$$= \frac{4.75\ L/hr}{73.5\ L}$$
$$= 0.065\ hr^{-1}$$

$$t\frac{1}{2} = \frac{0.693}{Kd} \qquad \text{(Eq. 31)}$$
$$= \frac{0.693}{0.065\ hr^{-1}}$$
$$= 10.66\ hr$$

Given the half-life and the desire to choose a dosing interval that is between one and two half-lives for vancomycin, a logical approach would be to use a convenient dosing interval of 12 hours and a trough concentration of 10 mg/L and Equation 17.1 to solve for a dose.

$$Dose = \frac{(Cpss\ min)(Vd)(1 - e^{-Kd\tau})}{(S)(F)(e^{-Kd\tau})}$$
$$= \frac{(10\ mg/L)(73.5\ L)(1 - e^{-(0.065)(12)})}{(1)(1)(e^{-(0.065)(12)})}$$
$$= 868.4\ mg\ every\ 12\ hr$$

This dose would usually be rounded off to a reasonable amount and 1000 mg would probably be given every 12 hours. The trough concentration on this new dose could be confirmed by using Equation 47 and inserting the appropriate values.

$$Cpss\ min = \frac{\dfrac{(S)(F)(Dose)}{Vd}}{(1 - e^{-Kd\tau})}(e^{-Kd\tau})$$

$$= \frac{\dfrac{(1)(1)(1000\ mg)}{73.5\ L}}{(1 - e^{-(0.065)(12)})}(e^{-(0.065)(12)})$$

$$= \frac{\dfrac{13.6\ mg/L}{(1 - 0.46)}}{}(0.46)$$

$$= 25\ mg/L\ (0.46)$$

$$= 11.5\ mg/L$$

Alternatively, the expected trough concentration could have been calculated by simply using a ratio of the new dose to the old dose. This technique of using a ratio of doses to calculate the new concentration is appropriate as long as the dosing interval and time of sampling has not changed.

$$Cpss\ Desired = \frac{Desired\ Dose}{Current\ Dose} \times Cpss\ Current$$

$$= \frac{1000\ mg}{868\ mg} \times 10\ mg/L$$

$$= 1.15 \times 10\ mg/L$$

$$= 11.5\ mg/L$$

Note that any difference between the plasma concentrations calculated by the two methods is due to rounding-off errors and not to any other assumptions.

References

1. Alexander MB. A review of vancomycin. Drug Intell Clin Pharm. 1974; 8:520.

2. Kirby WMM et al. Treatment of staphylococcal septicemia with vancomycin. N Engl J Med. 1960;262:49.

3. Banner WN Jr, Ray CG. Vancomycin in perspective. Am J Dis Child. 1984;183:14.

4. Cunha BA, Ristuccia AM. Clinical usefulness of vancomycin. Clin Pharm. 1983;2:417.

5. Rotschafer JC et al. Pharmacokinetics of vancomycin: observations in 28 patients and dosage recommendations. Antimicrob Agents Chemother. 1982;22:391.

6. Blouin RA et al. Vancomycin pharmacokinetics in normal and morbidly obese subjects. Antimicrob Agents Chemother. 1982;21:575.

7. Mollering RC et al. Vancomycin therapy in patients with impaired renal function; a nomogram for dosage. Ann Intern Med. 1981;94:343.

8. Farber BF, Mollering RC Jr. Retrospective study of the toxicity of preparations of vancomycin from 1974 to 1981. Antimicrob Agents Chemother. 1983;23:138.

9. Edwards DJ, Pancrobo S. Routine monitoring of serum vancomycin concentrations: waiting for proof of its value. Clin Pharm. 1987;6: 652–4.

10. Fitzsimmons WE, Postelnick MJ. Rational use of vancomycin serum concentrations: Update on infectious disease for the hospital pharmacist. Macmillan Health Care Information. Florham Park; 1988;2:1.

11. Newfield P, Roizen MF. Hazards of rapid administration of vancomycin. Ann Intern Med. 1979;91:581.

12. Cook FV, Farrar WE. Vancomycin revisited. Ann Intern Med. 1978; 88:813.

13. Karchmer WA. Staphylococcal endocarditis: Laboratory and clinical basis for antibiotic therapy. Am J Med. 1985;78:116–27.

14. Krogstad DJ et al. Single dose kinetics of intravenous vancomycin. J Clin Pharm. 1980;20:197.

15. Nielsen HE et al. Renal excretion of vancomycin in kidney disease. Acta Med Scand. 1975;197:261.

16. Lindholm DD, Murray JS. Persistence of vancomycin in the blood during renal failure and its treatment by hemodialysis. N Engl J Med. 1966;274:1047.

17. Ayus JC et al. Peritoneal clearance and total body elimination of vancomycin during chronic intermittent peritoneal dialysis. Clin Nephrol. 1979;11:129.

18. Paton TW et al. Drug therapy in patients undergoing peritoneal dialysis: Clinical pharmacokinetic considerations. Clin Pharmacokinetics. 1985;10:404–26.

19. Morse GD et al. Comparative study of intraperitoneal and intravenous vancomycin pharmacokinetics during continuous ambulatory peritoneal dialysis. Antimicrob Agents Chemother. 1987;31:173–7.

20. Morse GD et al. Overestimate of vancomycin concentrations utilizing fluorescence polarization immunoassay in patients on peritoneal dialysis. Ther Drug Monit. 1987;9:212–5.

21. Lanese DM et al. Markedly increased clearance of vancomycin during hemodialysis using polysulfone dialyzers. Kidney Int. 1989;35:1409–12.

22. Pollard TA et al. Vancomycin redistribution: dosing recommendations following high-flux hemodialysis. Kidney Int. 1994;45:232–7.

23. Freeman CD et al. Vancomycin therapeutic drug monitoring: Is it necessary? Ann Pharmacother. 1993;27:594–8.

24. Schadd UB et al. Clinical pharmacology and efficacy of vancomycin in pediatric patients. Pediatr Pharmacol Ther. 1980;96:119.

25. Vance-Bryan K et al. Effect of obesity on vancomycin pharmacokinetics as determined by a bayesian forecasting technique. Antimicrob Agents Chemother. 1993;37:436–40.

26. Leonard AE, Boro MS. Vancomycin pharmacokinetic parameters in middle-aged and elderly men. Am J Hosp Pharm. 1994;51:798–800.

Appendix I: Nomograms for Calculating Body Surface Area

Nomogram for Calculating the Body Surface Area of Children[a]

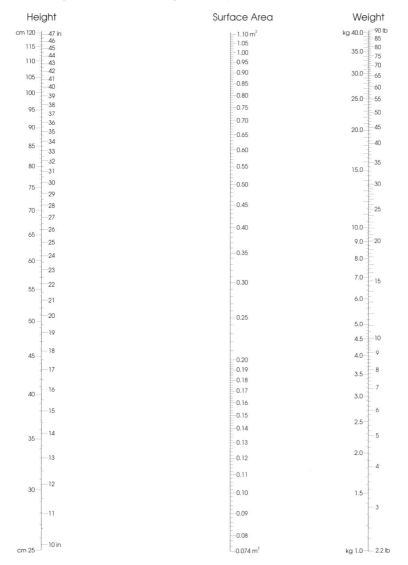

| Height | Surface Area | Weight |

[a] From the formula of DuBois and DuBois. Arch Intern Med. 1916;17:863: $S = W^{0.425} \times H^{0.725} \times 71.84$, or $\log S = 0.425 \log W + 0.725 \log H + 1.8564$, where S = Body surface area in cm^2, W = Weight in kg, H = Height in cm.

Nomogram for Calculating the Body Surface Area of Adults[a]

Height	Surface Area	Weight

[a] From the formula of DuBois and DuBois. Arch Intern Med. 1916;17:863: $S = W^{0.425} \times H^{0.725} \times 71.84$, or $\log S = 0.425 \log W + 0.725 \log H + 1.8564$, where S = Body surface area in cm^2, W = Weight in kg, H = Height in cm. Reprinted with permission from the publisher. Lontmer C., ed. Geigy Scientific Tables. 8th edition. Volume 1: Basle: Ciba-Geigy. 1981:226-27.

Appendix II: Common Equations Used Throughout the Text

The following is a list of equations which are frequently used in pharmacokinetic calculations. They are grouped together according to specific dosing situations. For a complete discussion, refer to the text and figures cited next to each equation. Although some of the equations may appear complicated, most are simple rearrangements of basic equations which can be broken down into one or more of the following components:

$$\frac{(S)(F)(Dose)}{Vd}$$
The change in plasma concentration following a dose (ΔCp).

$$\frac{(S)(F)(Dose/\tau)}{Cl}$$
Average steady-state concentration.

$$(e^{-Kdt})$$
Fraction remaining after time of decay (t).

$$(1 - e^{-Kdt})$$
Fraction lost during decay phase *or* fraction of steady state achieved during infusion.

Single Dose (Absorption Time or $t_{in} \leq \frac{1}{6} \, t\frac{1}{2}$)

$$Loading \; Dose = \frac{(Vd)(Cp)}{(S)(F)}$$
Part I: Equation 11; Figure 21

$$Incremental \; Loading \; Dose = \frac{(Vd)(Cp \; Desired - Cp \; Initial)}{(S)(F)}$$
Part I: Equation 12

$$Cp^{\circ} = \frac{(S)(F)(Loading \; Dose)}{(Vd)}$$
$$= (Change \; in \; Concentration)$$
Part I: Equation 49; Figure 21

$$Cp_1 = \frac{(S)(F)(\text{Loading Dose})}{Vd} (e^{-Kdt_1})$$

$$= \left(\begin{array}{c} \text{Change in} \\ \text{Concentration} \end{array} \right) \left(\begin{array}{c} \text{Fraction Remaining} \\ \text{After Time of Decay } t_1 \end{array} \right)$$

Part I:
Equation 50;
Figure 21

Half-Life (t½) and Elimination Rate Constant (Kd)

$$Kd = \frac{Cl}{Vd}$$

Part I:
Equation 27

$$t\tfrac{1}{2} = \frac{(0.693)(Vd)}{Cl}$$

Part I:
Equation 32

$$Kd = \frac{0.693}{t\tfrac{1}{2}}$$

8: Metho-
trexate,
Equation 8.4

$$t\tfrac{1}{2} = \frac{0.693}{Kd}$$

Part I:
Equation 31

$$Kd = \frac{\ln\left(\dfrac{Cp_1}{Cp_2}\right)}{t}$$

Part I:
Equation 28

Single Dose (Absorption or $t_{in} > \tfrac{1}{6}\, t½$)

$$Cp_2 = \frac{(S)(F)(\text{Dose}/t_{in})}{Cl} (1 - e^{-Kdt_{in}})(e^{-Kdt_2})$$

$$= \left(\begin{array}{c} \text{Average} \\ \text{Steady-State} \\ \text{Concentration} \end{array} \right) \left(\begin{array}{c} \text{Fraction of} \\ \text{Steady State} \\ \text{Achieved After} \\ \text{Time of Infusion } t_{in} \end{array} \right) \left(\begin{array}{c} \text{Fraction Remaining} \\ \text{After } t_2 \\ \text{Time of Decay} \end{array} \right)$$

$$= \left(\begin{array}{c} \text{Change in} \\ \text{Concentration} \\ \text{at the End of a} \\ \text{Short Infusion} \end{array} \right) \left(\begin{array}{c} \text{Fraction Remaining} \\ \text{After } t_2 \\ \text{Time of Decay} \end{array} \right)$$

Part I:
Equation 53;
Figure 24

Continuous Infusion

At Steady State

$$\text{Maintenance Dose} = \frac{(Cl)(Cpss\ ave)(\tau)}{(S)(F)}$$

Part I:
Equation 16

$$Cpss\ ave = \frac{(S)(F)(Dose/\tau)}{Cl}$$

Part I:
Equation 35;
Figure 22

$$= \text{Average Steady State Concentration}$$

Decay From Steady State

$$Cp_2 = \frac{(S)(F)(Dose/\tau)}{Cl}\ (e^{-Kdt_2})$$

Part I:
Equation 51;
Figure 22

$$= \left(\begin{array}{c}\text{Average}\\\text{Steady-State}\\\text{Concentration}\end{array}\right)\left(\begin{array}{c}\text{Fraction Remaining}\\\text{After } t_2\\\text{Time of Decay}\end{array}\right)$$

NonSteady State

$$Cp_1 = \frac{(S)(F)(Dose/\tau)}{Cl}\ (1 - e^{-Kdt_1})$$

Part I:
Equation 37;
Figure 19

$$= \left(\begin{array}{c}\text{Average}\\\text{Steady-State}\\\text{Concentration}\end{array}\right)\left(\begin{array}{c}\text{Fraction of}\\\text{Steady State}\\\text{Achieved } t_1 \text{ Time}\\\text{After Starting Infusion}\end{array}\right)$$

Decay From NonSteady State

$$Cp_2 = \frac{(S)(F)(Dose/\tau)}{Cl}\ (1 - e^{-Kdt_1})(e^{-Kdt_2})$$

Part I:
Equation 41;
Figure 19

$$= \left(\begin{array}{c}\text{Average}\\\text{Steady-State}\\\text{Concentration}\end{array}\right)\left(\begin{array}{c}\text{Fraction of}\\\text{Steady State}\\\text{Achieved } t_1\\\text{Time After}\\\text{Starting Infusion}\end{array}\right)\left(\begin{array}{c}\text{Fraction}\\\text{Remaining}\\\text{After } t_2\\\text{Time of Decay}\end{array}\right)$$

Multiple Dose
(Consistent τ and Dose): Steady State

Absorption or $t_{in} \leq t\frac{1}{2}$

$$Cpss_1 = \frac{\frac{(S)(F)(Dose)}{Vd}}{(1 - e^{-Kd\tau})} (e^{-Kdt_1})$$

Part I:
Equation 48;
Figure 26

$$= \frac{\left(\begin{array}{c} \text{Change in} \\ \text{Concentration} \end{array}\right)}{\left(\begin{array}{c} \text{Fraction Lost in} \\ \text{Dosing Interval} \end{array}\right)} \left(\begin{array}{c} \text{Fraction} \\ \text{Remaining} \\ \text{After } t_1 \\ \text{Time of Decay} \end{array}\right)$$

$$= \left(\begin{array}{c} \text{Steady-State} \\ \text{Peak} \\ \text{Concentration} \end{array}\right) \left(\begin{array}{c} \text{Fraction Remaining} \\ \text{After } t_1 \\ \text{Time of Decay} \end{array}\right)$$

Absorption or $t_{in} > \frac{1}{6} t\frac{1}{2}$

$$Cp_2 = \frac{\frac{(S)(F)(Dose/t_{in})}{Cl}(1 - e^{-Kdt_{in}})}{1 - e^{-Kd\tau}} (e^{-Kdt_2})$$

Part I:
Equation 57.
1: Amino-
glycoside
Antibiotics
Figure 1.1

$$= \frac{\left(\begin{array}{c} \text{Average} \\ \text{Steady-State} \\ \text{Concentration} \end{array}\right)\left(\begin{array}{c} \text{Fraction of} \\ \text{Steady State} \\ \text{Achieved After } t_{in} \\ \text{Time of Infusion} \end{array}\right)}{\left(\begin{array}{c} \text{Fraction} \\ \text{Lost in a} \\ \text{Dosing Interval} \end{array}\right)}\left(\begin{array}{c} \text{Fraction} \\ \text{Remaining} \\ \text{After } t_2 \\ \text{Time of Decay} \end{array}\right)$$

$$= \left(\begin{array}{c} \text{Steady-State} \\ \text{Peak Concentration} \\ \text{at End of} \\ \text{Short Infusion} \end{array}\right)\left(\begin{array}{c} \text{Fraction Remaining} \\ \text{After } t_2 \text{ Time of Decay} \end{array}\right)$$

Multiple Dose
(Consistent τ and Dose): NonSteady State

Absorption or $t_{in} \leq t\frac{1}{2}$

$$Cp_2 = \frac{(S)(F)(Dose)}{Vd} \frac{}{(1 - e^{-Kd\tau})} (1 - e^{-Kd(N)\tau})(e^{-Kdt_2})$$

Part I:
Equation 55

$$= \left(\begin{array}{c} \text{Change in} \\ \text{Concentration} \\ \hline \text{Fraction Lost in} \\ \text{Dosing Interval} \end{array}\right) \left(\begin{array}{c} \text{Fraction of} \\ \text{Steady State} \\ \text{Achieved} \\ \text{After N Doses} \end{array}\right) \left(\begin{array}{c} \text{Fraction} \\ \text{Remaining} \\ \text{After } t_2 \text{ Time} \\ \text{of Decay} \end{array}\right)$$

$$= \left(\begin{array}{c} \text{Steady-State} \\ \text{Peak} \\ \text{Concentration} \end{array}\right) \left(\begin{array}{c} \text{Fraction of} \\ \text{Steady State} \\ \text{Achieved} \\ \text{After N Doses} \end{array}\right) \left(\begin{array}{c} \text{Fraction} \\ \text{Remaining} \\ \text{After } t_2 \text{ Time} \\ \text{of Decay} \end{array}\right)$$

Mass Balance

$$\frac{(S)(F)(Dose/\tau) - \dfrac{(Cp_2 - Cp_1)Vd}{t}}{Cp\ ave} = Cl$$

Part I:
Equation 58

Creatinine Clearance (Cl_{Cr})

$$\begin{array}{c} Cl_{Cr} \text{ for Males} \\ (mL/min) \end{array} = \frac{(140 - Age)(Weight)}{(72)(SrCr_{ss})}$$

Part I:
Equation 63

$$\begin{array}{c} Cl_{Cr} \text{ for Females} \\ (mL/min) \end{array} = (0.85)\frac{(140 - Age)(Weight)}{(72)(SrCr_{ss})}$$

Part I:
Equation 64

where: Age in Years Weight in kg SrCr in mg/dL

$$\begin{array}{c} Cl_{Cr} \text{ for Children} \\ (mL/min/1.73\ m^2) \end{array} = \frac{(0.48)(Height\ in\ cm)}{SrCr_{ss}}$$

Part I:
Equation 68

$$Cl_{Cr} \text{ for Children} = (Cl_{Cr}\ mL/min/1.73\ m^2)\left(\frac{BSA}{1.73\ m^2}\right)$$

Part I:
Equation 69

$$BSA \text{ in } m^2 = \left(\frac{Patient's\ Weight\ in\ kg}{70\ kg}\right)^{0.73} \left(1.73\ m^2\right)$$

Part I:
Equation 17

Nonlinear Equations (Phenytoin)

$$(S)(F)(Dose/\tau) = \frac{(Vm)(Cpss\ ave)}{Km + Cpss\ ave}$$

10: Phenytoin
Equation 10.5

$$Cpss = \frac{(Km)[(S)(F)(Dose/\tau)]}{Vm - (S)(F)(Dose/\tau)}$$

10: Phenytoin
Equation 10.6

Time Required to Achieve 90% of Steady State ($t_{90\%}$)

$$t_{90\%} = \frac{(Km)(Vd)}{[Vm - (S)(F)(Dose/day)]^2} [(2.3\ Vm) \\ - (0.9)(S)(F)(Dose/day)]$$

10: Phenytoin
Equation
10.13

Has Steady State Been Achieved?

$$90\%\ t = \frac{[115 + (35)(Cp)][Cp]}{(S)(F)(Dose)}$$

10: Phenytoin
Equation
10.14

Days on current maintenance regimen must exceed 90% t value to assure that steady state has been achieved. Dose is in mg/day normalized to 70 kg.

Adjustment For Plasma Protein Binding (Phenytoin)

Adjustment For Serum Albumin If $Cl_{Cr} > 25$ mL/min

$$Cp_{Normal\ Binding} = \frac{Cp'}{\left((1 - 0.1)\dfrac{Patient's\ Albumin}{4.4\ gm/dL}\right) + 0.1}$$

10: Phenytoin
Equation 10.1

Adjustment For Serum Albumin If $Cl_{Cr} < 10$ mL/min

$$Cp_{Normal\ Binding} = \frac{Cp'}{\left((0.48)(1 - 0.1)\dfrac{Patient's\ Albumin}{4.4\ gm/dL}\right) + 0.1}$$

10: Phenytoin
Equation 10.2

Cp' = Patient's phenytoin level. Patient's albumin concentration in gm/dL.

Appendix III: Glossary of Terms and Abbreviations

Ab: See Amount of Drug in the Body.

Accumulation Factor: $1/1 - e^{-Kd\tau}$ or the degree to which a maintenance dose will accumulate when steady state is achieved.

Adjusted Body Weight: A weight for dosing drugs in obese patients which is between ideal body weight and total body weight (see Equation 67).

Administration Rate (R_A): The average rate at which a drug is administered to the patient.

Alpha (α): a) Fraction of the total plasma concentration which is free or unbound (see Equation 6). b) The initial half-life in a two compartment model, usually representing distribution (see Figure 9).

Amount of Drug in the Body (Ab): The total amount of active drug which is in the body at any given time.

Average Steady-State Concentration (Cpss ave): The average plasma drug concentration at steady state (Equation 35).

Beta (β): a) Second decay half-life in a two compartment model, usually representing elimination. b) The fraction of total plasma concentration which is bound to plasma proteins.

Bioavailability (F): The fraction of an administered dose which reaches the systemic circulation.

Body Surface Area (BSA): The surface area of a patient, as determined by weight and height (see Equation 17 and Appendix I).

Bolus Dose: A model for rapid input of a dose into the body or an individual dose usually given by intravenous injection.

BSA: See Body Surface Area.

CAPD: See Continuous Ambulatory Peritoneal Dialysis.

Cl: See Clearance.

Cl$_{adjusted}$: Clearance of a patient which has been adjusted or altered for the presence of a disease state such as renal failure (Equation 24) or heart failure.

Cl$_{CAPD}$: Drug clearance by peritoneal dialysis.

Cl$_{Cr}$: See Creatinine Clearance.

Cl$_{dial}$: Drug clearance by dialysis (see Equations 76–81).

Cl$_m$: See Clearance, metabolic.

Cl$_{pat}$: Drug clearance of patient, usually associated with decreased renal function (see Equations 73–82).

Cl$_r$: See Clearance, renal.

Clearance (Cl$_t$ or Cl): Total body clearance is a measure of how well a patient can metabolize or eliminate drug. It is used to calculate maintenance doses (Equation 16) or average steady-state plasma concentrations (Equation 35).

Clearance, metabolic (Cl$_m$): A measure of how well the body can metabolize drugs. The major metabolic organ is usually the liver.

Clearance, renal (Cl$_r$): A measure of how well the kidneys can excrete unchanged or unmetabolized drug. It is usually assumed to be proportional to creatinine clearance.

Cp: See Plasma Concentration.

Cp': Plasma concentration measured in patients with altered plasma protein binding (see Equations 7, 8, 10.1).

Cp^0: The initial plasma concentration at the beginning of a decay phase, usually following a loading dose (see Equations 26 and 49).

ΔCp: Change in plasma concentration resulting from a single dose.

Cp desired: Plasma concentration desired following an incremental loading dose (see Equation 12).

Cp free: Unbound or free plasma concentration (see Equation 9).

Cp$_{Normal\ Binding}$: Plasma concentration that would be observed or measured if patient's plasma protein binding is normal (see Equations 8 and 10.1).

Cp$_{initial}$: Plasma concentration present in patient before incremental loading dose (see Equation 12).

Cp$_{t_{in}}$: Plasma concentration at the end of a short infusion or at the end of absorption (see Equation 52).

Cpss ave: Average plasma concentration at steady state (see Equation 35).

Cpss max: The maximum or peak concentration at steady state, when a constant dose is administered at a constant dosing interval (see Equation 43).

Cpss min: The minimum or trough concentration at steady state, when a constant dose is administered at a constant dosing interval (see Equations 46 and 47).

Creatinine Clearance (Cl$_{Cr}$): A measure of the kidney's ability to eliminate creatinine from the body. Total renal function is usually assumed to be proportional to creatinine clearance (see Equations 61–64, 68).

Dosing Interval (τ): The time interval between doses when a drug is given intermittently.

Dry Weight: Weight of patient before excessive fluid gain.

Dwell Time (T$_D$): The time between instillation and removal of a peritoneal dialysis exchange volume.

e^{-Kdt}: Fraction remaining at the end of a time interval.

1 $-$ e^{-Kdt}: a) Fraction lost during a dosing interval at steady state, if $t = \tau$. b) Fraction of steady state achieved during a constant infusion "t" hours after starting the infusion.

Elimination Rate Constant (Kd): The fractional rate of drug loss from the body or the fraction of the volume of distribution which is cleared of drug during a time interval (see Equation 27).

Elimination Rate (R$_E$): The amount of drug eliminated from the body during a time interval (see Equations 13 and 14).

Extraction Ratio: Fraction of drug which is removed from the blood or plasma as it passes through the eliminating organ.

F: See Bioavailability.

First-Pass: Drug removed from the blood or plasma, following absorption from the gastrointestinal tract, before reaching the systemic circulation (see Part I: Figure 2).

First-Order Elimination: A process whereby the amount or concentration of drug in the body diminishes logarithmically over time. The rate of elimination is proportional to the drug concentration (see Part I: Figure 15).

Half-Life (t½): Time required for the plasma concentration to be reduced to one-half of the original value (see Equations 31 and 32 and Part I: Figure 15).

Half-life, alpha (αt½): Initial decay half-life usually representing distribution of drug into the tissue or slowly equilibrating second compartment in a two-compartmental model (see Part I: Figure 9).

Half-life, beta (βt½): Second decay half-life; usually represents the elimination half-life. Half-life, beta for most drugs can be calculated using the elimination rate constant. (See Part I: Figure 9 and Equations 31 and 32).

IBW: See Ideal Body Weight.

Ideal Body Weight: Body weight used as an estimate of non-obese weight (see Equations 65 and 66).

Incremental Loading Dose: An adjusted loading dose required to achieve a desired plasma concentration (Cp desired) when a pre-existing plasma concentration (Cp observed) is present. (Also see Loading Dose and Equation 12).

Initial Volume of Distribution (Vi): Initial volume into which the drug rapidly equilibrates following an intravenous bolus injection.

Iterative Search: A trial and error process to determine patient-specific pharmacokinetic parameters when direct solutions are not possible due to the nature of the pharmacokinetic model being resolved.

Kd: See Elimination Rate Constant.

Kd$_{adjusted}$: Elimination rate constant which has been adjusted or altered for the presence of a disease state such as renal failure (see Equation 29).

Kd$_{dial}$: Elimination rate constant representing both the patient's drug clearance and the drug clearance by dialysis (see Equation 76, 77).

Km (Michaelis-Menten Constant): Plasma concentration at which the rate of metabolism is occurring at half the maximum rate.

K$_{metabolic}$ (K$_m$): The elimination rate constant calculated from the metabolic clearance and the volume of distribution (Cl_m/Vd) (see Equation 29).

K$_{renal}$ (K$_r$): The elimination rate constant calculated from the renal clearance and the volume of distribution (Cl_r/Vd) (see Equation 29).

Linear Pharmacokinetics: Assumes the elimination rate constant is not affected by plasma drug concentration and that the rate of drug elimination is directly proportional to the concentration of drug in plasma.

ln: Natural logarithm using the base 2.718 rather than 10 which is used for the common logarithm or log.

Loading Dose: Initial total dose required to rapidly achieve a desired plasma concentration (see Equation 11).

Maintenance Dose: The dose required to replace the amount of drug lost from the body so that a desired plasma concentration can be maintained (see Equation 16).

Mass Balance: The process of comparing drug administration rate (R_A) to the rate of change of drug in the body ($(\Delta Cp)(Vd/t)$) in order to estimate drug elimination rate (R_E).

(N): The number of doses that have been administered at a fixed-dosing interval (see Equations 54 and 55).

One-Compartment Model: Assumes that drug distributes equally to all areas of the body. Most drugs can be modeled this way if sampling during the initial distribution phase is avoided.

P_{NL} or P': Plasma protein concentration. P_{NL} refers to the normal plasma protein concentration and P' refers to the plasma protein concentration of the specific patient (see Equations 7, 8).

Pharmacokinetics: Study of the absorption, distribution, metabolism, and excretion of a drug and its metabolites in the body.

Plasma Concentration (Cp): Concentration of drug in plasma. Usually refers to the total drug concentration and includes both the bound and free drug.

R_A: See Administration Rate.

R_E: See Elimination Rate.

S: See Salt Form.

Salt Form (S): Fraction of administered salt or ester form of the drug which is the active moiety.

Sensitivity Analysis: The practice of examining the relationship between a change in either clearance or volume of distribution and the corresponding change in the calculated plasma concentration. (See Part I: Interpretation of Plasma Drug Concentrations: Sensitivity Analysis.)

SrCr: Serum Creatinine Concentration.

Steady State: Steady state is achieved when the rate of drug administration is equal to the rate of drug elimination (see Equations 13 and 14 and Figure 10).

$t^{1/2}$: See Half-Life.

$t_{90\%}$: Time required to achieve 90% of steady state for phenytoin on a fixed dosing regimen in a patient with known values of Vd, Vm, and Km (see Equation 10.13).

Tau (τ): See Dosing Interval.

$\tau-t_{in}$: Time from end of infusion to trough concentration when using a short infusion model.

TBW: See Total Body Weight.

T_d: Time of Dialysis (see Equations 76–81).

T_{in}: Time required for drug to be infused or absorbed (see Equations 52, 53, 57, and 1.5).

Tissue Concentration (C_t): Concentration of drug in the tissue.

Tissue Volume of Distribution (Vt): Apparent volume into which the drug appears to distribute following rapid equilibration with the initial volume of distribution (see Part I: Figure 9).

Total Body Weight: Total weight of a patient usually used for obese patients (see Equations 65 and 66).

Two-Compartment Model: Comprised of an initial, rapidly equilibrating volume of distribution (Vi) and an apparent second, more slowly equilibrating volume of distribution (Vt). (See Part I: Figure 9).

Unbound Vd: Volume of distribution based on the free or unbound plasma concentration (see Equation 82).

Vd: See Volume of Distribution.

Vi: See Initial Volume of Distribution.

Vm: Maximum rate at which metabolism can occur.

Vt: See Tissue Volume of Distribution.

Volume of Distribution (Vd): The apparent volume required to account for all the drug in the body if it were present throughout the body in the same concentration as in the sample obtained from the plasma (see Equation 10).

90% t: Duration of therapy on a fixed dosing regimen which must be exceeded to assure that a measured phenytoin concentration represents steady state (see Equation 10.14).

Index